PLAGUE
DOCTORS

PLAGUE DOCTORS

Responding to the AIDS Epidemic in France and America

JAMIE L. FELDMAN

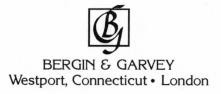

BERGIN & GARVEY
Westport, Connecticut • London

Library of Congress Cataloging-in-Publication Data

Feldman, Jamie L.
    Plague doctors : responding to the AIDS epidemic in France and
America / Jamie L. Feldman.
        p.   cm.
    Includes bibliographical references and index.
    ISBN 0–89789–385–9 (alk. paper)
    1. AIDS (Disease)—United States.   2. AIDS (Disease)—France.
3. Medical anthropology.   4. Social medicine.   I. Title.
    [DNLM: 1. Acquired Immunodeficiency Syndrome—ethnology—France.
2. Acquired Immunodeficiency Syndrome—ethnology—United States.
3. Attitude of Health Personnel.   4. Cross-Cultural Comparison.
5. Epidemiologic Methods—France.   6. Epidemiologic Methods—United
States.   WD 308 F312p 1995]
RA644.A25F46   1995
362.1'969792'00944—dc20
DNLM/DLC
for Library of Congress   94–43601

British Library Cataloguing in Publication Data is available.

Library of Congress Catalog Card Number: 94–43601
ISBN: 0–89789–385–9

First published in 1995

Bergin & Garvey, 88 Post Road West, Westport, CT 06881
An imprint of Greenwood Publishing Group, Inc.

Printed in the United States of America

The paper used in this book complies with the
Permanent Paper Standard issued by the National
Information Standards Organization (Z39.48–1984).

10 9 8 7 6 5 4 3 2 1

Copyright Acknowledgment

The author and the publisher gratefully acknowledge permission to use the following:

Chapter 12, "French and American Differences," is an adapted version of: Feldman, Jamie. "The French Are Different: French and American Medicine in the Context of AIDS." *Western Journal of Medicine* (special issue: "Cross-Cultural Medicine: A Decade Later"), 157, no. 3 (September 1992): 345–349. Reprinted by permission of the *Western Journal of Medicine*.

To my father, the late Gerald Feldman, who taught me to ask, "How does it work?" and to all people living with AIDS.

Contents

Illustrations

Acknowledgments

Many people have been instrumental in the development and realization of this research. Drs. Clark Cunningham, Paula Treichler, Edward Bruner, and the late Demitri Shimkin, of the University of Illinois, Urbana–Champaign, contributed their expertise and support throughout the project. Dr. Diane Gottheil and the Medical Scholar's Program made the education of this physician-anthropologist possible and fostered the interdisciplinary spirit behind this research. My appreciation goes also to Dr. Atwood Gaines at Case Western Reserve University and Dr. Barbara Koenig at the University of California, San Francisco. I am indebted to Dr. William Ferguson and the Department of Family Practice at Lutheran General Hospital, who made available both time and resources. My deepest thanks go to my family, for their infinite patience, and to my husband, Douglas Hulick, for his unshakable faith. Finally, I wish to acknowledge the time and trust granted to me by my informants, particularly the physicians of the Rousseau and Northlake clinics.

This study was funded primarily through a generous grant from the National Science Foundation. Additional support was provided by the Graduate College and Medical Humanities and Social Sciences Program in the College of Medicine, University of Illinois, Urbana–Champaign.

1

Introduction

Well before AIDS, one already knew that illness and medicine are invested
on a symbolic map, objects of a construction of meaning as much as of an
elaboration of knowledge. From this point of view AIDS seems to
constitute, for the researcher in social science, the opportunity of an almost
too perfect demonstration.

Herzlich and Pierret (1988, 48)

This book is about acquired immunodeficiency syndrome (AIDS). No single work
can begin to encompass its worldwide impact, for AIDS pervades social, economic,
ethical, historical, and medical aspects of our lives. Instead, I have deliberately chosen
the biomedical moment as my focus and in doing so, have created an ethnography of
medicine as much as an ethnography of AIDS. The reader might recognize the
experience of her mother's cancer, or her patient's heart disease in these pages. And
yet . . . AIDS is different. How the medical community defines these differences and
responds to them lies at the heart of this book.

Epidemics in general, and AIDS in particular, give social scientists an
unparalleled opportunity to examine the interaction of institutional practices, social
values, and cultural assumptions in a given place and time, particularly those of
medicine. Western *medicine*, or *biomedicine*,[1] has been defined as an objective
science of the chemical and physiological functions and malfunctions of the human
body (Ohnuki-Tierney 1984). Within the last ten years, however, we have begun to
recognize that biomedicine, like non-Western medicines, is also a system of beliefs
and practices intrinsically linked to its larger sociocultural context, and a legitimate
object of anthropological research (Kleinman 1980; Wright and Treacher 1982;
Lindenbaum and Lock 1993).

This book examines how members of the French and American medical
communities, composed of clinical and research sectors, construct their models of

AIDS. The recent and well-documented emergence of the AIDS epidemic allows a more detailed analysis than historical counterparts such as polio and syphilis, as well as being an intense focus of larger social concern. I will concentrate on how these models emerge through discourse, that is, spoken or written utterances here united by the common context of medical science. Additionally, I will explore how medical understanding of AIDS is expressed in clinical and laboratory practice and subsequently communicated within and outside the medical community. This comparative study is grounded in participant observation conducted in two clinics involved with AIDS, French and American, as well as interviews with other medical professionals outside these clinics. The primary goal is to develop a comparative, ethnographically based understanding of how medical models of AIDS emerge and change.

Why examine biomedical models of AIDS from a cultural perspective? Because AIDS is first and foremost a phenomenon of the human body, it falls into the realm of medicine and in large part is defined by medical discourse. *AIDS*, though now used as a distinct name for a particular disease, is technically an acronym devised by members of the medical community—"*a*cquired *i*mmunodeficiency *s*yndrome."[2] As Treichler notes, "Rather the very nature of AIDS is constructed through language and in particular through the discourses of medicine and science" (1987, 263). Herzlich and Pierret, in their discussion of the media's contribution to the construction of AIDS, observe that especially in the first two years of the epidemic clinicians and researchers were the true authors of all the pronouncements emitted by the press (Herlizch and Pierret 1988, 10). Thus, in order to examine AIDS as a social phenomenon, one must examine how AIDS is understood within the biomedical community.

More important, the narratives generated by the medical community are communicated to those outside of medicine and often take on the role of "authoritative tellings," which occupy dominant positions and often represent a state-sanctioned (if not state-promoted) "official line" (Bruner and Gorfain 1984). At the 1987 AIDS conference in Washington, D.C., a petition was circulated, drawing 1,300 signatures, recommending that no political or public health statements be made unless scientific consensus had been reached (Hodgkinson 1987). Additionally, a French study on lay understanding of AIDS and its transmission laid the blame for public misunderstanding at the feet of the medical community for not stating the facts—telling the authoritative story—more clearly (Moatti et al. 1988). To understand how people in the larger society perceive, fashion and act upon AIDS, it is imperative that we understand how medical models are constructed and communicated.

No one study can begin to encompass the totality of AIDS, even within one segment of society. With this work, I hope to fill three substantial gaps in social science research on AIDS. First, this study focuses exclusively on the medical community and its discourses, rather than embedding it within a study of public policy or overall social behavior. Second, being an ethnographic study, the data were obtained directly from medical personnel within a medical context. As a physician as well as an anthropologist, I had access to a range of data not generally accessible to the ordinary ethnographer, such as similarities in treatment to other diseases. Finally, I examine AIDS as a "constructor," a medium and context for the construction of other aspects of the medical experience, such as health care systems and professional identity. All of these research goals, in turn, benefit from the integral cross-cultural comparison.

The amount of published research on biomedical aspects of the AIDS phenomenon is overwhelming, with more than 10,000 scientific papers alone in print as of 1986 (Whippen 1987). Previous research on social aspects of AIDS is voluminous, and a full review of the literature would require a book in its own right.[3] In regards to AIDS and the medical community, however, many studies focus on political or historical accounts of the epidemic—Patton (1985), Altman (1986), Shilts (1987), Grmek (1990), and McCombie (1990) are all examples of this approach.[4] Many analyses of the involvement of the medical community with AIDS are subsumed in larger examinations of public policy regarding AIDS and health care in general (Shulman and Mantell 1988; Bayer 1991; Steffen 1993) and behavioral responses of persons with AIDS (Velimirovic 1987) or populations "at risk" (Pollak 1988; Desenclos, Papaevangelou, and Ancelle-Park 1993; Galavotti and Schnell 1994). Works on educational efforts and public understanding often involve references to the medical community (Moatti et al. 1988; Golden and Anderson 1992).

Research on representations of AIDS constitutes another important approach to the sociocultural aspects of AIDS and medicine. Herzlich and Pierret's study (1988) of French newspaper representations of AIDS provides a remarkable analysis of how the media has shaped interpretation at various stages of the epidemic. Cook and Colby (1992) use a similar approach in their study of American television coverage. Gilman (1987), like Herzlich and Pierret, utilizes print media in order to examine how sufferers from AIDS and syphilis have been represented in various parts of the world. Watney (1988) also concentrates on depictions of the person with AIDS, particularly their impact and implications for homosexual identity. Once again, the role of the medical community is addressed only indirectly in these works.

Until recently, few studies addressed the attitudes or behavior of the medical community directly, outside of analyzing past events, such as the history of transfusion-associated AIDS (Sapolsky and Boswell 1992) and issues surrounding refusal to treat persons with AIDS (Fox 1988b—one among many). More recently, a number of direct studies of the medical community have emerged. Bosk and Fraser (1991) examine the impact of AIDS on medical residents, as do Koenig and Cooke (1989) in one of the few ethnographic studies. Friedland's sensitive discussion of clinical care and AIDS (1989) emerges out of his experience as a codirector of an AIDS center rather than a formal study. Norton and colleagues (1990), in comparison, utilized a survey instrument in analyzing general physicians' language about AIDS.

Within the past few years, a number of historically oriented papers have been published, examining how biomedicine, in terms of epidemiology has defined AIDS and guided research (Feldman 1992a; Oppenheimer 1992; Packard and Epstein 1992). Treichler (1987, 1992a, 1992b) presents several analyses of biomedical discourse, exploring the many metaphors utilized by the medical community, based primarily on visual media and printed materials. Like others, she, too, is concerned with representation, of the gay male body, of women, of the Third World. Patton (1990) examines multiple models of AIDS, including scientific ones, and their relationship to social stereotypes, power, and education. Murray and Payne (1989) examined how medical classification of AIDS "risk groups" developed and how it influenced the way AIDS has been investigated. Rothman and Edgar (1992) compare scientific approaches to cancer drug trials and AIDS drug trials, with a focus on underlying disease models. In all these works, however, data come from published material and not ethnography. Only Koenig and Cooke, mentioned previously, and Farmer and Kleinman (1989), in their article on the importance of illness narratives in caring for AIDS patients, utilize ethnographic data in reference to physicians.[5]

Thus, those works that do focus specifically on physicians and researchers almost exclusively utilize published materials, such as scientific papers and educational pamphlets. This study, in contrast, incorporates data from clinical practice into the analysis as well and, unlike previous studies, is based on direct participant observation rather than written material. Ethnographic data are vital to understanding medical discourse and practice, AIDS or otherwise, because written materials represent only a small fraction of what physicians and researchers say and do in their professional lives. To examine written materials without, at some point, taking into account the ethnographic data is to analyze the end product without exploring the process of production. In a less theoretical view, ethnography also allows us to address physicians and researchers as human beings rather than mere representatives of a generically powerful institution called "Medicine."

Another unusual aspect of this study lies in its comparative nature. While several studies incorporate cross-cultural epidemiological or other quantitative data, few utilize comparative ethnographic data in any systematic way.[6] Medical discourse is also social discourse, unified not only by the context of medicine but by the context of the society. A comparative study of medical discourse on AIDS thus becomes essential for three reasons. First, it substantially increases the amount and breadth of available data. Second, it enables us to distinguish what is common to medical culture from what is particular to a society. Finally, the comparative approach allows us to explore the interaction of medical and social realities as they are constructed through discourse and how local differences in biomedicine emerge through this interaction. In this way, one may gain insight into not only differences in biomedical systems but the cultures themselves, as played out in the context of biomedicine.

While it is now well accepted for Westerners to study differences in the biomedical practices of culturally distant places such as Japan (Ohnuki-Tierney 1984), biomedicine is generally perceived by them as uniform across the Western world, particularly North America and Western Europe. A notable exception is the research compiled by Robert Hahn and Atwood Gaines (1985) demonstrating the heterogeneity of biomedicine, particularly across medical specialties. Such direct qualitative research into biomedical practices is rare in France due to the resistance of physicians toward the involvement of social scientists either in the clinic or in medical school (Herzlich 1985). On either side of the Atlantic, few researchers outside of Payer (1988) and, more recently, Gaines (1992) have explored possible biomedical differences between Western nations such as France and the United States, perpetuating the assumption of uniformity. This study challenges that assumption, highlighting culturally based differences not only in health care delivery, but in how each medicine constructs the interaction between disease and the human body.

There are significant reasons for choosing France and the United States as the sites of this study. Though AIDS is now found worldwide, the highly visible initial research, and the medical discourse surrounding it, was mainly localized in the United States and France. An additional incentive to examining the French-American axis lies in the recent history of conflict between two French and American research teams over the discovery of the Human Immunodeficiency Virus (HIV), the virus believed to cause AIDS. Although the patterns of transmission are similar in both countries, there are some differences in their overall experience with the AIDS epidemic, involving epidemiological differences as well as the structure of health care delivery. Thus, the potential is present for socioculturally based differences between the two biomedicines in their approach to AIDS.

Medical discourse does more than simply construct models of disease. It serves to interpret experience encompassed in the act of doing medicine (Hahn 1985). AIDS, because of its puzzling biomedical traits and its powerful sociocultural impact, generates a wide variety of discourse within the medical community, with understandable differences between clinicians and laboratory researchers. Discourse by medical professionals on AIDS can serve other sociocultural purposes, particularly that of reconstituting cultural and professional identity. Through narrative and commentary, medical personnel involved with AIDS explore and shape the field of medicine, its relationship to other aspects of society, and their own professional, personal, and cultural identity (Friedland 1989). As I discovered, AIDS often acts as a generative medium for discourse on a diversity of topics not directly related to the functioning of the human body. Focusing on the key symbol of biology, Gaines reaches a similar conclusion about medical discourse:

Biology serves to unite disparate themes such as professionalism, competence, scientism, progress and objectivity. It also serves to summarize them as well. It serves as the focus and validation of its work and establishes group and self-identity. (1987, 21)

Therefore, above and beyond the possibilities of French-American distinctions, we can aim to understand the biomedical construction of AIDS, as object and as process, and through AIDS, increase the understanding of biomedicine as a cultural system.

In the end, this book is not just about AIDS or even just about medical culture. It is about the means of understanding—how we as human beings make sense of our world, our experiences, our selves. The discursive tools that physicians and researchers use to construct AIDS may well be the ones Californians use to talk about earthquakes, or taxi drivers about traffic. In the process of examining AIDS and medicine, I hope to shed some light on larger issues of communication, construction, and the relationship between discourse and practice.

The book is broken down into four basic sections. Part I, "Theory, Method, and Context," begins with an overview of the theoretical framework and methodology of the research. It is not meant as an exhaustive review of anthropological theory but as a means of establishing a relevant framework for the material that follows. This section also establishes the context for the AIDS epidemic and both French and American biomedical systems, as well as descriptions of the two clinics that served as fieldwork sites. The biomedical knowledge needed to interpret clinical and research discourse is presented in this section, as well as in an appended glossary.

Parts II and III compose the main body of the study, exploring how AIDS is constructed by—and constructive of—the medical community in both countries. Part II, "Constructing AIDS," shows how the medical community uses a variety of techniques to make AIDS a knowable disease that can be recognized and acted upon, while the expected course of the disease is reshaped in every medical encounter. These medical constructions of AIDS regularly encounter lay models, such as those of patients, that may share a similar terminology but ultimately require continual negotiation between physicians, researchers, and laypersons.

Just as AIDS is constructed through medical discourse, other constructions are being made simultaneously and inseparably from those of AIDS, such as the nature of AIDS patients, medical practice, health care systems, and the identity of French and American medical professionals involved with AIDS. In Part III, "AIDS as Constructor," AIDS is demonstrated as a medium for talking about, and thus refashioning, a wide variety of experiences encompassing the medical, the social, and that vast area of overlap between the two.

Finally, Part IV, "Medical Differences, Different Medicines," explores the differences between French and American biomedicine in the context of AIDS. Though they share many commonalities, the two biomedicines are not the same—not in structure, social relations, or physiological concepts. The context of AIDS not only reveals these differences but is transforming them. Many of these differences are not specific to AIDS, but AIDS instead may act as a medium for expressing what makes French and American medicine distinct.

This study is an ambitious one because it aims to develop understanding of AIDS and the medical community in situ, rather than isolated from its social, historical, or political contexts. The analysis of clinical discourse, for example, is conducted in reference to practice, both of which are in reference to larger frameworks of meaning. Of course, it is impossible to contemplate all the permutations and interconnections simultaneously. One can only represent experience, not reproduce it. At best, I can evoke that experience while contributing to anthropological understanding of the biomedical world.

NOTES

1. Because the focus of this study is on biomedicine only, the terms *biomedicine* and *medicine* will be used synonymously.

2. The French acronym, "SIDA," translates similarly.

3. I have included an extensive bibliography, containing references from bench and medical sciences, humanities, and social science. For the most up-to-date scientific/medical references, I suggest the following journals: *AIDS*, *AIDS Patient Care*, *AIDS Care*, *AIDS Research and Human Retrovirus*, and for epidemiologic information, *Morbidity and Mortality Weekly Reports*. There does not exist a social science or humanities journal dedicated exclusively to AIDS—at least not yet. However, AIDS articles can be found commonly in: *Medical Anthropology*, *Social Science and Medicine*, and numerous critical theory and cultural studies journals. The "AIDS and Anthropology Research Group" newsletter provides information and networking resources. Support group newsletters such as *Positively Aware* and *AIDS Treatment News* are excellent resources as well. Finally, there are a considerable number of databases and discussion groups available via computer, mainly through Internet. The latest information, including scientific data, will often hit Internet before other media sources.

4. There exist several excellent anthologies combining epidemiologic, historical, sociological and political approaches to the AIDS epidemic. These include *AIDS: The Burdens of History* (1988) and *AIDS: The Making of a Chronic Disease* (1992), both edited by Elizabeth Fee and Daniel Fox; *AIDS and Contemporary History* (1993), edited by Virginia Berridge and Philip Strong; *The Meaning of AIDS* (1989), edited by Eric Juengst and Barbara Koenig; *Culture and AIDS* (1990), edited by Douglas Feldman, and *A Disease of Society* (1991), edited by Dorothy Nelkin and colleagues.

5. Fox, Aiken and Messikomer (1991) do provide an invaluable ethnographically oriented look at AIDS and nursing.

6. Farmer and Kleinman (1989) being a rare example.

Part I

THEORY, METHOD, AND CONTEXT

2

Cultural Constructions—Choosing among Stories

The world as we know it is a set of stories that must be chosen among in order for us to live life in a process of continual re-creation.

Walter Fisher (1987, 65)

THEORETICAL CONSIDERATIONS

As I indicated in the Introduction, the main goal of this research is to develop a comparative, ethnographically based understanding of how biomedical models of AIDS emerge and change, primarily through discourse. Inherent in this goal are certain assumptions about biomedical knowledge and the nature of the world, as well as the relationships between culture and discourse. To study the emergence of biomedical models assumes that biomedicine, at the very least, is culturally informed rather than based purely on an objective reality—hence, the place for ethnography in this research. This goal also allows that different biomedicines may exist and can be compared. Another assumption is that diseases such as AIDS exist as models within biomedicine and that these change not simply through the mechanisms of scientific discovery but also through the mechanism of discourse. The question then becomes, What theoretical framework best suits the nature of this goal, laden as it is with these assumptions?

The approach I have taken here has its roots in Geertzian interpretive anthropology and its branches in a variety of related perspectives loosely grouped under the term *cultural constructionism*. It is Geertz, in his seminal work *The Interpretation of Cultures* (1973), who promulgated four key ideas that form a foundation for constructionists. First, anthropological analysis is interpretation or, more precisely, the interpretation of other people's interpretations. Anthropology is then "not an experimental science in search of law but an interpretive one in search of meaning" (1973, 55). Second, these interpretations, both those of the informant and those of the anthropologist, are constructed rather than discovered. Third, cultural analysis is intrinsically incomplete: One can never know the whole truth of the matter. Finally, culture can be examined as an assemblage of texts, "imaginative works built out of social materials" (1973, 449), to be read as a meaningful assemblage in relation to a specified context. Emphasizing interpretation and construction over the discovery and inscription, Geertz opens up the concept of culture to what is fluid, ambiguous, and changeable in human interaction. Geertz does not, however, deny that objective reality exists.

Constructionists, who vary widely in their approaches, generally take Geertz one step further by elaborating on the ideas of construction and culture as text, incorporating concepts from the fields of linguistics, literary criticism, philosophy and the sociology of knowledge.[1] From a constructionist point of view, an objective reality may or may not be "out there," but what we know of it is a construction, continuously fashioned by active participants forming interpretations in a particular social and historical context. As Rabinow and Sullivan (1979, 5) summarize: "Interpretation begins from the postulate that the web of meaning constitutes human existence to such an extent that it cannot be meaningfully reduced to constitutively prior speech acts, dyadic relations, or any predefined elements." Thus, there is no preexisting pattern or rules from which meaning—personal, scientific, anthropological—is deduced. Reality is always mediated by human experience or, as Black (1979) states, "the world is necessarily a world *under a certain description.*"

In anthropology, the focus of interpretation is often considered to be *social structure, ethnicity,* or *culture,* each term itself problematic. "If 'culture' is not an object to be described, neither is it a unified corpus of symbols and meanings that can be definitively interpreted. Culture is contested, temporal, and emergent" (Clifford 1986a, 19). In other words, culture is an ongoing process of meaning, to be understood through interpretation.[2] I have yet to find an adequate definition of *culture,* but borrowing from Bruner (1986b), I would state that culture is a process by which human beings understand themselves and their lived experiences (including the natural world and interactions with others) and which produces and is produced by people's expressions of these experiences.

A constructionist approach to anthropology is thus not limited to the realm of traditional social relationships. Rather, it involves all forms of knowledge, including knowledge of a material world. According to this view, knowledge is fashioned within a particular sociocultural context—giving rise to the phrase "cultural construction"—and is thus contested, temporal, and emergent as well (Berger and Luckmann 1967; Kuhn 1970; Foucault 1972; Knorr-Cetina 1981). A material object, such as a table, is considered constructed because our knowledge of it is continuously being constructed and reconstructed by people. We cannot "know" the table independent of such interactive interpretations. Truth then becomes highly problematic, no longer "what is" but "what is constructed at a given time and place for a given audience." As Fleck (1979, 100) defines it, truth is "an event in the history of thought." A constructionist approach is not the only useful approach to AIDS; rather, it opens up a range of meanings that would not be available with another theoretical perspective.

The constructionist framework, disturbing as it can be to our desires for a stable, knowable reality, has several advantages for the present venture. First, unlike earlier functionalist or structuralist accounts, individual persons here are not passive receptacles for social relations or reproducers of an underlying sociocultural pattern but are active creators at the center of anthropological understanding (Bruner 1986a). This in turn has important implications for appreciating the various power relationships between ethnographer and informants, driven home when those informants are well-read, well-published clinicians and researchers of international status. Second, change is intrinsic to the system, part of the process of ongoing construction rather than an external force imposed on a static society. This is especially crucial in the context of AIDS, where the accepted definition of the disease has changed four times in twelve years.

Additionally, if we accept knowledge as something constructed and embedded within a given context, then scientific knowledge is no longer exempt from anthropological study as somehow being closer to reality, outside of culture. More simply, Geertz takes anthropology out of the realm of science, and constructionists bring science into the realm of anthropology. As Brandt (1985, 5) observes, "A 'social construction' reveals tacit values, it becomes a symbol for ordering and explaining aspects of human experience. In this light, medicine is not just affected by social, economic, and political variables—it is embedded in them." Finally, this framework, with its emphasis on culture as text, allows us to begin to explore the processes of construction, how human beings give meaning to their sensory experience through what they say and what they do—discourse and practice.

By the term *discourse,* I mean spoken or written utterances occurring in a particular context and directed, however vaguely, at a particular audience. Debate over the distinctions between spoken and written discourse has been ongoing, but for my purposes, they will be treated as equivalent. Discourse is a fundamental way in which we as human beings construct meaning, or, to paraphrase Foucault (1972), there is no knowledge without discourse and discourse can be defined by the knowledge that it constructs. In the constructionist view, language, perception, and knowledge—including scientific knowledge—are elaborately intertwined (Ortony 1979, 1). Discourse does not stand alone, but arises out of and participates in a web of interacting discourses. As Bakhtin describes:

The living utterance, having taken meaning and shape at a particular historical moment in a socially specific environment, cannot fail to brush up against thousands of living dialogic threads, woven by socio-ideological consciousness around the given object of an utterance; it cannot fail to become an active participant in social dialogue. (1981, 276–277)

Thus the meanings that emerge from discourse are fluid but not arbitrary, being constrained by their context, which includes a host of other such meanings.

There are many forms of discourse, but one singularly powerful type is that of narrative. On its most general level, narrative may be seen as a discursive process of organizing events—one might say interpretive events—into a meaningful whole. The key words again are *process* and *meaning*. Because narrative is a process and not a static object, it can yield incomplete, less than fully coherent meanings. In fact, a narrative might not always look like the stereotypical story with distinct setting, characters, and organized plot but may instead be fragmentary, have multiple authors, and be conflated with other stories. I would agree with Bruner and Gorfain's assessment: "In our theoretical perspective, narration refers to a process rather than an entity; to discourse rather than a text; to interpretation and feeling rather than the abstract sequence of events" (1984, 57–58). Metaphors are an integral part of narrative, and nonnarrative, discourse, a means of creating new meanings through the juxtaposition of old ones.[3]

How do narratives relate to models, given that the aim of all this theory is to examine medical models of AIDS? I use the term *model* in its broadest sense, being a description or pattern used to help visualize something that cannot directly be observed. Models are used both to predict and to represent phenomena, often simultaneously (Susser 1973). By description alone, narratives and models have much in common. Louis Mink (1978, 144) observes, "The cognitive function of narrative form, then, is not just to relate a succession of events but to body forth an ensemble of interrelationships of many different kinds as a single whole." Narratives make models. Scientific knowledge, as Kuhn (1979, 415) points out, is based on models of nature, not nature itself. The interactive, similarity-creating process seen at work in metaphor can be detected in the role of models in the scientific enterprise. Other forms of discourse and their relation to narrative will be defined as they are encountered in the data.

I do not mean to suggest that discourse is the sole method of cultural construction. The domain of practice, including that of ritual and performance, is an equally dynamic component of the constructionist framework (Bruner 1986a). To make the scope of analysis manageable, I focus primarily on discourse. This means that I take for granted the strong links between discourse and laboratory and clinical practice, as seen, for example, in the inscription of data, the interpretation of results, or the discussing and writing of treatment plans. As Knorr-Cetina (1981) describes, scientific practices are constituted by the manipulation of meaning within the laboratory. These practices, in turn, construct scientific arguments, which then enter into discursive interaction through written communication. The Gallo-Montagnier dispute over the identity and discovery of HIV is an example of such an interaction, carried out in a series of journal articles over many years (J. Feldman 1992c). Indeed, because discourse and practice are interrelated though not identical, it can be productive to regard practice as one might a text, constructive as well of its own themes and metaphors. This concept will be brought out as we examine the practices of AIDS treatment.

In bringing the constructionist approach to bear on the field of biomedicine and AIDS, I am able to more clearly focus the assumptions outlined at the beginning. Thus, biomedicine is here viewed first and foremost as a cultural system, a system of meanings grounded in a particular array of social institutions and interpersonal interactions (Kleinman 1980, 24). This in turn suggests that there is not one universal biomedicine but many related biomedicines, "created and grounded in local cultural knowledge and history, and expressed as biology" (Gaines 1987, 22). Diseases, the entities that physicians designate and ascribe to a patient's particular set of experienced symptoms, are not preexisting objects but models fashioned within the cultural system of biomedicine. They emerge out of social interaction and change over time, becoming invested with new meaning and involved in different patterns of social behavior (Fleck 1979; Wright and Treacher 1982; Herzlich and Pierret 1988). As Rothman and Edgar note, "Science comes in a variety of models, and the process by which one or another subsumes a particular area of medicine is determined not by immutable canons of research but by historical and social contingencies, or, if you will, by metaphor" (1992, 205). AIDS is no different in this regard. The name itself—"acquired immunodeficiency syndrome"—is descriptive rather than etiologic in character, defining a particular set of clinical symptoms as a biomedical entity, a disease. So the very name began as a conscious construct of medical discourse, a means of signifying an otherwise amorphous, little understood concept (Treichler 1987).

Discourse is then central to the creation of meaning in biomedicine. The models made by physicians and medical researchers are both models "of " a perceived disease and models "for" structuring and behaving toward that disease in the future (Geertz 1973, 93–94).[4] David Tracy has observed, "We do not first experience or understand some reality and then find words to name that understanding. We understand in and through the languages available to us, including the historical languages and science" (1987, 48). The particular importance of narrative discourse in biomedicine has recently been emphasized by both physicians and social scientists. Jared Goldstein (1990), a family practitioner, talks about the creation of therapeutic knowledge through narrative in the clinical setting, and Arthur Kleinman (1988) stresses the importance of patients' illness narratives in the clinical treatment of AIDS. Suzanne Poirier and Daniel Brauner (1988) have examined the case history as a rigidly structured form of narrative. Kathryn Hunter (1991) further asserts that clinical medicine is an interpretative activity exercised through narrative, quite distinct in character from any of the physical sciences. She additionally reminds us that "doctors' stories" are not patients' stories, and as we shall see quite clearly with AIDS, the two are fundamentally distinct, even irreconcilable, in the meanings they fashion.

While the physical sciences might not utilize narrative in the same way or to the same extent as clinical medicine, they are by no means devoid of the discursive process. Like the clinician's disease, the scientist's fact is made, not discovered. Bruno Latour and Steve Woolgar (1979, 236) define *scientific activity* as "the construction and sustenance of fictional accounts which are sometimes transformed into stabilized objects." As was seen in the dispute over the initial isolation of HIV, the virus involved in AIDS, this transformation is achieved through the work of narrative, competing in a type of marketplace replete with its own set of investments and credits (Latour and Woolgar 1979, 242–243; J. Feldman 1992c). Scientific narratives, often published as journal articles, are not extracted from scientific events, but as Mink (1978, 147) observes, "rather an event is an abstraction from a narrative."

Once a fact is created, it then becomes divorced from its constructive origins, becoming that which has always been true. Accordingly, I utilize *fact* to mean an event or explanation that is held by the vast consensus of the audience to be valid and coherent and that is generally presented as given, without need of further proof. Biomedicine is hence doubly constructed, deriving, as Starr (1982) notes, much of its authority through its intimate ties with the privileged discourse of physical science in addition to its clinical knowledge.

Although it would be equally accurate to speak of medical or scientific discourses, I find it simpler at times to refer to it as if it were the product of a single actor and directed towards a homogeneous audience, such as examining differences between physician and patient narratives. I do not intend to imply that the Word in medicine is uncontested and uniform—far from it. However, it is often presented and accepted as such, even within the field of medicine itself. The use of the plural *discourses* emphasizes the multivocality of medical talk and particularly the disparity with its attempts at a uniform narrative. The case of AIDS has dramatized controversy both within the medical community and in the continuing interplay between medical and public policy concerns, thus amplifying the dissonance in the medical narrative of AIDS. By looking at how medical professionals talk about AIDS, one can begin to elucidate the various discourses that interact to construct the "facts" of the AIDS epidemic.

Referring to diseases as narratives or social constructions does not make them any less valid or effective as a way of approaching the world. The work of physicians and researchers and the pain of patients are not any less real. Rather, this approach allows us to accept them as something made by actively interpreting human beings. We create our world as much as, if not more than, the world creates us.

The relationship between knowledge and reality—historical, material or social—continues to be problematic. A pervasive criticism of constructionism is that it denies, or at the very least ignores, the existence of a material reality (Winkler 1992). In my view, the strength of constructionism lies in its appreciation that our knowledge of reality is mediated by human interpretation situated within a particular context. As Rabinow and Sullivan observe, "Understanding is entirely mediated by the procedures that precede it and accompany it" (1979, 12). These interpretations (or more radically, "constructions") of reality have a profound impact on real people living real lives. There would have been no research or treatment for AIDS had it not been constructed as something different, a disease apart from other diseases. Unlike Sontag (1978), I do not accept that metaphor is something that we can remove from medicine or science, anymore than we can remove it from other areas of understanding. It is *how* we understand. Interpretive discourse—be it metaphor, narrative, or commentary—does not invalidate biomedicine but empowers it: "Of course, where AIDS is concerned, science can usefully perform its interpretive part: we can learn to live—indeed, *must* learn to live—as though there were such things as viruses" (Treichler 1987, 290). This study is intended to look at that interpretative part, both demonstrating and elucidating the constructive processes within it.

Two other well-recognized disadvantages to a constructionist approach concern the issues of structure and verification. Constructionism does an excellent job of making structure problematic but has not yet developed a way to make it useful. Pappas notes: "In anthropology a number of approaches, including symbolic interactionism, correctly view social life as action accomplished by purposive, knowledgeable actors, but deal with structure as a vague context. . . . Institutions appear as if they were little more than backdrops against which action is negotiated and meaning formed" (1990, 199). Given that constructionism generally regards institutions themselves as being continuously fashioned, we are left in the unenviable position of analyzing the interaction of one or more emergent, fluid constructions (institutions) with another (biomedicine/AIDS). Yet there is little doubt that we must attempt it, for how can one seriously examine biomedical discourses without accounting for the context of medical education, the system of health care delivery, the funding of laboratory research?

The solution comes from recognizing the constructed nature of anthropological research itself. Since I am looking at biomedical discourses of AIDS, and not, for example, the institution of medical education, I can choose to regard AIDS as if it were under continuous construction compared with the institutions that serve as its context. I am not implying that these institutions are static—indeed, as we shall see, the experience of AIDS acts to re-create these "structures" as well. However, for at least this analysis, I would define *structure* as a slowly changing support for sociocultural activity, analogous to the role of bone in the human body. Bone is constantly being destroyed and remade, changing in form and density in response to various stressors, yet the body overall varies relatively little in height over its lifetime. This definition may not be universally applicable, but I find it both useful and valid in many circumstances—which leads to the next problem: verification.

Given that cultural accounts, like the scientific accounts discussed previously, are themselves fashioned interpretations, then how are they to be evaluated? Are all accounts equal? This dilemma has been present as long as there has been interpretive and constructionist theory. Rabinow (1977, 14) gives a succinct analysis of the problem, along with a clue to its handling: "Ultimately a good explanation is one which makes sense of the behavior. But to agree on what makes sense necessitates consensus; what makes sense is a function of one's readings; and these in turn are based on the kind of sense one understands." Cultural accounts are evaluated based on anthropological sense, utilizing the forms of persuasion that Kuhn (1970) first outlined for scientific accounts, albeit in perhaps a more reflexive manner. No account solves all the problems it defines, and since different versions identify different problems, accountability depends on which problems are deemed to be more significant. As Clifford (1986, 110) remarks, "Whereas the free play of readings may in theory be infinite, there are, at any historical moment, a limited range of canonical and emergent allegories available to the competent reader (the reader whose interpretation will be deemed plausible by a specific community)." What is deemed plausible by a particular community is, of course, subject to change—whether that community is made up of anthropologists, literary critics, or physicians.[5]

Walter Fisher, in *Human Communication as Narration* (1987), developed a working model for assessing narrative rationality based on the concepts of "coherence" and "fidelity." Coherence is defined in whether a story hangs together in terms of internal structure, conformity with stories told in other discourses, and the reliability of its characters as narrators and actors. Fidelity is generally described as attentiveness to both logic and values, derived and maintained in a particular community. Fisher's model is both a "model of" how people assess their world through narrative and "model for" analyzing narratives themselves, be it the stories told by our other-of-the-moment ("otherness" being an emergent construction as well) or stories told by ourselves as ethnographers. In this way, theoretical considerations evolve into methodological ones.

METHODOLOGICAL CONSIDERATIONS

If we accept anthropology as something other than a scientific enterprise, we are no longer restricted to methodologies based on the goals of predictability and reproducibility.[6] Still, anthropologists must account for the way they produce their narratives in a way that is meaningful to their community. Oddly enough, the language and concepts of scientific method, such as *data set* and *representative population*, are still used as a means of talking about methods in some orderly fashion, and it is in this sense that I utilize them.

Biomedicine encompasses not only the clinical domain of doctors treating patients but a research component that draws on a number of biological disciplines as well as epidemiology. Thus, I include the discourse of both researchers and clinicians as being within the scope of my study. A *clinician* is here defined as a physician whose primary activities revolve around caring for patients and conducting clinical trials. A *researcher* is defined as someone with an advanced degree, not necessarily a physician, whose primary activities involve laboratory or epidemiological research, with little direct patient care. A *physician* is, quite simply, a person holding the MD degree.

Clinicians and researchers do share a fundamental approach to interpreting the world, that of scientific method and biomedical practice, so the concept of a "medical community" generating a "medical discourse" is, to a limited extent, a valid one (Snow 1963; Latour and Woolgar 1979). As I noted above, biomedicine is intertwined with nonclinical science, to the point that a large portion of medical school, two years in the United States, is devoted to learning the "basic sciences"—usually anatomy, physiology, microbiology, immunology, and biochemistry. Not only are clinical medicine and physical sciences linked in training; more tellingly they are linked in the discourse of the medical community (Hunter 1991). In the context of AIDS, as we shall see, this link is reinforced and celebrated. Nevertheless, while the informants in this study represent both the clinical and research branches of the medical community, their discourses are not identical nor produced in identical contexts. Differences, where appropriate, will be explored.

The two primary methods of data collection in this study were participant observation and semistructured interviews with informants. With regard to participant observation, several studies have demonstrated that an ethnographic approach to studying discourse, performance, and meaning in biomedicine is entirely viable. Helen Schwartzman's (1984) study of narrative in a mental health center, is one example. She notes that stories are triggered by everyday conversation in therapy sessions, at coffee breaks, or during chats in the hall, as well as by the researcher's interviews. Latour and Woolgar (1979) and Knorr-Cetina (1981) approach the construction of scientific knowledge in a laboratory setting in a consciously ethnographic manner. Robert Hahn (1985) bases his portrayal of the work and world of an internist on five months of accompanying him on daily rounds, consultations, office visits and night and weekend call. In Good and DelVecchio Good's (1993) study of learning medicine at Harvard, Byron Good participated in the preclinical years of the New Pathway program. These studies, among others, demonstrate that participant observation can be a profitable technique for approaching both the research and clinical aspects of the biomedical system.[7]

My choice of sites for participant observation evolved out of the selection of informants. French informants, all living in Paris, were initially chosen in 1986, after a survey of the literature on AIDS and HIV, including not only articles in scientific journals but also articles in social science journals, newspapers, and the popular press. As I quickly discovered, the vast majority of AIDS cases in France are located in and around Paris, as well as most of the associated treatment and research. In 1987, I contacted those people with a history of involvement with AIDS, either clinically or in the laboratory, and most of them agreed to meet with me. The few—no more than five—refusals I had were based on lack of time or interest on the part of the potential informant. These initial informants in turn introduced me to others working in the lab or the clinic, increasing my total number of 1987 informants to thirty-three over a period of two and a half months. While some observation, usually over three to seven days, took place at the various clinic and research sites of my informants, most of the data from this period are from interviews, quite similar in style to those done in 1990–1991.

I returned to Paris in the fall of 1990 and renewed contact with as many of my former informants as I could. A number of the younger 1987 informants—mainly doctoral students working in the labs and resident physicians—had left the field of AIDS altogether or had moved on to other labs/clinics and were generally untraceable. Those with the longest history of involvement with AIDS were still in the field and able to meet with me, again introducing me to new colleagues. Of my twenty-six French informants in 1990, exactly half had participated in my 1987 study. The emphasis during this four-month period of research was on participant observation rather than interviews, resulting in data slanted toward the clinical. One particular Paris clinic, at Hôpital Rousseau,[8] was chosen on the basis of my good relationship with its director (one of my 1987 informants), its large AIDS/HIV patient population (over 2,000), and its involvement with AIDS since the beginning of the epidemic.

Informants and sites in the United States were chosen in a similar manner, beginning in 1988 with another survey of the literature as preliminary contact with informants at the Fifth International AIDS Conference in Montreal in 1989. Unlike France, however, neither AIDS cases nor AIDS treatment and research are clustered predominantly in one city in the United States but have several different loci, each with its own epidemiologic history. With this in mind, I chose Chicago as the main site for participant observation, given the similarity to Paris in the size and demographic pattern of the epidemic (see Chapter 3). Additionally, institutional links, strong personal contacts, and its central location made Chicago the best candidate for a primary site. The particular clinic, Northlake, was selected on the basis of its similarities in patient population to the one in Paris, and as in Paris, the focus was on the clinical rather than bench research. Some interviews were conducted at other Chicago clinics as well, achieving a total of twelve Chicago informants in all.

In and of itself, however, Chicago would hardly give me the broadest range of data, nor the most historically sensitive perspective. Five additional sites—Houston, New York City, Atlanta, Washington, DC, and San Francisco—were chosen on the basis of having a large number of AIDS cases and a strong history of AIDS clinical treatment or laboratory research. This enabled me to represent some of the regional diversity present in American medicine vis-à-vis AIDS. Obviously, clinicians and researchers in areas without large AIDS caseloads produce discourse on AIDS. However, as seen in the Montreal abstracts (*Fifth International Conference on AIDS* 1989), most widely disseminated laboratory and clinical research comes from the larger AIDS centers, as does discourse directed at the lay public through the media.

In the five secondary sites, individuals rather than institutions were selected as potential informants, though many of those institutions are heavily committed to AIDS treatment or research. The number of informants per site ranged from four to eight. Among those potential informants contacted, the few refusals were, again, on the basis of lack of time or interest. A number of people at one highly productive and influential lab could not participate due to institutional, rather than individual, concerns. As was the case in France in 1987, only a modest amount of observation was done at these sites, with the majority of data coming from interviews with informants. Time spent at secondary sites varied from five to ten days each; the overall time of the US portion of study ran from January to August 1991 and involved a total of forty-one informants.

The aim of this process was not to generate a statistically representative population but to allow access to a solid amount and breadth of data, forging a moderate path between the intensive single life history and the quantitatively oriented large population studies. Numerical or statistical information was gathered only in regard to adequately representing the context of encountered medical discourse, such as the age, sex, professional status, and specialty of the speaker (usually my informants), the approximate size and type of audience, and the organizational setting. These data are presented in the Appendix, the following chapter, and where needed, in subsequent chapters.

My own biomedical experience, which at the time included two years of basic medical sciences as well as a variety of clinical clerkships (including Infectious Disease), enabled me to participate more fully in the cultural systems of French and American biomedicine than previous ethnographers. My status as medical student eased my initial access to informants, though as one French physician asked of my research, "Don't you think it's a bit incestuous?" At both sites, I was able to fill the niche of a senior medical student, initially accompanying physicians when seeing patients, then later seeing some patients in a limited capacity on my own. At the Chicago site, I also accompanied the physicians on hospital rounds, since—unlike the situation in Paris—the Chicago doctors handled inpatient as well as outpatient care. Additionally, I attended all presentations and meetings involving clinic physicians. Thus, I was able to participate in a way that few anthropologists have been able to do in the study of biomedicine. Through participation, I contributed to the work of the site and of my informants, as well as gaining from their knowledge and experiences. This more equitable relationship tended to improve my acceptance at a site, open up communication, and thus increase the amount and quality of data.

There are disadvantages to this level of participation, mainly the difficulty of distancing myself from the biomedical culture in order to be able to make anthropological interpretations. Indeed, at both sites, the longer I was there, the more enmeshed in the daily activities of the clinic I became. I was penciled into the schedule for seeing patients, and certain patients became "my patients." Fortunately, distancing one's self from the focus of study—generally the patient and his story—is also part of biomedical training, and I was able to counter "going native" by limiting the number of patients I saw on my own to four a day and by having one day a week in which I did not participate in the clinic at all but conducted interviews, did preliminary analysis, or simply observed. Furthermore, I was able to distance myself from the American biomedical culture by doing the French half of the study first. I thus came into the Chicago clinic trained to diagnose and treat AIDS in the French manner. If nothing else, my constant note taking served as a daily reminder of my ambiguous status at both sites, and one French medical student went so far as to label me "the spy."

Like participant observation, the interview has been a standard research tool of anthropologists. Interviewing techniques have varied greatly, from intensive loosely structured protocols to highly structured, "standardized" ones. Additionally, the verbal interaction that occurs in an interview has often been categorized as something entirely different from discourse, more akin to a set of stimuli and responses. In order for interviewing to be considered an appropriate methodology for a constructionist framework, one must see it as a form of discourse produced by two active speakers. Elliot Mishler (1986) has developed an alternative model of interviewing consistent with the Geertzian values of interpretation and meaning rather than the scientific values of quantification, experimental control, and reproducibility. Mishler's model of interviewing rests on four key propositions: that interviews are speech events, that their discourse is constructed jointly by the interviewer and the informant, that analysis is based on a theory of discourse and meaning, and that the meanings of both questions and answers are contextually grounded (ix).

The advantages of Mishler's model converge, not coincidentally, with the advantages of the constructionist theory outlined above. The concept of standardization—in both interviewers and their questions—becomes highly problematic, not only in terms of whether it is achievable but also in terms of whether it is desirable. If the discourse produced by an interview is always affected by the presence of a particular interviewer and the context of the interview itself, then why not acknowledge and explore these differences? This perspective opens up the methodology of interviewing and the analysis of interviews to a variety of techniques, including those oriented toward narrative. As Mishler points out, if one treats the interview as discourse, then narratives should be pervasive unless suppressed by an overly structured protocol or discarded as problematic:

We are more likely to find stories reported in studies using relatively unstructured interviews where respondents are invited to speak in their own voices, allowed to control the introduction and flow of topics, and encouraged to extend their responses. Nonetheless, respondents may also tell stories in response to direct, specific questions if they are not interrupted by interviewers trying to keep them to the "point." (69)

Interviews were audiotaped and lasted from twenty to ninety minutes, averaging about forty-five. They were conducted at the clinic, office, or lab of the informants at their convenience, which sometimes necessitated talking in hallways or a quiet corner. Because I was interested in specific narratives, namely those constructing AIDS, I developed a basic list of open-ended, adaptable questions designed to elicit this type of discourse; for example, "How did you get started working with AIDS/HIV?" By no means were interviews limited to these questions, however, as the informants' responses sparked other questions and responses of my own, varying from informant to informant. My very presence, as an American, as a medical student, as an anthropologist, and as I was sometimes labeled, as a reporter certainly influenced what topics were brought to the mind of the informants and how these topics were expressed. This is probably one reason why references to the United States and French-American relations were common, at least on the part of my French informants.

The power relationship inherent in the ethnographic situation is somewhat modified in this study, because I was often younger, with less medical training than my informants, who in turn were literate people from my own country and a country considered equally as "civilized" as my own. My power lies only in the sanction I have to interpret their words, which are really "our" words. "Actors communicate their interpretations to others by means of shared symbol systems, and together the parties to an interaction negotiate a common definition of their circumstance" (Karp and Kendall 1982, 263). Thus, my interpretations are based on a set of discourses negotiated between myself and my informants.

This is especially true of my interactions with French informants, both during the interview and in daily clinical work. At the clinic, I spoke French 90 percent of the time, necessitated by the need to communicate with receptionists, nurses, patients, and interns, most of whom did not speak English. However, the majority of informants, including the post residency physicians, spoke at least a moderate amount of English and were able to help me out of rough linguistic spots. Most interviews were conducted in English or a mixture of English and French, after I explained to informants that it would be helpful in speeding later transcription. Some interviews were conducted completely in French at the request of those informants who felt uncomfortable speaking English, and no interviews were canceled due to the informant's preference in language. In addition to practical concerns, I felt that if any translation must be made, it should be made by the informant. In this way, the informant has some control over the means of expression, choosing the translation he or she deems most appropriate. Sometimes, of course, we would run into "untranslatable" ideas. In these cases, both French and English would be used and we would together attempt to hammer out a reasonable approximation in English. The following excerpt provides one such example:

Informant: I had never thought that one of the reasons that we had such big advance in the research in the AIDS field was that because of the confrontation of different aspects, different . . . *c'est l'observation, le même phénomène et différente éclairage.* You have understood?
Myself: A little bit.
Informant: It's the observation of this phenomenon with different . . . [*overlap*]
Myself: Points of view.
Informant: Points of view. *Éclairage* is light.
Myself: Okay.
Informant: Different types of light . . .

In this way, too, the interviews generated a negotiated text.

Full transcriptions were done of the interviews by myself and a hired transcriber whom I trained. The style of transcription is quite simple, unlike that utilized by Mishler or many sociolinguists. I made little attempt to represent the speech stream in detail, with all its pauses and stutters. Rather, I wanted an accurate, readable representation of the words that were spoken, by whom they were spoken, in the order in which they were spoken. Pertinent paralinguistic phenomena—laughing, hitting the table, sighing—were also noted. This style of transcription both reflects and structures the priorities in my analysis of the data produced from both interviews and field notes.[9]

A number of specific procedures of discourse or narrative analysis have been developed, such as those of Labov and Waletzky (1967), Cicourel (1974), and Agar (1986). However, many of these focus intimately on how things get said—who speaks first, who interrupts whom, what the linguistic structures are—rather than what is said. Of those approaches that do focus on the words themselves, most are practical only for handling small amounts of discourse at a time, on the order of sentences or perhaps a single narrative. My primary goal is not to analyze all discourse but discourse on AIDS, to understand not so much how it gets done but what it does.

Thus, in Mishler's terms, I am most interested in the ideational function of discourse, "referential meanings—that is, content,—expressed through 'themes' and their relations to each other" (1986, 87). The conventions of literary criticism are useful in this regard: symbols, metaphors, characterization, plot, setting. What does this story mean and how does it interact with itself? With other such stories? With its social, cultural and historical surroundings? In this way, my analytical approach shares similarities with the levels of dialogic narration presented by Bruner and Gorfain (1984) who state, "If we ask where the dialogic is located, the answer is in the discourse, in the discourse about the story, about society, and about the self" (60). Thus, I look for my answers in discourses of AIDS, of biomedicine, professional identity, and cultural identity, spoken by clinicians and researchers with me, with colleagues, with patients. These spoken narratives are viewed as complementary discourse, even commentary, on the body of written discourse, often in the form of standardized journal articles. Since such articles tend to minimize the multivocal nature of medical discourse (Knorr-Cetina 1981), my emphasis on the spoken reintroduces diversity into the data. Interpretation can be systematic but not routinized, not if one wishes to avoid the typing, coding, and counting strategy common to many sociologic studies. The process of interpretation need not be made explicit to be effective, as can be seen in Schwartzman's (1984) work.

I am not entirely disinterested in the "how" of discourse analysis, particularly as it helps to understand the meanings that emerge from it. The concept of coherence, used by Walter Fisher (1987) and in a slightly different way by Agar (1986), describes a means of evaluating how a discourse, usually a narrative, interacts with itself and other discourses. Agar sees ethnographic data as being composed of "strips," that is, interviews, actions, events or anecdotes. A strip, in turn, is composed of smaller "segments." Agar then outlines three levels of coherence: how segments relate with other segments, how segments relate to the strip, and how interpretations of the strip relate to understandings of other segments and strips. While I will not use Agar's terminology to break down my own data, as it seems to create a rather static classificatory scheme, I will draw on his model of coherence, as well as that of Fisher, described earlier. Of course, some data are interpreted as simply information provided in response to my questions, such as, "How many doctors work at this clinic?" To paraphrase Freud, sometimes a cigar is just a cigar. More important, material from the interviews will be examined in conjunction with the data gained through participant observation itself. Thus, the analyzed discourse is situated within its clinical or laboratory setting, rather than divorced from the context of its production.

To summarize, analysis of the data, including physician-patient encounters, is based on interpretation of discourse in light of the cultural context, focusing on common symbols, metaphors, and models of AIDS; professional identity; medicine in general; and French/American culture. These, in turn, are discussed in the context of medical and laboratory practices, as well as the relationships between lay and biomedical discourse. Change is integral to this analysis, provided through comparison of the 1987 and 1990–1991 data, as well as in the informants' understandings of changes over time throughout the AIDS epidemic. Discourse, interpretation, and context are considered as an interwoven system of construction rather than distinct structural entities. Finally, a comparison of the French and US data, sensitive to the differences in how the health care system is structured in each country, is incorporated in the discussion as a whole. Again, before this interpretation is possible, we must know the context of the discourse, including the history of the AIDS epidemic, the textbook definitions of HIV and AIDS, and their adjunct tests and treatments, as well as the structure of the biomedical community and health care delivery in both countries.

NOTES

1. Much interpretive and constructive theory has emerged out of the work of several philosophers including Hans-Georg Gadamer, Wilhelm Dilthey, Paul Ricoeur, and George Herbert Mead. Other seminal works in this field include Blumer, *Symbolic Interactionism* (1969); Whorf's *Language, Thought and Reality* (1956), Bourdieu's *Outline of a Theory of Practice* (1977); and multiple works by Michel Foucault and Mikhail Bakhtin. Rabinow and Sullivan (1979), cited below, provide an overview of this development of interpretive theory as utilized in the social sciences, as does Skinner (1985). My purpose is here to present a basic theoretical framework for the research that follows rather than to attempt a review of constructionist theory.

2. To put it visually, cultural interpretation is more like navigating a river in a wobbly canoe than studying an amoeba under a microscope.

3. Discussion on the definition and role of metaphor dates back to Aristotle at the least and is beyond the scope of this study. My view of metaphor is derived mainly from that of Max Black (1962, 1979), who concluded that there can be no hard and fast criteria for defining a metaphor. Rather, metaphors are recognized by the users of the language in a particular context. Thus, as has been said of pornography, you can't define metaphor, but you know it when you see it.

4. In Snow's view (1963), the scientist's motives are both of understanding and controlling the natural world.

5. This review by no means sums up the debate on constructionism; rather, it distills from the literature what is germane to the present project. For more detailed discussion of the issues involved see: Gaines (1991), Treichler (1992b), Ortony (1979), and Lakoff and Johnson (1980).

6. Michael Lynch (1993) makes a detailed and powerful argument against analyzing scientific knowledge in terms of epistemology. Likewise, he argues that attempts to develop a "science of society" are equally problematic. "To say that the social sciences are 'merely practical' or 'merely literary' enterprises begs the question, What else can they be?" (311).

7. Other important studies include: Bosk's *Forgive and Remember: Managing Medical Failure* (1979); Strauss's *Social Organization of Medical Work* (1985), Koenig's, "The Technological Imperative in Medical Practice: The Social Creation of a 'Routine' Treatment" (1988).

8. This name is a pseudonym, as is Northlake, the name I use for the Chicago clinic.

9. In keeping with these priorities, excerpts from transcripts or field notes cited in the body of this study have been made more readable by the elimination of repeated and half-started phrases, as well as the most awkward grammatical mistakes. My goal has been to render spoken language readable, without entirely losing its spoken "flavor." Additionally, specific references to institutions and individuals, except in regard to well-publicized events, have been altered using pseudonyms or generic phrasing (eg, "Cook County Hospital" to "the public hospital").

3

Surveying the Contextual Ground

Discourse cannot occur in a vacuum. It is always situated within a given context, enabling a particular set of meanings to emerge. Context not only is the immediate microenvironment in which the discourse takes place but intersects the historical, political, and structural spheres of social interaction. Thus, in order to understand the themes emergent in French and American biomedical discourse on AIDS, it is necessary to explore its context in the largest sense of the term. A major advantage of analyzing discourse on AIDS, as opposed to other diseases, is that its history as a disease is quite short, spanning barely more than a decade. In addition, the historical context of AIDS is incredibly rich, with a wealth of written material covering the entire course of the epidemic. The history of the epidemic has already been the subject of several books, including those by Jacques Leibowitch (1985), Randy Shilts (1987), Dominique Lapierre (1990) and Mirko Grmek (1990), as well as several historically-oriented anthologies (Fee and Fox 1988, 1992; Berridge and Strong 1993). Monika Steffen (1993) provides an excellent overview of the development of AIDS policy in France, while Daniel Fox (1988a, 1988b, 1992) analyzes similar issues on the US side. An extensive discussion of the historical and political context of AIDS in France and the United States is beyond the scope of this study,[1] but relevant factors will be addressed in each section.

The most accessible way of surveying the contextual ground is to begin with an overview of present-day biomedical knowledge and treatment of HIV infection and AIDS,[2] including epidemiologic material. This discussion also provides a vocabulary, in terms of both biomedical references and historical events, for lay readers unfamiliar with biomedical language in general and the AIDS epidemic in particular.[3] A brief examination of the structural considerations in the French and American systems of health care and biomedical research will follow. The final section will focus on the organization of the Paris and Chicago clinics and their daily operations, which directly impinge on clinical discourse.

AIDS THE DISEASE: MEDICAL DEFINITIONS AND EPIDEMIOLOGY

Though, as Treichler (1987) notes, it is difficult to distinguish between scientific and nonscientific conceptions in terms of "factuality," scientific conceptions—the "facts"—are also an intrinsic part of medical discourse, often forming both context and text. One must know the facts in order to interpret the discourse that constructs them. Unfortunately, facts rarely hold still, especially when they are facts about AIDS. The following overview of the course of HIV infection and the epidemiologic pattern of the disease is, from a biomedical point of view, already out-of-date, but these conceptions were the ones generally in place during the time of my field research in 1990–1991.[4]

AIDS, clinically speaking, is a syndrome, a combination of signs and symptoms that forms a distinct clinical picture. AIDS thus manifests itself in a variety of ways, which are, according to the above definition of a syndrome, different combinations of the same general signs and symptoms. The Centers for Disease Control (CDC) first outlined a surveillance case definition in 1982, used primarily for epidemiologic rather than clinical purposes and which was modified first in 1983 (see Table 3.1). In 1985, after discovery of HIV and the development of the enzyme-linked immunosorbent assay (ELISA) antibody test, the CDC published a new classification of the manifestations of AIDS, which was used by many to determine what constitutes a "case," both clinically and epidemiologically. The case definition and classification system was modified again in 1987 (Table 3.1) and was adopted by the World Health Organization (WHO) for international use.

The 1987 classificatory scheme, presented in Table 3.2, is based on the concept of AIDS as an infection by the HIV virus. CDC Group I refers to those infections that manifest as an acute mononucleosislike sickness accompanying seroconversion. Seroconversion, the new presence of HIV antibodies in a person's serum, is taken as a sign that the patient is infected with the virus and is recognized via the ELISA antibody test.[5] Group II infections are asymptomatic seroconversions. Note that persons in Group II are thus defined as having a disease, even though they are not experiencing an illness, that is, a sociopsychologically defined departure from health (Ohnuki-Tierney 1984). Group III infections are characterized by diffuse lymphadenopathy (swollen lymph nodes), fever, weight loss, and oral candidiasis (a fungal infection). This constellation of symptoms was, and occasionally still is, referred to as ARC, AIDS-related complex. It is now considered a precursor to "full-blown AIDS," Group IV. The CDC lists five types of Group IV infection. Type A is known as "slim disease," and is marked by persistent fever, weight loss, and diarrhea.[6] Type B is a neurological form of the disease involving dementia and changes in behavior and motor skills. Type C is characterized by opportunistic infections, such as *Pneumocystis* pneumonia, and is common in the United States and Europe. Type D AIDS is associated with secondary malignancies such as Kaposi's sarcoma (KS), and non-Hodgkin's lymphomas. Type E consists of less common

Table 3.1
CDC AIDS Definitions, 1982, 1987

1982

"The CDC defines a case of AIDS as a disease, at least moderately predictive of a defect in cell-mediated immunity, occurring in a person with no known cause for diminished resistance to that disease. Such disease include KS, PCP and serious OI (opportunistic infections). These infections include pneumonia, meningitis, or encephalitis due to one or more of the following: aspergillosis, candidiasis, cryptococcosis, cytomegalovirus, nocardiosis, strongyloidosis, toxoplasmosis, zygomycosis or atypical mycobacteriosis; esophagitis due to candidiasis, cytomegalovirus or herpes simplex virus; progressive multifocal leukoencephalopathy; chronic enterocolitis due to cryptosporidiosis; or unusually extensive mucocutaneous herpes simplex of more than five weeks duration."[a]

1987 (includes 1985 modifications)

In the face of a positive ELISA and Western blot test for HIV antibodies, the following diseases indicate a presumptive diagnosis of AIDS: CMV retinitis, KS, disseminated mycobacterial disease, PCP, cerebral toxoplasmosis, lymphoid interstitial pneumonia and/or pulmonary lymphoid hyperplasia in a child under thirteen years.

The following diseases, plus a positive HIV antibody test, indicate a definitive diagnosis of AIDS: multiple or recurrent bacterial infection in a child under thirteen years, disseminated coccidiomycosis, HIV encephalopathy, disseminated histoplasmosis, isosporiasis with diarrhea greater than one month, lymphoma of the brain, Non-Hodgkin's lymphoma of the B cell type, mycobacterial disease other than *M. tuberculosis*, recurrent *Salmonella* bacteremia, "slim disease."

Without a positive HIV antibody test but no other cause of immunodeficiency, the following diseases indicate a definitive diagnosis of AIDS: esophageal candidiasis, extrapulmonary cryptococcosis, cryptosporidiosis with diarrhea greater than one month, CMV in organ other than liver, spleen, or lymph node, herpes simplex bronchitis, pneumonia or mucocutaneous ulcer of greater than one month, disseminated *Mycobacterium avium* complex or *M. kansasii*, PCP, progressive multifocal leukoencephalopathy, toxoplasmosis of the brain, lymphoid interstitial pneumonia in patient under thirteen years.[b]

---

[a] From Centers for Disease Control (1982b, 508).

[b] Adapted from Centers for Disease Control case definition (1987, 15S).

forms that do not fit into any of the above categories. Depending on the study, a "case" may consist of either both Group III and IV infections or Group IV infections only.

Table 3.2
CDC Classification System for HIV Infection, 1986

Group I: Acute infection

Group II: Asymptomatic infection
    A. Normal lab findings
    B. Abnormal lab results including: anemia, leukopenia, lymphopenia, drop in CD4 count

Group III: Persistent generalized lymphadenopathy
    A. Normal labs
    B. Abnormal labs

Group IV: Other diseases
    A. Constitutional symptoms including: prolonged fever, diarrhea, weight loss
    B. Neurological symptoms
    C. Opportunistic infections (includes case-defined AIDS)
    D. Secondary cancers
    E. Other pathologies

Adapted from Centers for Disease Control (1986, 35: 334–339).

    The 1987 CDC classification system of HIV infection was designed to count cases and predict trends in the epidemic on a population basis. It was not intended either as a diagnostic tool or as a prognostic schema. Yet in the United States, clinicians, governmental agencies, and community activists have adopted it for both these purposes, resulting in continuing controversy over what exactly constitutes a case of AIDS. The French clinician informants only used the CDC system when collecting epidemiologic data for WHO or in writing articles for medical journals.

    In 1991, after my field research had ended, the CDC proposed a new classification system, based primarily on positive serology and the number of T4, also known as CD4, lymphocytes in the blood, the immune system cells believed to be initially targeted and destroyed by the virus (Nowak 1991). This "CD4 count," as it is called, has been in use for prognostic and treatment purposes on both sides of the Atlantic since about 1984, increasing in use as the process of lymphocyte typing and counting has become more accurate. The initial proposal was modified to incorporate symptoms into the classification and was adopted in 1993 (Centers for Disease Control 1992a; see Table 3.3). The new classification system, while not explicitly a "staging" system, is both descriptive and prognostic, to be used in guiding treatment decisions (5).

The most startling change is that a person may be totally asymptomatic and still be classified as having AIDS, stage A3. This definition of AIDS will now include many people that had previously been defined as not yet having AIDS. For example, the 1993 US case estimates using the 1987 definition ranged from 52,000 to 61,000. Applying the 1993 definition, the estimates ranged from 95,000 to 118,000 (CDC 1992b, 18). This carries implications for the US health care system, to be discussed below.

The World Health Organization has yet to adopt the CDC case definition. The CDC definition is internationally problematic if only due to its reliance on CD4 counts, which are far from globally available. In their guidelines for clinical management (World Health Organization 1991), for example, WHO refers only to symptomatic and asymptomatic HIV infection. The WHO Collaborating Group proposed a new staging system in 1993 (without reference to the CDC proposals), which utilizes a similar combination of clinical and laboratory data but is based on four rather than three clinical stages—asymptomatic, early, intermediate, and late. Unlike the CDC system, CD4 counts are supplemental rather than essential, and this proposal is explicitly intended for classifying patients into hierarchical stages of disease progression. It does not, however, define a case of "AIDS." As will be seen, the differences between the two new systems are linked to differences in the structure of health care and in approaches to AIDS between the United States and Europe. The WHO International Collaborating Group proposal, unlike the new CDC definition, has yet to be formally adopted, and neither system was yet in place during the time of this study.

Another classification system for HIV infection does exist, used nearly exclusively by the US military and developed by Robert Redfield and associates at the Walter Reed Army Hospital in 1986. Unlike the CDC system, the Walter Reed system was designed from the start as a diagnostic and prognostic tool to predict the course of the disease in an individual as well as in a population. It is thus a staging system, quite similar in structure to staging systems used for various cancers, and forms a basis for treatment decisions in individual patients. Its focus is on CD4 counts and biochemical data rather than the various clinical manifestations that make up the 1987 CDC system (see Table 3.4).

As will be seen, treatment for HIV infection and AIDS varies between France and the United States, and indeed from site to site within the United States. However, some very generalized approaches have been developed over the past decade. After the patient has been diagnosed with HIV infection, usually through the ELISA and confirmatory Western blot tests, he or she is given a full checkup and an initial CD4 count is made. If that count is above a certain level (which varies) and the patient is experiencing no symptoms, he or she is merely observed every six months

Table 3.3
CDC Classification for HIV Infection and
AIDS Case Definition, 1993

	(A) Asymptomatic or Acute HIV or PGL[a]	**(B)** Symptomatic Not (A) or (C)	**(C)** AIDS Indicator Conditions
CD4 > 499/mm³ **CD4 > 28%**	(A1)	(B1)	(C1) **AIDS**
CD4 200-499/mm³ **CD4 14-28%**	(A2)	(B2)	(C2) **AIDS**
CD4 < 200/mm³ **CD4 < 14%**	(A3) **AIDS**	(B3) **AIDS**	(C3) **AIDS**

AIDS indicator conditions include the following:

Candidiasis (bronchi, trachea, lungs)
Candidiasis, esophageal
Cervical cancer, invasive
Coccidiomycosis, extrapulmonary
Cryptosporidiosis, chronic intestinal
Cytomegalovirus disease (other than retinitis)
Cytomegalovirus retinitis
Encephalopathy, HIV-related
Herpes simplex: chronic ulcers, bronchitis, pneumonitis, esophagitis
Histoplasmosis, disseminated or extrapulmonary
Isosporiasis, chronic intestinal
Kaposi's sarcoma

Lymphoma, Burkitt's
lymphoma, immunoblastic and/or brain
Mycobacterium avium complex or *M. kansasii*, disseminated or extrapulmonary
Mycobacterium, other species
Pneumocystis carinii pneumonia
Pneumonia, recurrent
Progressive mulitfocal leukoencephalopathy
Salmonella septicemia, recurrent
Toxoplasmosis, brain
Wasting syndrome of HIV

[a] persistent generalized lymphadenopathy
Adapted from Centers for Disease Control (1992a, 1–19).

Table 3.4
Walter Reed Staging System for HIV Infection

Stage	HIV Antibody	Lymph- adenopathy	CD4 Count	Skin Sensitivity	Thrush	OI
WR0	–	probable	or	possible	exposure	0
WR1	+	0	> 400	normal	0	0
WR2	+	+/–	> 400	normal	0	0
WR3	+	+/–	< 400	normal	0	0
WR4	+	+/–	< 400	partial	0	
WR5	+	+/–	< 400	partial/ complete	+	0
WR6	+	+/–	< 400	partial/ complete	+/–	0

Notes: "Skin sensitivity" refers to delayed skin hypersensitivity response, much like an allergy skin test, which helps to determine the functioning of certain elements of the immune system. "Thrush" is another name for oral candidiasis, a common fungal infection in AIDS. "OI" stands for the presence of opportunistic infections.

Adapted from Redfield, Wright and Tramont (1986, 131–132)

to a year, with repeated testing of the CD4 count. When the count drops to a certain level or the patient experiences symptoms, antiviral therapy is begun, usually with AZT (formerly called azidothymidine; now called zidovudine), though other antiviral drugs such as DDI (also known as dideoxyinosine or didanosine) and DDC (formerly known as dideoxycytidine; now called zalcitabine),[7] may also be used. The time from infection to the first clinical symptoms of the disease may be ten years or longer. When the CD4 count drops to 200/mm^3—this seems to be universal—prophylaxis against *Pneumocystis carinii* pneumonia (PCP) is begun, usually with inhaled aerosolized pentamidine or the antibiotic Bactrim, taken in the form of pills.

After this point, treatment varies considerably, depending on the type of infections and/or neoplasms developed by the patient. The most common infections, besides PCP, are various forms of tuberculosis; cytomegalovirus (CMV) retinitis, an infection of the retina; esophageal candidiasis, a fungal infection of the throat; and toxoplasmosis, an infection that affects the brain and occurs more commonly in France due to differences in food storage and preparation. Once a patient has had an opportunistic infection, he or she will generally remain on medication to prevent recurrence, if possible. The most common cancers seen in persons with AIDS are Kaposi's sarcoma and lymphoma, usually of the non-Hodgkin's type.[8] Kaposi's sarcoma, if confined to the skin, usually has a more indolent course than lymphoma, is found more commonly among homosexual men with HIV, and can occur in patients with relatively high CD4 counts. Thus, though treatment for both types of cancer can include chemotherapy, KS is often left alone or treated locally with radiation. With all this, survival of persons in the United States with 1987 CDC-defined Group IV AIDS has doubled since the start of the epidemic, from a matter of months to about two years in some populations (Bartlett 1992; Jacobson et al. 1993). A few people infected with HIV at the beginning of the epidemic have yet to develop symptoms. A few people with AIDS have survived, though are generally quite sick, for ten years. Most people with AIDS die.

AIDS is a global epidemic but affects different parts of the world differently, particularly in terms of caseload and demographic patterns. In West and Central Africa, the prevalence of AIDS and HIV infection is suspected to be quite high, but lack of access to antibody test materials and inconsistent reporting make the actual numbers difficult to assess. Men and women are affected in equal number, with transmission of HIV occurring mainly through heterosexual intercourse, perinatal (mother-fetus) transmission, and transfusions with HIV-infected blood, demonstrating what has been called a "Pattern Two" epidemiologic picture (Von Reyn and Mann 1987). Additionally, the picture is complicated in West Africa by the prevalence of another virus, HIV-2, which can also cause AIDS.

The United States and Western Europe, in contrast, have been considered "Pattern One" areas, with men being affected with HIV more often than women, transmission more commonly occurring in the context of male-male sexual activity and/or intravenous drug use. Most Pattern One countries, however, are experiencing a rise in HIV infection in women and, through perinatal transmission, in children, thus increasingly blurring the distinctions between the two epidemiological "patterns." Despite broad, general similaritpies, there are some notable differences in the specific configuration of the epidemic in France and the United States.

According to WHO figures as of March 1987, France had 1632 reported AIDS cases, the greatest number for all Europe, averaging 29.7 cases per million population (WHO Collaborating Centre on AIDS 1987). In contrast, the United States had 35,219 cases, averaging 148 cases per million (quoted in *Liberation* June 1, 1987, 4–5). By March 1990, France reported 9,718 cases, for a cumulative incidence rate of 173.2 cases per million population, giving France the highest total caseload and the second-highest cumulative incidence rate in Europe (WHO Collaborating Centre 1990a). The United States, in March 1991, reported a total of 166,913 cases, for an annual rate of 168 per million population (CDC 1991) and a cumulative rate approaching 834 cases per million. Because of the over fourfold difference in the cumulative incidence of AIDS between the two countries, one suspects that American physicians would speak of AIDS as a more immediate and threatening health problem than French clinicians, especially in hard-hit urban areas.

Approximately half of all French AIDS cases are located in and around Paris, while most of the remaining cases occur along the southern coastal region. In contrast, New York City alone accounts for approximately 19 percent of all American cases—nearly the same absolute number of cases as all of Europe—with most of the rest spread among ten urban centers (Direction Générale de la Santé 1990; CDC 1991—see Table 3.5). Note that Paris and Chicago have similar caseloads of about 4,500 apiece. Thus, the AIDS epidemic in France is mainly confined to one area, while it is geographically more dispersed in the United States. Still, a provincial physician in France and a rural/small urban physician in many parts of the United States are unlikely to have yet encountered AIDS in their daily practice. The epidemiologic character of the epidemic differs to a moderate extent as well. The ratio of men to women with AIDS in France is 5.8 to 1; in the United States, it is 9.1 to 1. In France, 52 percent of cases occur in gay or bisexual men, 19 percent among IV drug users (IVDUs) and 10 percent in heterosexual men and women without histories of IV drug use. The percentages in the United States are similar for the first two categories, 57 and 19 percent respectively, but only 5 percent reported heterosexual cases (Direction Générale de la Santé 1990; CDC 1991). In Italy and Spain, in contrast to France, IV drug users make up a large (up to 66 percent) proportion of AIDS cases, and this proportion continues to increase in much of Europe (WHO Collaborating Centre 1990b). Thus, while homosexual men still constitute the greatest population at risk in France, the experiences of Italy and Spain, both France's immediate neighbors, may sensitize the French medical community to AIDS in the drug-using population. A similar contrast exists within the United States itself, between the predominantly homosexual/bisexual caseload in San Francisco and the spiraling numbers of affected IV drug users in the New York City area. IV drug users have a reputation for being noncompliant and generally difficult patients, an idea accentuated further by the AIDS epidemic (Newmeyer et al. 1989). As the proportion of persons with AIDS who are IV drug users grows in certain areas, medical discourse in those areas may utilize different metaphors than in areas with another makeup of cases.

It is interesting to note that while US statistics often show a breakdown of numbers according to race, French statistics do not. Rather, the French record the number of cases in people coming into France from Africa and the Caribbean, usually immigrants (Direction Générale de la Santé 1990). In 1987, 5 percent of AIDS patients diagnosed in Europe originated from thirty African countries, and this percentage was closer to 13 percent earlier in the epidemic. Fifty-seven percent of these patients were living in Europe before the onset of the first symptoms (WHO Collaborating Centre 1987). In France in 1986, 11 percent of patients came from equatorial Africa (CDC 1986), and while the percentage has decreased somewhat, it

Table 3.5
French and American AIDS Statistics, 1990–1991

Reported AIDS Cases

United States (March, 1991)[a]
	Total	171, 876
	Men	153, 695
	Women	18, 181

France (June, 1990)[b]
	Total	9, 718
	Men	8, 297
	Women	1, 421

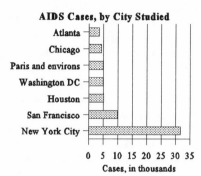

AIDS Cases, by City Studied

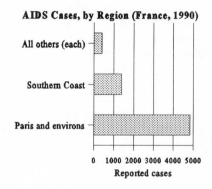

AIDS Cases, by Region (France, 1990)

Breakdown of Cases by Exposure Category

United States

male homosexual/ bisexual contact	57%
intravenous drug use	19%
heterosexual contact	5%
transfusion	2%
hemophilia	1%
other/undetermined	4%

France

male homosexual/ bisexual contact	52%
intravenous drug use	19%
heterosexual contact	10%
in persons of African or Caribbean origin	6%
transfusion	6%
children	3%

---

[a]All US data adapted from Centers for Disease Control (1991)
[b]All French data adapted from Direction Générale de la Santé (1990) and WHO
Collaborating Centre on AIDS (1990b)

is this feature of AIDS in France, this awareness of Africa, that sets the French medical perspective somewhat apart from the gay-oriented view common to the United States (Leibowitch 1985). Additionally, immigrants and travelers with HIV infection from other European countries are not uncommon and were encountered on a regular, if infrequent, basis at the Paris clinic. Thus, the diverse character of the AIDS epidemic in France is often a result of international encounters, while the diversity in the US epidemic stems from that found within its own borders.[9]

HEALTH CARE IN FRANCE AND THE UNITED STATES

France, unlike the United States, has a nationalized system of health care, one that is organized and administered uniformly on the national level by Securité Sociale and financed through employee/employer payroll contributions to various Sickness Insurance Funds (SIFs).[10] The governing board of the main SIF includes union and employer representatives plus two representatives from the Ministry of Social Security. Approximately 80 percent of the public, those who work for a yearly salary, pay into this main fund, while the agricultural fund covers another 9 percent, and a third fund covers self-employed persons, about 6 percent of the population. Finally, the last 5 or so percent are the unemployed poor, who are covered by Securité Sociale and legally required local funds (Fielding and Lancry 1993). Supplemental private insurance provides additional coverage for the self-employed, who have a lower reimbursement rate, and for coverage of the extensive copayments integral to the French system.

One drain on the system comes, at least in theory, from non-European Community visitors and immigrants who have yet to pay into the French system and carry no applicable health insurance of their own.[11] At the Paris AIDS clinic, these were most often Americans and people from African countries.

Under the French national health system, patients pay their doctor directly and then apply to the local Social Security office for a refund, usually 75 percent of the cost. The physician, in turn, must agree to abide by the authorized fees (Wilsford 1991). Securité Sociale pays for 80 percent of hospitalization and 100 percent for long or complicated illnesses. Medications are covered as well, ranging from 40 to 100 percent reimbursement. Almost all of the medications used to treat HIV infection and its severe complications are reimbursed fully, including AZT and other antivirals, as well as intravenous antibiotics. Finally, Securité Sociale covers disability benefits, up to two thirds of the person's former salary, provided over a number of years if necessary. Patients may choose any physician they wish, as long as the doctor has agreed to the national fee schedule—which encompasses over 85 percent of physicians (Ardagh 1987). Patients may also change doctors whenever they wish.

About 57 percent of all French physicians are in primary care fields (Fielding and Lancry 1993). The majority of these are general practitioners, *médecins de ville*, working in private, meaning nonsalaried, practice. These doctors cannot admit or follow their patients in the hospital and, in the case of AIDS, cannot prescribe certain medications, including AZT. They have generally little power or prestige in the French medical community (Baszanger 1985). A little more than a third of French doctors are employed on a salary basis in hospitals and, except for medical residents, are all specialists, with general internal medicine considered a specialty (Wilsford 1991). Thus, the American medical term *attending physician* has no meaning in the French context. Patients in the hospital are followed by the appropriate hospital-employed specialist. Eighty percent of all French hospitals are public hospitals, which includes all academically associated medical centers. Thus, public hospitals in France tend to have the most highly trained personnel and most advanced technology.

With the recent increase in the number of doctors in France, from 86 to 210 per 100,000 persons between 1965 and 1983, many clinicians are facing stiff competition for patients and a decrease in income. Although the average yearly income is about 250,000 francs ($45,000), many practitioners in industrial areas earn less than half that figure. In addition, many health service physicians work up to sixty-hour weeks and even take on additional part-time jobs to supplement their income (Ardagh 1987). For the hospital-based physician, finding a position and advancing in one's career are both difficult propositions. The position of department head, known as *chef de service*, is a lifetime appointment, and the *chef* exerts near-total control over the organization and makeup of his service, to the bane of younger physicians (Escande 1975). Other than time-limited junior staff positions, the number of long-term salaried positions is strictly controlled. In the university hospitals, there must be an academic opening as well as a physician's opening in order for a new senior physician to be hired. As a consequence, doctors may sometimes find themselves unemployed or with little hopes of advancement. This very situation led to a physician's strike around 1989 (Rozenbaum 1990, personal communication).

Finally, there exists no single French medical association comparable in size and power to the American Medical Association (AMA). Rather, there are three more moderately sized associations, generally affiliated with a particular political viewpoint, and a host of smaller associations. Well under 40 percent of private practice physicians, as of 1984, belonged to any medical association (Wilsford 1991, 100). Thus, as Wilsford points out, the medical community in France is fragmented in the face of a unified central administration, leading to bureaucratic control of the health care system and devaluation of traditional prerogatives of physicians. Discourse of French physicians, as will be shown later, revolves more intently around issues of bureaucracy and governmental control than that of American physicians.

The American health care system may hardly be said to constitute a "system" at all but rather consists of a number of highly variable and loosely related institutions. Better than 50 percent of Americans purchase private health insurance of variable cost and coverage, either as individuals or through group plans at their workplace. A number of health programs, such as Medicare for the elderly, are administered, at least in part, by the federal government but do not form a cohesive whole in any sense, being administered, funded, and overseen separately (Wilsford

1991). Some, but not all, who cannot afford private insurance participate in Medicaid, a joint federal-state program, with eligibility and coverage varying from state to state. Approximately 37 million people have no form of health insurance at all, and generally few medications of any kind are covered by insurance (Wilsford 1991).

The physician in the United States has historically been an independent agent, working alone or in a group practice, although this is changing with the rise of HMOs (health maintenance organizations) and similar prepaid plans. With the exception of physicians in the nationalized military and prison systems, the physician is almost never an employee of a hospital and is reimbursed by the patient or insurer on a fee-for-service basis (Starr 1982). On the average, American doctors earn more than twice their French counterparts, over $100,000 a year as of 1982 (Wilsford 1991). There are no general practitioners in the United States, at least not in the same sense as French generalists, with the possible exception of family practice doctors, who constitute only 7 percent of all American physicians. Rather, there are classes of specialties considered as "primary care"—general internal medicine, pediatrics, and sometimes obstetrics/gynecology. Under these categories are a number of affiliated subspecialties, and over 60 percent of US physicians fall into a specialist or subspecialist category (Fielding and Lancry 1993).

The vast majority of hospitals in the United States are private, either for-profit or not-for-profit. Only a few hospitals are run by city, state, or federal organizations, such as those of the Veterans Administration. In order to attract physicians into admitting patients and make enough money to continue to operate, American hospitals attempt to provide the latest technological equipment while limiting the admission of uninsured or poorly reimbursing Medicaid patients. In the case of AIDS, the direct financial burdens of patients on both the hospital and the physician's private practice are an important element in American clinical concerns. Again, physicians are not employees of the hospital but utilize their facilities by gaining admission privileges at a particular set of hospitals. Unlike the case in France, American physicians in any specialty may gain admitting privileges and prescribe any nonexperimental medication approved for use in the United States.

About 50 percent of all American physicians belong to a single, large organization, the American Medical Association (Starr 1982). Although not as monolithic an organization as in the past, it still acts as a powerful force in determining health care policy in the United States. Thus, in contrast to the French situation, the medical community is unified in the face of a fragmented central administration, retaining a high level of power in determining the structure of health care (Wilsford 1991). However, recently, the challenge to this power has come from third-party payers, insurance agencies, state governments (who must provide a portion of Medicaid coverage), health care consumer groups, and those parts of the federal government that administer the large Medicare and Medicaid programs. This change is reflected in the discourse of American physicians, who find their therapeutic decisions being increasingly controlled by financial concerns and the dictates of third-party payers.

There are a number of other differences in the two health care systems, mostly concerning the roles of nurses, pharmacists, and ancillary medical personnel, but these will be discussed when encountered in the data. The other half of the health care equation lies in biomedical research, the organization of which also differs in both countries.

BIOMEDICAL RESEARCH

French researchers, too, are caught up in their formidable bureaucratic system. Most medical research, not only on AIDS, is government sponsored through the Centre National de la Recherche Scientifique (CNRS) or the Institut National de la Santé et de la Recherche Medicale (INSERM), both state-run organizations. Research units of these organizations are found throughout the country and may or may not be affiliated with a university. In other words, CNRS and INSERM not only direct funding but organize and administer much of the biomedical research in France, with researchers becoming members of these institutions.

Even the Institut Pasteur, a private research institution and center for postgraduate teaching, receives over 40 percent of its funding from the government. Some researchers, as mentioned previously, rely on private funding alone, but on the whole, this is rare. There is stiff competition among young PhDs to gain a tenured position at either CNRS or INSERM. If a person is not accepted, he or she must look for a private position, completely outside of the French university system, which includes the Pasteur. The prospects are comparatively bleak. Unlike the United States, few private industries, including the small French pharmaceutical industry, have well-endowed departments for research and development (Ardagh 1987). Thus, the incentive, especially for younger researchers, is to produce and publish significant results as quickly as possible.

Once accepted into the system, funding—which provides technical equipment and personnel but not researcher salaries—for particular research projects remains problematic, even for those working on AIDS. Until recently, many of my research informants complained of not receiving oft-promised financial support from the government. Nontenured French researchers, therefore, have an even greater impetus than their American counterparts to publish spectacular results as quickly as possible, while tenured scientists have less need to tackle controversial topics such as AIDS. Since the government increased funding for AIDS,[12] along with its rise in scientific prestige, many established researchers have entered AIDS research, while doctoral and postdoctoral students feel they have little choice but to work at least temporarily in the AIDS field.

In the United States, research is less centralized than in France, though the government subsidizes a vast amount of research through grants to individuals, groups, and institutions. Federal institutions such as the National Science Foundation (NSF) direct funding but do not directly provide organization, materials or personnel for the research, while others, such as the National Institutes of Health (NIH), may do both. In general, the researcher in the United States, like the physician, is an independent agent whose grants must be reviewed and renewed on a regular basis. As Harden and Rodrigues (1993) note, the lengthy peer-review process at NIH inhibited swift distribution of funding to researchers, particularly in the early years of the epidemic. Since 1989, governmental agencies such as NIH and the Food and Drug Administration (FDA) have developed community-based and "fast-track" trials to help accelerate the pace of research (Fox 1992).

Universities are either private or organized on the state level, and thus many PhDs are not employed by federally organized institutions but by individual universities. The American university-based researcher has incentives to explore controversial areas of research if, and only if, governmental or private funding agencies recognize that area as important. A lack of federal interest was important early in the AIDS epidemic (Shilts 1987), but according to some of my informants, the pendulum has swung the other way, favoring AIDS research at the expense of other fields.

A large amount of biomedical research is done in the private sector, through industrial research and development. Pharmaceutical companies often invest major sums of money in exploring and marketing new medications and, unlike those in France, employ a significant number of PhD-level researchers to accomplish this. The drawback in terms of AIDS has been that, until recently, relatively small numbers of American patients have been affected by the disease, so there was little profit incentive for drug companies to invest in AIDS research. As the cases have multiplied, so has the participation of drug companies, to the point that some physicians and community activists have accused the industry of reaping exorbitant profits off of desperately ill people. The drug companies counter that they are simply recouping their research investment. The complicated ties between pharmaceutical companies, drug development, and health care in the United States are generally unknown in France. The result is that many of the major AIDS medications come out of American research, but once developed, access by American patients is problematic. French clinicians, on the other hand, often must rely on American antivirals research, but when the drug is finally made available in France, it is usually available to all French patients.

LOCAL CONTEXT: ORGANIZATION OF THE PARIS AND CHICAGO CLINICS

Accounting for the local context, the everyday environment of discourse, is equally important as the more global surroundings. Elements involved in the local context of a clinic include patient mix, number and types of physicians, the role of nurses and allied health care workers, physical setting, the daily organization of activities and lastly, the nature of the relationships—formal or informal—between all those participating in the life of the clinic. Differences and similarities between the Paris and Chicago clinics may serve as later markers of the distinctiveness of AIDS-related medicine and contrast French versus American approaches to clinical care. Since informants from both these clinics will be referred to often in the body of this study, a list of their names (pseudonyms) and clinic positions is provided in Table 3.6.

Table 3.6
Staff of Rousseau and Northlake Clinics

Rousseau (Paris)	**Northlake** (Chicago):
Chef de Service	Clinic Director
Dr. Bernard	Dr. O'Neill
Senior Physicians	Attendings
Dr. Farsi	Dr. Fields (also head of AIDS research)
Dr. Martine	Dr. Westin
Dr. Lefevre	
Médecins de ville (attachés)	Associated Attendings
Dr. Cohen	Dr. Landry
Dr. Bertrand	Dr. Goldstein
Dr. Cartier	Dr. Donaldson
Dr. Soulis	Dr. Norman
three others	Dr. Greco
Residents (three at a given time)	Infectious Disease Fellows
	Dr. Campbell
	Dr. Holtzman
	Dr. Peters

The Paris Clinic: Rousseau

The Paris clinic, now located in the university-affiliated Hôpital Rousseau, has been in existence in one form or another since 1982, nearly the beginning of the epidemic. It is thus the oldest of several similar clinics, and it is dedicated exclusively to treating HIV infection. Fortunately for my research, a patient database is maintained on the clinic's computer system and enabled me to perform demographic and epidemiologic breakdowns of its approximately 2,000 patients (see Table 3.6). The breakdown by transmission group is somewhat misleading, since the clinic has not officially been accepting any new patients since 1990 and thus does not reflect the higher rate of new cases among nonhomosexual patients.

The most interesting statistic is the significant percentage—13.6 percent—of foreign-born patients, not only from former French colonies (which continue to have ties with France) but from the United States as well. Although certainly forming a minority of their patients, doctors in the Rousseau clinic were exposed to the experience of AIDS outside their national, even continental boundaries. Additionally, many of the clinic's patients travel outside of Europe, to North Africa, the Middle East, or Asia, which expands on this international experience. For example, during an interview with one of the clinic physicians, we were interrupted by a phone call from Oman, a small country on the Arabian peninsula. The physician then explained to me that a French patient of the clinic had traveled with a friend to Sri Lanka, where he experienced several epileptic seizures and was put on emergency flight back to France. The patient had then gone into a coma on the plane and was hospitalized in Oman. The call had been from the patient's friend, asking the physician to advise the local doctors, who had never before encountered an AIDS patient. The rest of the world seems more of an immediate factor when, as happened to me, your patient brings in X-rays from Katmandu, Nepal.

The Rousseau clinic was staffed by four senior physicians, one of whom, Dr. Bernard, was the *chef de service*. Seven other general practitioners from the community, called *attachés*, worked part-time in the clinic, anywhere from one to three days a week—a most unusual arrangement for a French medical service. At the beginning of the epidemic, many of these physicians had contacted Dr. Bernard for advice concerning their AIDS patients. He and the general practitioners began meeting on an informal basis and in 1985 established a more formal group of fifteen generalists interested in AIDS. These physicians have a strong relationship with Dr. Bernard and received additional training through him before starting work at the clinic as part of an experimental program. Three residents, changing every six months, rounded out the physician staff, along with an occasional medical student. Additionally, two psychiatrists, a neurologist, and an ophthalmologist consulted at the clinic on a regular basis, ranging from every day to once or twice a week. Treatment for Kaposi's sarcoma was handled by the clinic doctors, but patients with lymphoma were referred to an oncologist outside the clinic.

Allied health staff consisted of a psychologist and five nurses. There were no phlebotomists, respiratory therapists, physical therapists, or other ancillary personnel common to US medical clinics, and these are rare in French hospitals in general. The nurses were responsible for administering aerosolized pentamidine treatments (prophylaxis for PCP), intravenous antibiotics, and intravenous chemotherapy and performing all blood draws. They did not see patients into offices or check any vital

Table 3.7
Patient Population at the Rousseau Clinic in Paris

Number of Patients[a]

Total	2284
Men	1983
Women	301

Only 1,000-1,200 of the total are followed regularly

Breakdown by Exposure Category[b]

Homosexual	1,026	hemophiliacs	0
Bisexual[c]	171	partner at risk	84
IV drug user	203	undetermined[d]	100
single transfusion	19		
mult. transfusion	15		

Geographical breakdown (based on 2,284 patients)

Living in Paris	1,230
Living in suburbs (100km radius)	614
Living outside Ile-de-France	440

National origin

This is based on country of origin, not where patient presently lives. Unless otherwise noted, all non-French have present address in France. Based on 1,345 patients for whom this information is given.

Total French	1,162	Total North, South and Central	
Total non-French	183	Americans	63
Total other European	53	Total Asia,	
Total Africa,		including Middles East	22
including North Africa	42	Pacific islands, Australia, NZ	2
		Soviet Union	1

Fourteen most common nationalities of non-French patients

1. United States	6. Lebanon	11. Guadeloupe
2. Italy	7. Argentina	12. Morocco
3. Algeria	8. Brazil	13. Congo
4. Portugal	9. Colombia	14. Spain
5. Tunisia	10. Germany	

[a]All data were derived from clinic's computer database as of November 25, 1990
[b]Based on total of 1,618 patients for whom this information is given
[c]Not usually distinguished from homosexual
[d]Heterosexual transmission accounted for by the last two groups

signs. In fact, none of the nurses carried stethoscopes, standard equipment for American nurses. The nursing staff held weekly meetings separately from the physicians and did not participate routinely in case discussions. Clinic doctors, however, verbally acknowledged "the special work" of the nurses on a daily basis and often stated that working with AIDS patients was hardest on them. One nurse was trained as a TEC, *technicien d'études cliniques*, to collect and organize the data for clinical trials. The trials themselves, however, were coordinated by one doctor who had recently finished residency, in consultation with the *chef*.

Most patients came to the clinic as referrals, already knowing their HIV-positive status. Fifty to sixty patients a day came in for office visits, *consultations*, with the senior physicians, *attachés*, or visiting specialists. About twenty to thirty patients a day came into the *hôpital de jour* (HDJ), an area of the clinic serving outpatients, consisting of five beds separated by dividers and run mainly by the residents. The *hôpital de jour* handled routine outpatient needs, such as scheduled labs, renewing of prescriptions, intravenous antibiotics and chemotherapy, and diagnostic procedures including lumbar punctures and skin biopsies. Additionally, patients with new or urgent complaints generally came in through the HDJ.

Residents checked vital signs on all these patients, as well as performed the histories and physicals needed for many of the therapies used in treating HIV infection. Residents were overseen by one of the senior physicians (other than the clinic director), and I participated mainly in this area of the clinic. Patients often came alone to the clinic, but sometimes a lover, friend, or single family member—usually the mother—would accompany them.

If hospitalization was needed, approximately fifteen beds were available in the main hospital itself, on the general medicine and gastroenterology services. However, there was an agreement between the clinic and main hospital that clinic doctors did not follow their patients during hospitalization unless called in by the hospital physicians. This is somewhat unusual in France, and my clinic informants seemed unhappy with the situation. If there were no beds at the main hospital, or the patient had a condition best treated at a hospital with a different range of specialties, he or she could be admitted to another hospital. Thus, unlike the case in Chicago, there were no hospital rounds as part of the daily routine.

Patients could also receive some hospital-style treatment, such as intravenous antibiotics, at home through a program called *Hôpitalization à Domicile* (HAD), literally "hospitalization at home." This type of program, unusual in France, was overseen by nurses and functioned as a cross between American-style home health care and hospice programs.

The Rousseau clinic was not a physically imposing space, being rather small in comparison with many American hospital clinics. The floors were tile, the waiting room was a hallway with chairs, and the heating erratic. The equipment was serviceable rather than state-of-the-art, with reuseable glass thermometers and digital scales that one could find in most American department stores. Lumbar puncture equipment was assembled individually rather than coming in a prepackaged tray. Yet after the initial adjustment, I felt little lack for the medical necessities, with the exception of having to send patients to another hospital for an MRI (magnetic resonance imaging) scan.

The day at the Rousseau began at 8:30 A.M. with espresso and cigarettes in a tiny meeting room. Residents and senior doctors crowded around the table, reviewing the patients scheduled to come in that day. Recent journal articles and world and personal events were also prime topics for conversation, making this meeting a social gathering as much as an informational one. Patients would be seen generally from nine to noon, depending on the number of patients scheduled and the flow of HDJ patients, who did not have specific appointment times. Lunch, taken at the hospital cafeteria, was rarely shorter than an hour, and wine was not an uncommon accompaniment to the meal.[13] Though specific cases were rarely discussed over lunch, AIDS generally found its way into the conversation at some point. The afternoon was dedicated to patient care, and most of the staff left by six in the evening.

A physician staff meeting was held one morning a week, and all interested doctors, including those from the main hospital, were invited to attend. Three or four cases would be informally presented, sometimes to the point of a doctor simply asking, "What's going on with so-and-so?" A radiologist from the main hospital came to nearly all of these meetings, and several were dedicated to examining X-rays and CT (computerized tomograhpy) and MRI scans of patients with various AIDS-related ailments. The *chef* generally presided over these meetings, and often would bring in outside guests, such as palliative care experts, exposing the rest of the staff to new perspectives. Additionally, a "journal club"—a common fixture in American hospitals—was held once a week, in which senior physicians and residents would present relevant articles for discussion.

As several informants pointed out to me, the organization and atmosphere of the clinic were different from other hospital clinics in France. Patients often changed the paper on the beds in the HDJ themselves, and some checked their own weight and temperature before the resident could greet them. Patients, nurses and residents were on a first-name basis, and long-standing patients greeted the senior doctors by first name as well. Patients would bring gifts to the nurses or secretarial staff, such that there were consistently flowers on the front desk and a box of chocolates in the nurses' office.

More remarkable to me was the informality between residents and the senior physicians. Residents often came dressed in jeans and sweaters—not uncommon in other hospital settings in France, I was told—and were also on a first-name basis with all the senior physicians, including Dr. Bernard, something quite unusual in the rigidly hierarchical French system (Escande 1975; and according to all informants). Few formal case presentations were required of the residents, and they were not pushed to do procedures with which they felt uncomfortable, quite different from my own American experience as a medical student. The atmosphere was one of warmth, informality, support, and guidance through a complex medical experience.

The Rousseau clinic was different from other French clinics not only in atmosphere but in structure. The involvement of community general practitioners and the HDJ and HAD programs all were innovations almost unheard of prior to AIDS, along with the introduction of organized palliative care. In fact, the Rousseau clinic is structured in many ways like American AIDS clinics, be it through intentional adoption of some American practices (though only a few of the staff had ever been to the United States) or through independently arriving at similar solutions to similar problems.

The Chicago Clinic: Northlake

The Chicago clinic, part of the not-for-profit Northlake Hospital, has been in place since 1986 and shares a patient population comparable to the Rousseau clinic in terms of size and breakdown by transmission. Though exact data were impossible to obtain since the clinic did not keep computerized records, there were also some obvious differences between the two clinic populations. A greater percentage of the Chicago patients were male and lived within fifty miles of Chicago. A handful of patients came from other parts of Illinois and an even smaller number from other states, along with a few foreign-born, mainly Hispanic patients. The international diversity seen in the French clinic was countered by the internal diversity of the American clinic, represented by significant numbers of African-American and Hispanic patients. Like the French clinic, Northlake was attempting to limit the total number of new patients, but particularly uninsured or Medicaid-insured patients trying to transfer their care from the county's public hospital.

The Northlake clinic was run mainly by two full-time attending physicians, along with six part-time associated attendings, trained either in internal medicine or in infectious disease. The two full-time doctors also did some private practice work but devoted most of their time to the clinic, while the part-time attendings spent considerably more time on research, clinical duties on other medical services, or at their private offices. At any given time, three infectious disease fellows, postresidency doctors working on specialty training, shared a large responsibility for patient care and worked daily in the clinic, while two others did clinical work on a part-time basis. Residents were not involved with the clinic on any regular basis.

As was the case in Paris, there were a number of specialists affiliated with the Chicago clinic. A neurologist and hemophilia specialist saw patients in the clinic one to two days a week, as well as on a consultation basis. An ophthalmologist and oncologist saw clinic patients in their own separate offices in the hospital. All AIDS-related cancer care, including treatment for Kaposi's sarcoma, was handled virtually independently by the oncologist. Additionally, other specialists, such as gastroenterologists, were consulted through the hospital network and informal understandings with the clinic doctors.

The most distinctive aspect of the Northlake organization, in comparison to Rousseau, was the extensive role played by nurses and allied health workers. Many of the thirteen nurses at Northlake held higher-level nursing degrees—bachelor's or master's in nursing—as well as specialized clinical training. The clinical nurses not only administered routine treatments, such as aerosolized pentamidine, but checked vital signs and did preliminary history taking before administering such treatments. Nurses were also responsible for the administration of clinical trials. While the trials were designed by clinic-affiliated doctors or as part of multicenter studies such as the AIDS Clinical Trials Groups (ACTG), the nurses enrolled patients, recorded data, and handled problems associated with the running of the study, roles handled by residents or senior physicians at the Rousseau clinic. Additionally, the clinic staff included two phlebotomists, two respiratory therapists, two psychologists, and two social workers. The social workers, peripheral within the clinic structure at Rousseau, were an integral part of daily patient care and participated in all clinic activities not strictly limited to physicians.

As in France, most patients came to the clinic as referrals, knowing their HIV-positive status. Some continued to utilize their private community physician in addition to the clinic, while many others relied on the clinic for their total health care. Patients would come in for office visits as part of clinical trials, for regular checkups including laboratory work, and for new or urgent problems. The clinic did have an area set aside for administering intravenous medication, lumbar punctures and the like, but it was not as integral a part of the clinic routine as the HDJ in Paris. This area, in fact, was mainly overseen by nurses, not physicians. Seriously ill patients would be admitted to the hospital, usually on an internal medicine floor, but with the "HIV service" as the admitting service and a clinic doctor listed as the attending physician. Thus, unlike the situation at Rousseau, Northlake clinicians were responsible for inpatient as well as outpatient care, and hospital rounds were a part of the daily routine.

Home health care, run by nurses but overseen by clinic physicians, was another integral component of the clinic's activities, and many patients with acute problems were able to be treated in part or entirely at home. Additionally, Northlake Hospital in general maintained a home-based hospice program, with a floor in the hospital dedicated to palliative care. In contrast, terminally ill patients in Paris were cared for in the home or as regular inpatients, so that except for the role of the HAD, no formal hospice program existed at Rousseau. Many Northlake patients were part of the hospice program, and here, too, clinic doctors were responsible for overseeing their care.

A well-endowed, university-based hospital, Northlake strives for state-of-the-art medical care, and the clinic was no exception. All basic medical supplies, such as tongue depressors or procedure trays, came wrapped and prepackaged, and each exam room had its own electronic thermometer. The clinic itself took up about two thirds of a floor, with approximately ten exam rooms and five or six offices for doctors and nurses, plus a large conference room, considerably more space than at Rousseau. All diagnostic equipment, including MRI scans, were available at the hospital, though nonemergency scans sometimes took a week to work into the schedule. Thus, even Northlake was not exempt from technological glitches or occasional lack of supplies. The floors were carpeted, the waiting room filled with upholstered chairs, and colorful framed prints lined the walls.

The daily routine at Northlake began at 8:30 A.M. with patient appointments, lasting straight through until lunch. On the average, a doctor would see from five to ten patients a day, mostly in the mornings, slightly less on average than their Paris counterparts. Lunch was usually a half hour to forty-five minutes and was often taken individually or in small groups, depending on who had finished seeing their morning patients. This contrasts to the French doctors, who all went to lunch together, more or less shutting down the clinic for an hour. In the afternoon, some of the Northlake doctors, usually the part-time physicians, would work in the clinic, while one of the two full-time attendings would lead hospital rounds.

An average of about fifteen to twenty inpatients would be seen daily by "the team": the attending, at least two fellows, the clinic nurse specialist, and at least one of the social workers. The social worker, and sometimes the nurse, would often spend time with the patient apart from the team. Rounds took up the entire afternoon and not infrequently would last until seven at night. Hospital residents, unaffiliated with the clinic, would ask the team general questions on AIDS or discuss some particular aspect of a patient's care. It was here that the Northlake physicians would encounter a patient's friends, lovers, and family, a lesser part of the Rousseau experience.

Meetings and conferences seem to be a universal part of biomedical practice, and Northlake was no exception. The content and style of the meetings were quite different compared with those in Paris. A weekly staff meeting was held to discuss clinic functioning and patient problems. While one or two physicians were usually present, the meeting involved mainly nurses, psychologists, and social workers, and the discussion tended to focus on the financial, emotional, and social aspects of a patient's care. In fact, unlike Rousseau, there were no meetings where clinic physicians would present or discuss the medical aspects of individual cases. Rather, this was done informally during the day, as clinic doctors waited for patients, consulted charts, or looked at X-rays. A more physician-oriented meeting took place once a week to discuss a particular topic in HIV infection, usually with a clinic physician or hospital specialist giving an initial presentation. Sometimes outside speakers presented on topics such as African-Americans and AIDS, and alternative (nonbiomedical) health care. Finally, attendings and fellows participated in a hospitalwide infectious disease meeting, which sometimes involved AIDS-related case presentations.

The atmosphere at Northlake, like that at Rousseau, was one of warmth and collaboration. Nurses and physicians were on a first-name basis, as were the fellows and most of the attendings. However, one of the part-time attendings was also the head of AIDS research at Northlake, in addition to being one of the high-ranking infectious disease attendings, and neither the fellows nor myself ever addressed him by first name.[14] The basic relations between nurses, doctors, and patients at the clinic shared the same closeness that I observed in Paris but with less emphasis on gift-giving by patients.

Throughout this examination of the context of French and American medical discourse on AIDS, we have already encountered several differences that should alert us to variation in discourse and practice in both countries. The history of the epidemic, including the Gallo-Montagnier dispute and the French connection with Africa, forms part of this variation, as do aspects of the present AIDS epidemiology. The systems of health care and biomedical research, grounded themselves in cultural values, provide ample difference when they intersect medical experience with AIDS. Finally, the local, day-to-day context of the clinics themselves frames AIDS discourse as it demonstrates similarities and dissimilarities between the two biomedicines. As we shall see, there may be as much a unifying "culture" of AIDS medicine as there is a diversifying set of biomedical cultures.

NOTES

1. See J. Feldman (1993) for a more detailed discussion of these areas.

2. Technically, AIDS is now seen as the most advanced form of HIV infection. In general, I will use the term *HIV infection* or *HIV disease* when referring to the medically defined spectrum of the disease, which culminates in, and includes, "AIDS." I use *AIDS* when referring to (1) the advanced stage of HIV infection, (2) the disease historically (particularly in the pre-HIV era), and (3) the epidemic at large, including its social phenomena.

3. A glossary of medical terms and acronyms relevant to AIDS is provided at the end of this book.

4. This issue of AIDS in children is complex and outside the scope of this book. All the involved informants and clinics dealt only with adults.

5. Where the technology exists, ELISA results are confirmed by a second test, usually the Western blot technique.

6. This form of AIDS is more common in Africa but can also be found across the United States and Western Europe (Clumeck and De Wit 1988).

7. In 1991, DDI had recently been approved by the Food and Drug Administration, while DDC remained experimental until 1992. Stavudine, also known as d4t, was approved in 1994 for use in advanced HIV infection in those patients who have failed or are intolerant to other antiretrovirals.

8. These cancers are found at a much higher rate in AIDS patients than in the general population. AIDS patients may develop other cancers, including Hodgkin's lymphoma, but generally not at significantly different rates than non-AIDS patients. Recent studies suggest that cervical cancer, linked to infection with human papilloma virus (HPV), may also be more common among women with AIDS, as reflected in the 1993 CDC case definition.

9. As will be seen in subsequent chapters, this affects how AIDS is characterized in each country and interacts with their respective political contexts.

10. Employers pay approximately 13 percent on gross salary, while employees pay 7 percent (Fielding and Lancry 1993).

11. Approximately 1 percent of the population of France lacks health coverage, compared with approximately 15 percent in the United States (Fielding and Lancry 1993).

12. The research budget tripled between 1988 and 1989 (Steffen 1993). Several new agencies, or "structures," have been created as well, such as the Agence Nationale de Recherche sur le SIDA (ANRS), and Centre Interétablissement de Traitement et de Recherche Anti-SIDA (CITRAS).

13. The Rousseau residents usually ate with the physicians at the cafeteria rather than the usual *salle de garde*, a meal room set up explicitly for residents that exists at every French teaching hospital. The room is usually painted by the interns with a variety of satiric pictures of the *chefs de service*, often with sexual or scatological themes. Interns sometimes hold parties there and, according to my resident informants, will traditionally sing lewd or satiric songs poking fun at upper level doctors. There are a number of other rules and rituals governing behavior at the *salle de garde*, quite similar to an American college fraternity house. One of my resident informants told me of a new pediatric hospital deliberately built without a *salle de garde*. The interns there took over a room anyway, painted it, and restored the practice.

14. Dress of the entire staff was also more formal than I encountered in Paris, reflecting perhaps the more socioeconomically "upscale" environment.

Part II

CONSTRUCTING AIDS

4

The Building Blocks of AIDS

To disentangle, to decipher, to classify, to give a meaning to all this chaos, the first requirement is to understand what is happening. Medicine hastily must know, and reveal what it knows. Where, how, who, why, since when, and, as fast as possible, through whom does the evil come?

Dr. Jacques Leibowitch (1985, 9)

INTRODUCTION

AIDS the disease began as an inchoate collection of signs and symptoms recognized by a few physicians as being distinct from other diseases. Biomedicine, in turn, has been a way to "give meaning to all this chaos" through the discourse and practice of clinicians and researchers. As Oppenheimer (1992) remarks of epidemiology, "The content of this science, by providing and naming concepts (for example, 'risk groups'), made the epidemic potentially less frightening by making it appear more likely that the disease would eventually be understood and controlled" (52). The medical community uses a variety of techniques to make AIDS a knowable disease that can be recognized and acted upon, most notably naming, defining boundaries, and through analogies with other diseases. The expected course of the disease is shaped and reshaped in every medical encounter, creating a "new" AIDS over time. Yet, AIDS retains its ambiguity in the process, simultaneously known and unknowable for those who encounter it.

Medical constructions of AIDS do not stay within the medical community but regularly encounter lay models, such as those of patients. Though they may share a similar terminology, the models ultimately differ, requiring continuous negotiation between physicians, researchers, and laypersons. The gap is never completely bridged but becomes incorporated by all parties into the ongoing process of making meaning of AIDS. As Patton (1990) charges, science often serves, consciously or unconsciously, to administer all other discourses about AIDS.[1] Thus, in order to understand the complexity of AIDS as a social phenomenon, we must look at how the medical community builds its constructions of AIDS and then how these models compare and interact with those outside of medicine.

NAMING: THE DISEASE IS THE VIRUS, THE VIRUS IS THE DISEASE

Being able to understand things is incredibly important for physicians. If you get people and have them shut the door and talk to you, people will say "I can live with my patients dying as long as I know what they have."
Clinician, San Francisco

Naming is perhaps the first and most common step in making meaning of any experience. The naming process sets that experience apart and gives us a reference—"That's AIDS." Like many other new and unusual phenomena, what came to be known as AIDS went through a proliferation of names early on in the construction process: gay cancer, immunocompromise syndrome, gay-related immune deficiency (GRID). As we have seen, these names emerged out of a particular social and historical context, left their mark on the meaning of AIDS, and have now fallen by the wayside. The virus accepted to cause AIDS also went through a naming extravaganza, brought out in the Gallo-Montagnier dispute (J. Feldman 1992c). Ultimately, it too emerged with one name.

The name "acquired immunodeficiency syndrome" is purely descriptive, indicating no etiology, no prognosis. It simply defines a particular set of clinical symptoms, a syndrome, as a biomedical entity. This name was consciously decided upon by a committee, rather than arising out of idiosyncratic, informal usage as did most of the prior names (Grmek 1990, 32). It constructs three things about the nature of the disease: that it occurs after birth, that it involves deficits in the immune systems, and that it is not limited to any single group of people. As with HIV, AIDS emerged as the winner of a narrative contest about, in part, the nature of the disease. Although several members of the medical communities in France and the United States were unsatisfied with the name (Leibowitch, University of Illinois lecture 1988), it remains the sole name for the experience of both the disease of doctors and the illness of patients and, as we shall see, is invested with a great deal of meaning by both groups.

With the naming of HIV and its general acceptance as the primary cause of AIDS, another powerful construction was put into place. In lay discourse, HIV is often referred to as "the AIDS virus," inextricably melding the virus and the disease into a single entity. Clinicians and researchers do this too, but by quite a different route. Among American clinicians particularly, AIDS is becoming known as a part of "HIV disease" or "HIV infection." As one San Francisco physician remarked: "I hardly think about AIDS anymore, at least the medical, technical side of me doesn't. When I am thinking as a physician or as a nosologist, I think about HIV infection." Instead of the virus becoming the disease, as in lay discourse, the disease is becoming the virus, with the additional effect of further eliminating the possibility of other etiologies or co-factors from the construction.[2]

At Northlake, sometimes "HIV disease" or "HIV positive" was shortened to simply "HIV," particularly when the patient was sick but without a CDC-defined AIDS diagnosis, as in: "This guy's been HIV for four years now." As one Northlake doctor explained to his patient, "By having KS [Kaposi's sarcoma], you're no longer just HIV, you have AIDS." In French, *HIV disease* translates into a more cumbersome term, *maladie de VIH*, probably accounting for its lack of use at Rousseau, though in 1990 both clinicians and researchers would occasionally use the term when speaking in English.

Even before the term *HIV disease* was coined, however, the virus and the disease were often used interchangeably in medical discourse. John Crewdson, in a 1987 article about the isolation of HIV, quotes a CDC physician: "That we at CDC told NIH, 'You can't announce you've discovered AIDS, because the French already did.'" (Crewdson 1987, 22). The physician, of course, is referring to the discovery of the virus, not the disease. AIDS and HIV continue to be conflated with regularity on both sides of the Atlantic. Below are two French examples, the first from a physician and the second from a young lab researcher:

When you refer a patient to another center which was not used to working with HIV, it was quite common to have trouble with some [doctors]. They took some precautions which were not useful.

I like viruses, I would like to work on retroviruses, and why not AIDS?

The conceptual bond linking AIDS and HIV is so powerful that the two names have essentially become synonyms. The virus is the disease, the disease is the virus.

For laboratory researchers, who have little contact with AIDS patients, the virus acts as a name, a known and knowable entity signifying an unknown phenomenon. For the researcher particularly, to know the virus is to know the disease.

The only thing I know is gathering more and more information on HIV life cycle. We have different classes of drugs that we'll be working with, learning to manipulate in vitro and in patients, and I think we'll learn how to cure these patients of their HIV infection.

On a broader spectrum, I think AIDS, as a disease, while valid for treatment purposes—I think we should be dropping back and looking at the infection of the virus as the disease.

Despite the trend toward a new terminology of "HIV disease," AIDS remains the dominant name in medical and lay discourse. At Northlake, doctors intently address the question, "Is this the patient's 'AIDS defining illness?'" At Rousseau, a patient asks the resident, "Do I have AIDS?" When push comes to shove, it is still AIDS that retains the power in the process of naming. One clinician, even while emphasizing "HIV infection," acknowledged:

There's something powerful about the idea of AIDS that's not conveyed by HIV infection that remains important. To me, tied up in the concept of AIDS is fear of contagion, is our discomforts with sexuality, and our disapproval of some of the other behaviors associated with transmission, and even still some of the absence of control.

The power of naming should not be underestimated—the words themselves are the disease. As one French physician explained, "When you tell them [patients] they have the virus, you kill them."

BUILDING BOUNDARIES

For all the meaning to be found in the process of naming, it is perhaps the technique least used on a routine basis. I could go through an entire day at either the Paris or Chicago clinics without hearing the word "AIDS" more than a handful of times. In the laboratory, one might not hear "AIDS" mentioned in a week. There are instead myriad other ways in which AIDS is routinely constructed. These share the common characteristic of building boundaries, of sketching the outlines of AIDS utilizing smaller, more knowable elements of the medical experience. Such boundary markers include risk groups, modes of transmission, characteristics of HIV, patient symptoms, and clinical tests.

The delineation of risk groups is used epidemiologically to refer to subsets of the total population that experience a higher prevalence and/or incidence of the disease in question. Even before the discovery of HIV, epidemiologists and subsequently lab researchers were able to "name" AIDS by delineating the populations at risk. This construct is used in France and the United States, for one can find it both in the "two hemophiliac siblings, four homosexual males, four inhabitants of the Caribbean islands, and three Zairians" (Barré-Sinousi et al. 1985, 1737) of a French study and the initial "4-H list,"— homosexuals, hemophiliacs, heroin addicts, and Haitians—of the CDC (Treichler 1987). According to Herzlich and Pierret (1988), this naming of risk groups facilitated the progression of AIDS from a "medical mystery" to "a well-identified object" (11). AIDS is in this way constructed as the sum of risk groups, demarcating the boundaries of the disease through who is more likely to be affected. As discussed by Oppenheimer (1992) and Treichler (1987), which groups are designated "high risk" is dependent on social, cultural, and historical factors, creating social boundaries as much as disease boundaries. Unfortunately, the political and social consequences of such groupings tend to go unexamined prior to their adoption.

Construction of boundaries via risk groups, though more prevalent earlier in the epidemic, continues to be common among epidemiologists as well as clinicians. Clinicians use this interpretation most often when taking histories of AIDS patients, asking: "Have you ever used intravenous drugs?" "Are your sexual partners men or women?" "Have you recently received a transfusion?" and so on. At Rousseau in 1987, I noticed a basic checklist of risk factors[3] that the physician used during an initial consultation. With clinicians, then, the construction is not so much the sum of risk group populations but the discovery of to which risk group the individual patient belongs—a practice in keeping with Hunter's (1991) description of medicine as a "science of individuals" (28). By 1990, however, I encountered this delineation of risk groups less and less, with biological markers such as HIV-antibody status and T lymphocyte counts taking their place in the discourse at Rousseau.

At Northlake, clinicians did not directly attempt to place a patient in a particular group but rather focused on the patient's story of transmission by asking, "How do you think you were infected with HIV?" Questions regarding sexual orientation, specific sexual behaviors, history of transfusions, and history of intravenous drug use were for the most part relegated to the relevant parts of the standard medical history—transfusions as part of the past medical history along with exposure to sexually transmitted disease, intravenous drug use with questions about smoking and alcohol consumption, and finally sexual orientation with other questions regarding social relationships.

With the advent of biochemical markers, risk group information becomes relevant to the clinician not so much in relation to AIDS itself but in assessing and treating possible concomitant diseases, such as endocarditis (an infection of the heart) and hepatitis B, both common in intravenous drug users. As we shall see in the next chapter, "risk group" information is also used by clinicians to assess the impact on carrying out the medical care itself, regarding "easy" versus "difficult" patients, for example. In more generalized talk about AIDS, such as found in the context of an interview, French and American physicians and researchers still refer to risk groups on a regular basis, often redefining these groups to construct the boundary of AIDS beyond 1991:

The epidemic, over the next five to ten years, clearly is going to become one of socially disadvantaged individuals. It's going to move into minority communities, and become much more focused around—in this country at least—drug use. And it will become much more of a heterosexual disease than it has been in this country.

The second thing is that there will be a switch of the risk groups, the proportion of patients who were formerly IV drug addicts will be much more frequent. Certainly a lower incidence in homosexuals. . . . I think there is really a risk that the political involvement will lower with time. Because when it will be a disease just for Africans, for immigrants and for IV drug addicts, there will not be so much money.

The above examples, from an American clinical researcher and a French clinician, respectively, indicate that AIDS is demarcated by risk groups for both French and Americans, but the nature of those evolving risk groups is constructed differently. For the Americans, AIDS is delineated increasingly by heterosexuals, particularly intravenous drug users, the poor, and minorities. For the French, on the other hand, AIDS is a disease of immigrants, Africans, and drug users—immigration being a significant issue on the French political landscape.[4] Each construction arises out of its social, historical, and political context, in both instances retaining the emphasis on marginal groups in each society. Thus, while the technique of defining AIDS as the sum of its risk groups has become less formalized and is disappearing in the daily talk of the clinic, it is still a powerful element of medical discourse.

The boundaries of AIDS are also constructed by reference to the various means of transmission of HIV. This is different from talk about risk groups because it denotes specific events or behaviors rather than groups of people. In France in 1987, a clinician informant involved with HIV testing and counseling had arranged an evening seminar for other physicians in the hospital on educating the public about AIDS and invited me along. Only six physicians attended, all in their early to midthirties. Nearly half of the three-hour discussion was devoted to delineating all the possible means of transmission and their risk, with the stated aim of providing people with information that is both effective and correct. Various means of transmission were brought up, discussed, and assigned some form of risk value. Transfusions were given a small but real risk, while acupuncture, ear piercing, and tattooing, it was decided, had no risk under normal circumstances. The topic generating the most discussion was that of *baisser profonde*, or "French kissing." After much debate, it was decided that the actual risk remains uncertain and difficult to prove. As the organizing doctor remarked during the debate on French kissing: "People want to know 'yes' or 'no.' This is not possible. You must think in terms of 'the risk is acceptable' or 'the risk is not acceptable.'"

In this example, the care taken by physicians in outlining the means of transmission demonstrates three important points. First, the process of summing up all the means of transmission is one way physicians define AIDS. AIDS, the unknown entity, emerges out of this discussion as something bounded, something that can be apprehended. Second, the discourse that constructs these boundaries is not uniform but variable and rife with uncertainty. Last, there was a conscious determination to generate a uniform discourse, to reach a consensus. This was addressed in terms of minimizing "vagueness" and "contradictions" in how they, as physicians, talked to the public. Uncertainty itself did not seem to be especially problematic, as long as everyone had the same uncertainties. Listening to the discussion of these physicians was like seeing scriptwriters create a story, debating over plot, theme, and setting. The underlying goal is the same: to present a unified narrative aimed at a particular audience.

Interestingly enough, in 1990 the same physician, who had by then developed an entire educational resource center for AIDS, was again sponsoring a discussion on transmission and again invited me to attend. Unlike the first conference, this took place in a large, well-furnished auditorium at a new exposition center. The conference was attended by over a hundred people, most of whom were involved with health care.[5] One goal of this discussion was to draft a consensus text on the transmission of HIV, to be released to the public through the press. One speaker emphasized the need for "frank and open talk" about the uncertainties that still exist about transmission. Many of the questions brought up in 1987 remained active topics of discussion, including transfusions, sexual practices, and kissing. New means of transmission, such as insects and maternal-fetal interaction, were also evaluated. For the first time, I heard a real concern with transmission from patient to health care worker, though little about the reverse route, which has been highly publicized in the United States.[6]

Despite the passage of three years—a long time with regards to the history of AIDS—the discourse at the 1990 conference remained virtually identical to that in 1987. AIDS was being constructed as the sum of the means of transmission, and this construction was ascribed great importance, particularly for speaking with the lay public. The means of transmission, unlike the historically limited risk groups, are potentially limitless, covering the entire range of human behavior. The entire process is fraught with ambiguity. For example:

> *Questioner 1*: Can fleas transmit the virus?
> *Presenter*: The risk is null.
> *Questioner 1*: Me again. I ask why? Mosquitoes can transmit malaria. Why not AIDS?
> *Presenter*: There are no studies that show these insects transmit it. Why? You can ask why forever.

Still, as in 1987, a primary goal was the creation of a unified medical discourse, emerging through the process of a narrative contest focused on transmission.

The French are not alone in building AIDS from discourse on transmission. It was integral to several encounters at the Northlake clinic, usually in the context of discussing with patients the risks to family and friends. In one such case, Dr. Holtzman and I were seeing a female patient who was accompanied by her sister. The sister remarked that the patient had been nervous around her children. Dr. Holtzman then asked the patient if she felt nervous because of having HIV. The woman replied that she treated her one-year-old differently now, that she didn't pick him up as much and was careful that he doesn't eat anything off her plate. Dr. Holtzman replied, "We've been studying the virus for several years now, and we know that it is only transmitted by sex or intravenous needles, blood contact. Before, we weren't sure exactly how it was spread." He concluded by saying that studies have shown that there has been no transmission by touching or picking a child up, that she can hug and kiss him. He added, "You might not want him to drink from the same glass, though."

Here, an American clinician uses a narrative to demarcate the boundaries of AIDS with modes of transmission. As in the interchange among the French conference participants, AIDS retains a certain ambiguity: HIV is only spread by sex and blood, but perhaps sharing a drinking glass also transmits the virus. The process of constructing AIDS by transmission methods is unceasing, whether it occurs within the medical community or between the medical community and the lay public. There are always more potentially AIDS-transmitting situations, as many as there are people to talk about them. As a consequence, if to know the means of transmission is to know AIDS, then we will never fully know it.

Boundaries are not the sole province of clinicians. Oppenheimer (1992) notes that "bench" scientists have increasingly determined the definition of AIDS, redefining it "as a set of biomedical problems open to a chemical resolution in the form of drugs and vaccines" (63). The discourse of lab researchers tends to construct AIDS via HIV, and AIDS is thus sequenced, cloned, characterized, and constructed from the very experiments that researchers perform in search of a definition, as in these American and French examples.

We have characterized it to see whether we could figure out how the virus migrates, but more importantly, are there different types of strains that will biologically challenge any therapy. And what determines what virus infects one cell and one virus another.

I work on HIV-1. It is from Gabon. I try to clone it, to sequence it, to study the molecular biology of this virus.

Research discourse is hardly uniform. For example, some researchers construct an HIV that enters the body only via the CD4 lymphocytes, while others expand the interface between body and virus to include cells outside the immune system, such as those lining the intestine (Levy 1988). In 1987, as seen in the second example above, these constructions tended to focus on the traits of HIV itself, the boundaries emerging from experiments dealing with the sequencing of its ribonucleic acid (RNA) and the role of its proteins. In 1990, the emphasis seemed to be placed on delineating the interaction between the body and the virus, such as which antibodies, if any, help or hinder the virus entering cells, as shown in the first example.[7]

The process is one of constructing a valid narrative, in this case, a story where, inside a particular series of circumscribing events, one gets AIDS. These American and French excerpts are among a wide variety of narratives I encountered.

When I wrote the patent application [for a vaccine], amazingly enough, people were focusing on antibodies. So I reasoned that the HIV virus has molecular mimicry; that is, it mimics the immune system. . . . And reasoned that if we don't have cell-mediated immunity, we don't get better.

These days, we have evidence that cells which are not yet CD4 might be susceptible to HIV infection, and our project now is to try to define better which cells are susceptible to HIV infection and what is the effect of the infection on the differentiation pathway to CD4. So I think it is important to know if the virus can influence the pathway of differentiation. That might explain why patients cannot restore their immunity.

Unlike the case with risk groups, there seems no obvious distinction between French and American discourse, though this might be discovered with more intensive participant observation in the laboratory setting. In any case, a number of congruent and competing narratives are being fashioned in labs on both sides of the Atlantic, all of which attempt to give meaning to an amorphous entity, AIDS, by describing its knowable, biochemical boundaries. Though many pronounced differences exist between the discourse of clinicians and researchers, both define AIDS as the summation of its assigned attributes, be they viral proteins, risk groups, modes of transmission, or as is seen primarily with clinicians, the symptoms of patients.

Clinicians, in contrast with researchers, confront the disease on a daily basis. They must deal with patients in whom the disease is expressed, and thus their discourse tends to the clinical and the individual rather than the viral and the collective. AIDS becomes first and foremost the sum of symptoms. This is hardly surprising because, as noted previously, AIDS is medically distinguished as a particular cluster of symptoms. This model is constantly being reconstructed in assessing the patient. In this process particularly, AIDS emerges through interaction between patient and physician. For example, the clinician will ask, "Have you lost weight?" The patient in turn may suggest, "I have trouble breathing, and I tire easily." Thus, the construction of AIDS through its symptoms, born of interactive dialogue, is a powerful one for both the medical community and the general public.

In American biomedicine, students are taught to conduct a "review of systems" as part of taking a medical history. This review inquires about important additional symptoms related to every major organ system of the body. With AIDS, the review of systems is altered considerably, each time redefining the boundaries of AIDS and additionally distinguishing the practice of AIDS medicine from non-AIDS medicine. One sample, taken from an American guidebook on AIDS for physicians, is presented in Table 4.1. In these terms, AIDS is: fever, night sweats, fatigue, weight loss, change in vision, tingling in the extremities, difficulty breathing, and skin changes. Note that the symptoms themselves are present in many other diseases but taken together create a specific entity. The AIDS review is done routinely and replaces the standard lines of questioning to a large extent.

The French and American AIDS reviews are similar but not identical. All other things being equal, the Rousseau doctors tended to emphasize fatigue and sinus-related symptoms while those at Northlake more often stressed neurological symptoms. The French stress on fatigue may be related to the disorder *fatigué*, described by Gaines (1992) as a periodic "weighing down" from the daily struggles of life. Given the experience of living with AIDS and the doctor's secondhand encounters with that experience, it is not surprising that a French clinician might look for such a disorder more commonly in AIDS patients. The other differences suggest no similar explanations but may be due to variation in the prevalence of certain manifestations of AIDS, such as dementia.

Symptoms by themselves do not form the sole clinical boundaries of AIDS. AIDS has the unusual characteristic of being a disease encompassing other diseases. That is, a patient with AIDS is recognized by manifestations of other diseases, such as *Pneumocystis* pneumonia or toxoplasmosis (McCombie 1990). With some important exceptions, AIDS is not encountered firsthand—it is always mediated by

Table 4.1
Sample HIV Review of Systems

Each of these symptoms is associated with certain AIDS-related conditions. For example, "white patches in mouth" is suggestive of thrush (oral candidiasis).

Constitutional
Weight loss
Fever
Night sweats

Lymphatic
Lymphadenopathy

Head/Eyes/Ears/Nose/Throat
Sore or dry mouth
White patches in mouth
Acute unilateral vision loss
Sinus congestion

Respiratory
Dyspnea
Cough
Chest tightness/pain

Gastrointestinal
Dysphagia
Odynophagia
Anorexia
Nausea/vomiting
Constipation/diarrhea
Anorectal pain/sores

Genitourinary
Abnormal Pap smears
Painful sores
Vulvovaginal itch/discharge
Symptoms of STD
Decreased libido

Musculoskeletal
Myalgias
Arthralgias

Neurologic
Headache
Seizures
Focal symptoms
Ataxia
Poor memory
Trouble word-finding
Pain
Parasthesias

Skin
Rash
New lesions
New dermatoses
Bruising, petechiae

Adapted from E. Fisher (1993, 8–9).

another disease, sometimes several at once. This is borne out repeatedly in the definitions of AIDS given by my informants:

AIDS is an infection of the immune system by a virus that leads to destruction of the immune system, which allows for the development of multiple life-threatening infections and malignancies that people with normal immune systems don't usually get.

It's an infection of the T cells which results in a gradual but inexorable breakdown of the immune system, resulting in either opportunistic infections or in opportunistic neoplasms, which usually claims the life of the infected person over the years.

This definition also emerges from daily life in the clinic, particularly at Rousseau, which lacks the discourse on "AIDS- defining illness" found at Northlake. Talk often centers around recognizing and treating a patient's PCP or tuberculosis rather than assessing how the patient's "AIDS" is doing. Just as AIDS is manifested indirectly in the patient, so it is constructed indirectly in the discourse of the clinicians. As Dr. Martine at Rousseau recognized, one can almost forget about AIDS:"I notice that sometimes, when I see patients, it seems to me that I forget they are HIV positive. I treat them, I try to know what is wrong with them. Sometimes I think I forget they are HIV positive."

AIDS becomes then the sum of all its infectious and oncologic manifestations, to the point that AIDS itself almost disappears. The power of this construction is exemplified by one of the weekly staff meetings at Rousseau. Dr. Bernard raises the subject of there being a large number of patients with ongoing problems that have never gotten resolved who have been simply cycling between the day hospital, consults, hospitalization, and the town doctor. He then tells the story of one patient who has had a fever since May and a suspected mycobacterial infection. Bernard relates that cytomegalovirus (CMV) retinitis—a viral infection of the retina—was discovered in July and treated as the cause of the fever. After a week, the fever resumed. Next, sinusitis was discovered and treated, but again the fever returned. Bernard then exhorts everyone to behave less like *pompiers*, firemen, and to really go over and learn the history of the patient, not treat them simply blow by blow. Here the power of narrative is employed to underscore the search for means of treating AIDS as a whole rather than merely along its boundaries, as a series of infections or cancers. It is a daily struggle to develop AIDS and its management as a knowable, standardized entity.

There are two major exceptions from the rule of indirect construction, both of which have emerged in the discourse relatively recently. The first concerns syndromes considered to be a result of the direct action of HIV rather than being mediated by the destruction of the immune system. For example, some physicians will speak of "HIV enteropathy" in diagnosing a patient's diarrhea. Generally, this is a diagnosis of last resort, when no other causes can be attributed to the symptoms. The number and types of "HIV-opathies" vary considerably. The Rousseau clinicians used this type of diagnosis infrequently and would tend to attribute symptoms to an infectious cause that had yet to be located. Diarrhea was often diagnosed as CMV colitis, a diagnosis I heard only once at Northlake, while mental status changes were usually seen as a result of infection with CMV or toxoplasmosis, both of which can affect the nervous system. Fever was almost always attributed to tuberculosis or atypical mycobacteria. As Dr. Farsi explained:

He [Dr. Bernard] has always had the opinion that HIV-induced fever does not exist. So you have to look for an infection. If you look for an infection, you go until the end. If you don't find anything, you try an anti-tuberculosis or mycobacterial treatment.

At Northlake, on the other hand, direct HIV diagnoses were not uncommon: HIV encephalopathy (brain), HIV nephropathy (kidney), HIV adrenalopathy (adrenal glands), HIV enteropathy (intestines), HIV-induced fever. Clinicians did not agree on whether all of these were "really" due to the direct action of HIV, but all emerged out of the discourse on AIDS at Northlake. To a lesser extent, "HIV-opathies" are defined by practice; for a time, Northlake doctors performed additional laboratory tests on certain patients in an attempt to document HIV-induced hypoadrenalism.[8]

The second exception to the rule of indirect construction lies in both research and clinical discourse on markers, loosely defined as certain measurable biochemical characteristics in the body that stand in place of clinical observations (or other biochemical changes that cannot be measured).[9] For example, the first marker of AIDS or HIV infection is a positive ELISA test, demonstrating that the person has antibodies to HIV. We cannot clinically observe that a person is infected with the virus, at least until they become sick, but a positive ELISA test stands for this. As we shall see, the status of being seropositive has become part of the informal staging of the disease, but in and of itself, it does not equal AIDS for two reasons. In advanced cases of AIDS, the test may read negative, and clinicians will make the diagnosis of AIDS without a positive test as long as the appropriate symptoms are present. Thus, in the construction of AIDS as the sum of symptoms, a clinical marker takes precedence over a positive ELISA, a laboratory marker.

Second, in consultations I observed between patients and physicians, and among physicians themselves, the symptoms made the disease. Seropositivity made it more likely that a patient would develop symptoms, but he or she does not have AIDS, as seen in this 1987 explanation from a French physician:[10]

They [seropositive people] have to be followed, this is the first point. The second point is that we don't know how, when, why this patient will stay without disease for a long time and the other one will get AIDS or ARC in two months or two years.

All the clinicians I talked with, when in consultation with patients, clearly separated the state of being seropositive from the state of having AIDS, as in this Northlake example.

Patient: Am I AIDS or ARC or what?

Dr. Westin: There's no real term for the stage you're in, other than saying you're HIV positive and that you're having some symptoms related to that. You don't have AIDS.

Another marker is the CD4 lymphocyte count. Like the ELISA, it does not measure the virus directly but the body's biochemical activity in response to the virus, in this case, the destruction of the CD4 cells. Since the main research narrative on AIDS focuses on the CD4 cell as the primary target of HIV, it is sometimes constructed as a more direct link to the virus than clinical observations, especially when the patient has few or no symptoms. In discussing a case, at both Northlake and Rousseau, the first question clinicians usually ask is, "What is his CD4 count?" If the CD4 count is dropping quickly, the AIDS/HIV disease is seen as progressing. As Dr. Peters explained to a new patient:

HIV is a virus that infects mainly the helper or CD4 cells, a type of white blood cell responsible for fighting off infections. The helper cells are killed and decrease at a rate of about 100 a year; you start out with about 1,000. The number will fluctuate—700, then 900, then 600—but the overall trend is down. As the helper cells decrease, you are more likely to get what we call an "AIDS defining illness." These are malignancies or opportunistic infections that people with normal immune systems aren't affected by, like Kaposi's sarcoma or PCP, *Pneumocystis* pneumonia.

Note the change in discourse's emphasis from the CD4 count to the clinical manifestations once the numbers in the narrative are low. As we shall see in the discussion of staging, the association between CD4 count and AIDS is immensely powerful but recognized by clinicians as imperfect. Once the CD4 count in a particular patient reached a certain level, usually around 100 at Northlake and 50 at Rousseau, physicians reasserted clinical signs over lab markers in assessing the progression of the patient's disease.

Other biochemical measurements, including the level of HIV antigens, direct viral cultures, and viral deoxyribonucleic acid (DNA) recognition,[11] have all been used more or less routinely in the laboratory but only on an intermittent basis in the clinics. For the researcher, HIV may now be directly knowable, but as seen in the explosion of narratives on pathogenesis, AIDS itself remains elusive. For the clinician, AIDS remains primarily a disease that is defined indirectly, its symptoms manifested through other diseases. The obliqueness of AIDS is perhaps a clinician's ultimate challenge—challenging clinical skills, clinical stories.

The final set of boundaries are also clinically constructed, fashioning AIDS as the sum of its medical treatments and tests. Almost every patient with symptomatic disease, whether in France or the United States, takes several medications routinely, either to affect HIV, such as AZT and DDI, or to prevent or treat opportunistic infections—Bactrim, aerosolized pentamidine, acyclovir, and so on. Discourse about what medications should be part of this standard list again defines the boundaries of AIDS. In France, with its higher incidence of toxoplasmosis, antibiotics against this infection generally find their way onto the list. In the United States, adjunct treatments such as erythropoietin, a hormone to aid against anemia, are more common if only because of their greater availability. The construction of AIDS as the sum of its routine medications is reformulated with every patient, every day.

Reflexivity is not limited to anthropologists, and the clinicians at Northlake were certainly conscious of many of their constructions. In the clinic office hung a handwritten note on the bulletin board, headed "Proposed List of Maintenance Meds for HIV-Infected Persons." The list was in a variety of handwritings, indicating multiple authors, and included the following drugs: AZT, Bactrim (prevents PCP), fluconazole (anti-fungal), Rifabutin (experimental drug for atypical mycobaterial infection), Florinef (steroid to prevent sodium loss), vancomycin (antibiotic), steroids (adrenal steroids), acyclovir (antiherpesvirus drug), Lomotil (antidiarrheal), yohimbine (a supposed aphrodisiac), and Elavil (antidepressant). The list grew a little each month and included medications to treat both symptoms and HIV-associated diseases, touching nearly every organ system. In a sense, the construction of boundaries by medication is derivative of the summation of AIDS-associated diseases and symptoms described previously. The list also becomes a way of keeping track of medication successes, real and potential, as seen with Rifabutin. The inclusion of yohimbine underscores the recognized artificiality of this lengthy wish list—few patients could actually tolerate all these medications—and above all finding the humor in the complex, mutable world of AIDS.

The listing of diagnostic tests is used in the same way, and both French and American clinicians used this technique on a regular basis. A prime example is searching for the cause of a clinically unexplained fever, what my French informants term *le bilan de fièvre*. Their decision tree of tests involved was written on a chart inside the lab room adjacent to the day hospital, though there was considerable improvisation from this tree. The tests, along with their most likely diagnostic aim, included chest X-ray (looking for PCP, tuberculosis), blood cultures (bacterial sepsis), CT scan (toxoplasmosis), bronchoscope (PCP), and further down, bone marrow biopsy and gastric *tubage*, the last two used to look for tuberculosis bacteria in the bone marrow and swallowed phlegm in the stomach.[12] A common added first step was a sinus X-ray, rarely done at Northlake.

A diagnostic test list for fever was used daily at Northlake as well. For example, on rounds one day, we were discussing the case of a hospitalized patient with resolving infection of the mastoid bone but who continued to have fevers. Dr. Westin commented to the resident: "If the mastoid looks okay [on CT scan], then we'll give him the 'HIV-o-gram' for unknown fever—gallium scan, look for cryptococcal antigen in serum, bone marrow, etc." Though it differs in content—gallium scans were never used at Rousseau[13]—the discourse operates in the same way. Dr. Westin's coined phrase for this list, the "HIV-o-gram," caught on so well that a resident asked him whether it was a "real word." This is an excellent example of how a concept—the diagnostic boundaries of AIDS—is constructed through language and is transmitted on to the next generation.[14] Similar algorithms exist for evaluating diarrhea and neurological symptoms, as demonstrated in Fisher (1993, 18–23).

In review, the construction of boundaries appears to play a vital role in giving meaning to AIDS in both France and the United States. AIDS becomes defined through the summation of risk groups, modes of transmission, laboratory-based traits of HIV, symptoms, associated diseases, markers, and diagnostic tests. All of these boundaries overlap in discourse and are often used simultaneously. The separation between them is my construction, a device to aid understanding the process of building boundaries. Additionally, these boundaries, when taken together, can yield an incredibly rich picture of AIDS. A presentation at Northlake brought this point home.

Figure 4.1 AIDS: A Visualized Model

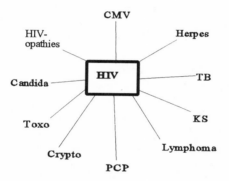

Dr. Fields led a two-hour meeting with the clinic nurses and doctors to discuss material presented at the recent AIDS Clinical Trials Groups (ACTG) Meetings, which serve to review this federally funded multicentric clinical research. A major part of the presentation focused on new studies of AZT in various subpopulations in relationship to the CD4 count. This was followed by discussions on DDI and DDC, at the time, two experimental antiretroviral drugs (which have since been approved). The focus then switched to new prevention strategies and treatments for opportunistic infections including cryptococcosis, resistant herpes, atypical tuberculosis, CMV retinitis, as well as HIV-induced pathology. The meeting ended with discussion of treatment of KS and lymphoma.[15] From this presentation and discussion, a visual model of AIDS emerges, constructed through discourse (see Figure 4.1).

When the boundaries are put together, as in Figure 4.1, a recognizable whole emerges, the whole of AIDS. Interestingly, this visual representation looks strikingly similar to the structure of a virus, with the genetic material at the center (HIV), and the supporting or identifying proteins (infections and cancers) forming an envelope around it.

The technique of defining boundaries can only go so far, however, in giving meaning to AIDS. Another technique, that of analogy, continues the process of constructing the unknown using the known, with subsequent powerful implications for the prognosis and treatment of AIDS.

ANALOGIES: "AIDS IS JUST LIKE ... "

Analogy is a powerful tool for making sense of human experience, as Allan Brandt (1988) demonstrates with historical analogies between sexually transmitted diseases at the turn of the century and present-day AIDS. From the standpoint of discourse, analogies are rooted in metaphor, such as: "Marriage is a roller coaster." In Black's (1979, 31) terms, metaphor mediates analogy. Analogy is among the most common techniques used by my informants to construct a set of medically and historically situated meanings for AIDS. Analogies with other viruses, for example, are especially common among researchers. In the Gallo-Montagnier dispute, references to leukemia viruses such as HTLV-I and feline leukemia virus (FLV), and the lentiviruses most often cited by the French, were utilized to construct a particular narrative about the cause of AIDS and a particular model of HIV. The leukemia virus references emphasized the targeting of T lymphocytes, while the lentivirus analogy stressed the slow, destructive effects of the AIDS virus (J. Feldman 1992c).

Other viruses and their associated diseases have come into play as well and are used by both researchers and clinicians. Smallpox and polio[16] viruses are often mentioned in the context of achieving a vaccine against HIV:

Now some remarkable things have happened with vaccines. We've been able to eliminate, for example, smallpox from the world. We've been able to eliminate polio from the Western Hemisphere in almost all places.

As in this excerpt, the analogy may be positive—we eliminated smallpox, we can eliminate HIV—or the analogy may construct a negative comparison, building a more problematic HIV.

Other viruses are used as reference points when talking about infectivity and progression to disease.

I reported at the first international conference that in excess of 10 percent of the people that were infected had developed the condition, which was an extremely high rate—polio, 1 in a 1,000 developed or died who were infected. With HIV, what has changed as we had more time to observe it, we're talking about upwards of three quarters or more of the people infected with the virus would die.

A Rousseau clinician, lecturing to the residents, used a similar analogy: "It's very reassuring to say, 'Well, it's a virus; like measles and the others, not everyone exposed to it gets sick.'" He then suggested that most people will eventually become ill: "In no other disease except rabies does everyone exposed get the disease." In fact, by 1990, rabies seemed to be a common viral analogy used by both French and Americans to describe the pathogenicity of HIV. AIDS is less like measles—easily prevented and treated—and more like rabies, despite how much people, lay and medical, would like it to be otherwise. Yet AIDS is even unlike the relatively unusual viral disease of rabies, despite its pathogenicity:

There is no other agent without therapy that has that [high level of fatality]—the only exception would be a Ebola virus, or Marburg virus, which are very unusual viruses that come out of Africa rarely. . . . Rabies, but rabies doesn't transmit very well through humans.

AIDS is thus constructed as even more exotic and deadly than Ebola virus and rabies.

Despite this proliferation of viral analogies, one stands out as being the most consistently powerful over time, that of hepatitis B. Hepatitis B virus (HBV) is an etiologic agent for hepatitis as well as liver cancer and is transmitted via blood, semen, and vaginal secretions. HBV infection, usually manifesting as hepatitis, is significantly more prevalent among homosexual men, intravenous drug users, and certain immigrant groups (mainly those from Southeast Asia), again, similar to HIV. Analogously, HIV is a significant factor in malignancies, the Kaposi's sarcoma and lymphomas of AIDS, and is also transmitted through blood, semen, and vaginal secretions. Both HIV and HBV infection may remain asymptomatic and undetected for years. Consequently, it is extremely common for laboratory researchers and epidemiologists to speak of HIV in terms of HBV. One French researcher began his career working on HBV, then changed viruses, commenting: "From hepatitis B to HIV is a short step. An enormous number of people who worked on hepatitis B—It's a blood-born virus, sex and blood and transfusions and drugs. I mean, it's like HBV." The use of HBV as a reference for AIDS dates to the beginnings of the epidemic, well before the isolation of HIV, as seen in the recollection of one American epidemiologist:

I had been working for the CDC for two decades now, and I was in the Phoenix part of CDC in June of '81 when AIDS first came forth. I was brought in straight away because of my interest in hepatitis B and the similarity in epidemiology.

Clinicians, too, forge strong discursive links between hepatitis B and AIDS, again dating back to the early days of the epidemic, pre-HIV.

My husband is also a physician, and in the fall of 1981, he was seeing the Kaposi's sarcoma patients because he was trained as an oncologist. And we were sitting in our kitchen one evening and talking about this disease, and he began to make the argument—that again was being made commonly by the front-line clinicians, not necessarily by experts—that the underlying unhealthiness that everybody agreed was the fundamental problem was transmitted like hepatitis B. And that was an absolutely riveting and terrifying concept.

As researchers and epidemiologists later described, the infectivity of HIV is considerably lower than HBV, thus allowing room for analogies with rabies. Yet even in 1990, hepatitis B remained a powerful analogy for both the Northlake and Rousseau physicians. For example, Dr. Lefevre incorporated it into a teaching session with the residents. He first mentioned the benefit of knowing if a patient has been exposed to HBV. A resident then asked why hepatitis B is prevalent in homosexual men, and Lefevre replied, "It's a venereal disease, that's all. The same means of transmission [as HIV], transfusions and sex." As Muraskin (1993, 110) observes, HBV served as a useful model of transmission for HIV/AIDS, yet did not serve a similar role in policy issues of testing, contact tracing, and social needs versus individual rights.[17]

The analogy with HBV goes further than its modes of transmission and is used in constructing the nature of HIV infection and its ultimate manifestation, AIDS. As seen in the interview excerpt below, it may also express broader themes about how AIDS fits in the natural world.

Its [HIV] replication results in the death of a cell, which many viruses do. It causes a chronic, lifelong infection just like the herpes virus, just like hepatitis B or hepatitis C do or the papilloma viruses can do. There is an immune response to this virus. . . . The immune response results in the humoral and cell-mediated immunity, just like other viruses. We can measure the infection, just like other viruses. The only difference is that this viral infection eventually destroys the immune system, which leads to the death of the patient, which is not totally different from other viruses. I mean, there are other viruses which can ultimately result in the death of the patient. . . . Chronic hepatitis B or chronic hepatitis C can result in the development of cirrhosis and the patient dying over twenty or thirty years, or they can develop liver cancer and die. So there's a million people infected with hepatitis B in the United States, and there's a million people infected with HIV in the United States. Both of those viruses are chronic plague-born viral infections. Risks of transmission are the same. The difference is that hepatitis B only causes chronic infection about 10 percent of the time and AIDS does it 100 percent of the time. The only difference is the target organ and the consequences of the effects on the target organ, i.e., the immune system that makes this disease different.

The discourse of this American infectious disease clinician relies heavily on analogy with hepatitis B and other viral diseases to construct a particular model of AIDS. AIDS here is a chronic, lifelong infection with HIV that results in cell death and yet still provokes an immune response. Its activity is measurable, its effects observable. It causes the death of the individual and at present infects a large number of people. AIDS is distinctive only its target organ—the immune system—and its level of fatality. Each of these constructions has implications for diagnosis and treatment, but more important for our immediate purposes is the overall theme of this discourse: AIDS is just like any other infectious disease. The consistent analogies with known infectious diseases like hepatitis B are integral to this model, constructing AIDS as something observable, measurable, and knowable.

For other informants, the use of analogies can build an AIDS that is knowable, yet still different and dangerous. To the clinician cited earlier, the idea that AIDS could be transmitted like hepatitis B presented a "riveting and terrifying concept." Hepatitis B has historically presented a risk to health care workers due to exposure to blood, most commonly through needle sticks. HIV now presents analogous risks—less infectious but more fatal. As the director of the Northlake clinic commented:

I think it [AIDS] has brought back some old things associated with medicine. There was a very brief period between the late '50's and the AIDS epidemic where there were very few dangerous infectious diseases left in the developed nations. Hepatitis B, but I mean, how much? Not very much. A little bit of TB, but I mean really contained. . . . There wasn't a lot of threat to health care workers, patients weren't dying from these things, everything was treatable. . . . So now there is risk again. Now there is a deadly infectious disease again.

Dr. O'Neill's narrative, which constructs the practice of medicine as much as the nature of AIDS, again creates AIDS as being like hepatitis B, especially in its risk to health care workers. AIDS thus represents a once-forgotten danger.

The bond between AIDS and hepatitis B emerges out of practice as well as discourse. At both Rousseau and Northlake, patients were routinely screened for exposure to HBV. At Northlake, the infectious disease fellows on the HIV service handled follow-up of the entire hospital's needle-stick exposures, which involved simultaneous determination of risk and intervention measures for both HBV and HIV.[18] As we shall see later, a discourse of risk plays an important role in the construction of medical practice in the context of AIDS.

Other diseases besides hepatitis act as important referents for AIDS. Surprisingly, syphilis is used rarely compared to hepatitis B, mainly to situate AIDS historically and construct its relatively chronic course.

Maybe it can be that the disease [AIDS] will be not so bad, like we saw with syphilis. You know that syphilis was a deadly disease in the beginning. . . . People used to die after sixty years, after forty years. It was a disease and not, you know, [snaps his fingers]. So maybe it will be the same [with AIDS].

What is more possible, that the virus will be in humans and they will get adapted, one to another, like what happened for syphilis. Syphilis was a really dreadful disease at the end of the fifteenth century in Europe. After, it became more chronic, but at the beginning, from what I've read, it killed people in a few months. [Then] people didn't die anymore, even before antibiotics.

Analogies with syphilis are part of American discourse as well and, like the above French examples, do not usually refer to the ties of both diseases with sexuality. It might be unnecessary in the sense that using an analogy with syphilis inherently implies the sexual connection.

I think many of [the] things that have been said at one time about syphilis are relevant to AIDS on the clinical level. In terms of manifestations and also in terms of what is AIDS, I think it's like syphilis, but even much more so it seems to me what is an unprecedented phenomenon where you have an essentially lethal infectious disease with a long latency period that spread very rapidly unbeknownst to the entire population that was being heavily affected by it.

In the above example, the nature of AIDS is constructed as through the analogy with historical syphilis: a lethal infectious disease with a long latency, sharing similar clinical manifestations.[19] At the same time, the speaker is constructing AIDS as something distinct from present-day syphilis in its lethality and rapid spread. As Allan Brandt (1988) notes in his own analogy with syphilis, "AIDS has threatened our sense of medical security. After all, the age of transmissible, lethal infections was deemed long past in the Western world" (426).

As we have seen before with the hepatitis analogy, not all members of the medical community use a disease analogy the same way and often develop larger themes while characterizing AIDS. When I asked Dr. O'Neill if AIDS is becoming a subspecialty of infectious disease, he replied:

I don't know if it is worthy of ever being categorized as a subspecialty if you look historically. I mean, TB is kind of the classic sort of subspecialty. Syphilis, syphology was sort of a big subspecialty. What happened to them? They're all part of ID [infectious disease]. It's [AIDS] really [just] infectious disease; it's just got a lot of baggage with it.

In this commentary, AIDS is constructed in reference to TB and syphilis as an infectious disease with "a lot of baggage with it." AIDS is temporarily something new but in essence is like every other infectious disease. Once again, AIDS is made knowable through analogy with something already known, though here it is not yet made part of regular medicine. As with hepatitis B, tests for syphilis also are an integral part of AIDS clinical practice.

Another extremely powerful disease analogy is that of tuberculosis, in part because of its high prevalence among AIDS patients. In clinic discussions at both Northlake and Rousseau, the topic of tuberculosis would come up repeatedly, either as a manifestation of AIDS or as an analogy for it.

Tuberculosis is going to be a bigger and bigger problem in HIV-infected people. Drug-resistant strains, transmission of TB within hospitals, transmission of TB to health care workers from HIV-infected patients, transmission to HIV-infected patients in hospitals from other patients with TB.

Probably the most dangerous part of the [AIDS] epidemic in my opinion is TB right now. The new TB epidemic is falling right on the heels of the AIDS epidemic, just as you would have predicted. . . . And then we are going to have people with AIDS who have drug-resistant tuberculosis who are unreliable—I mean, they have to be incarcerated. I see the potential for sanitariums being reopened.

In both of these American examples, the resurgence in TB in the United States is intrinsically linked to AIDS, carrying with it the same concerns about transmission (especially transmission to health care workers), drug resistance, and even the potential for confinement of infected persons. The *sidatorium* of the discourse of the political Far Right in France is a direct reference to the TB sanitoriums of the past.[20]

In medical discourse, analogies with tuberculosis help construct the diagnosis and treatment of AIDS, as seen in the following American and French examples.

I think we probably should move from those terms [AIDS] and start thinking in terms of HIV infection and HIV contained disease, much as we think about tuberculosis infection, skin test positivity in individuals, those persons who have tuberculosis, and those who have tuberculosis with clinical manifestations.

I think probably we will find a way of treating AIDS, and probably quite rapidly within the next ten years, we will have a treatment which probably kills the virus. But probably we will have to associate two or three different molecules to get results like we are doing for tuberculosis.

As we shall see later, this use of TB as a model for AIDS diagnosis and treatment can be encountered through the practice of treating these two diseases.

Tuberculosis, like hepatitis B, shares a number of clinical traits with AIDS.[21] It is an infection with a long latency period, so that people may be exposed and not develop active disease for years. It can affect many organ systems and is difficult to treat, requiring multiple drugs over several months, if not years. As has been seen historically in France, and more recently in the United States, drug-resistant strains of the bacterium can develop to the point of leading to fatal disease. Finally, tuberculosis has historically been more prevalent in poor, minority, and otherwise disenfranchised populations, and until the development of adequate medications in the last half century, was considered a fatal disease. As with hepatitis B, the analogy is not perfect. One American clinician explained:

The interesting thing that breaks down about that analogy [TB] is that the clinical diseases that constitute what we call AIDS are not the direct consequence of HIV infection. They are the consequence of the destruction of the immune system.

In this discourse, tuberculosis is known directly, but AIDS is known indirectly. Additionally, a significant proportion of the tuberculosis associated with AIDS is not pulmonary TB caused by the more common *Mycobacterium tuberculosis*, but by the so-called atypical *Mycobacteria* that affect the body systemically and have been more difficult to diagnose and treat. Thus, tuberculosis in AIDS, like AIDS itself, is distinct from other diseases—atypical, hard to categorize, and difficult to handle.

As with hepatitis B, tuberculosis analogies are used to construct a sense of danger associated with the practice of AIDS medicine, whether from HIV or exposure to tuberculosis itself.

We've done a lot of autopsy studies, and you grind up tissues. I've a wife, a child. I think my biggest fear would be transmitting it to somebody else. Tuberculosis also occurs, there's a fear of that. My response to both of those fears is to take sensible precautions.

AIDS has changed medicine in the same way bubonic plague changed medicine in the Middle Ages, or flu epidemic, or polio epidemic, or tuberculosis—it brings out some of its quirks. . . . I think what AIDS has done is it's focused medicine on what it would be like to practice medicine in a preantibiotic era, prevaccine era, when being a doctor was dangerous.

In this last example, as with others we have seen, multiple analogies are used to construct aspects of AIDS. As much as this discourse constructs AIDS, it uses AIDS to construct doctors and the practice of medicine.

As commanding as the links are between AIDS and tuberculosis, by far the most common analogy, both French and American, clinician and researcher, is with cancer. One of the earliest names for AIDS was, in fact, "gay cancer." Like tuberculosis, cancer is also a significant element of AIDS and, as such, became inextricably linked with AIDS in everyday clinic discourse at both Northlake and Rousseau.

A Northlake hallway discussion between Dr. Peters and the chief of medicine from another nearby hospital provides an excellent example of the cancer analogy at work:

Chief: How are these guys [*patients on the HIV service*]? Not all that sick?
Dr. Peters: They're some of the sickest people I've seen.
Chief: If there's a nuclear war, these guys wouldn't look as bad as we think now. I mean, they still have some white cells [*immune system cells*].
Dr. Peters: You can give tons of chemotherapy to cancer patients, and they don't seem to get nearly as sick. And they recover.

Nuclear war and its resultant cancers here provide a scale for assessing the level of sickness in AIDS patients, with the final analysis being that AIDS is worse than nuclear war, at least in its effects on the body. Cancer chemotherapy, with its side effect of severely depressing the white cell count—a condition called *leukopenia* or *neutropenia*—mediates the analogy.

Chemotherapy is a treatment for both cancer and cancers associated with AIDS. At the same time, antiviral treatment for AIDS is also often referred to as chemotherapy. Conflation between all of these chemotherapies is not uncommon and often occurs in lay discourse, as seen in the following interchange from Rousseau.

> *Doctor*: If the KS is not limited, you will need chemotherapy, and it will medicalize your life quite a bit. But if it is isolated, you need several sessions of radiation therapy, but it isn't serious. It won't affect your everyday life very much, I think.
> *Patient*: Will I have to stop work?
> *Doctor*: No, no. You come in once a week, in the morning, and a nurse would give you bleomycin, and that's it. We have many people on chemo, working. It's the hematological tolerance that's the problem.

The patient here appears to assume that chemotherapy for KS is like other cancer chemotherapy, which will take up time and cause disabling symptoms such as nausea. The doctor counters this implied narrative with a story of AIDS patients on chemotherapy who are well enough to work. KS chemotherapy, part of AIDS treatment, emerges as something different than cancer chemotherapy outside of AIDS. Comparison of cancer chemotherapy and AIDS chemotherapy, namely, AZT or other antiretrovirals, is found in American discourse as well.

So many of the chemotherapies that we use in cancer may prolong life, but you really don't really feel a lot better. So at least this is one where the therapy makes you both feel better, have more energy, stay more robust; you don't lose weight, you don't lose your hair. Basically, there are a lot of things about it that are positive benefits.

In the daily talk of the clinic, analogies with cancer were significantly more common at Northlake than Rousseau, be it with patients or among the physicians themselves. This may be a function of the history of involvement with AIDS in the American medical community. Cancer-oriented institutions have long been a part of AIDS treatment and research in the United States. A number of my American informants began their careers in oncology or related fields such as research on cancer drugs or animal tumor viruses. Research on opportunistic infections in AIDS has led to development of experimental drugs to be used for opportunistic infections in cancer patients, and vice versa. As one American researcher explained:

We've also done quite a bit of work with an antifungal agent, [name of drug], a conventional agent, giving it as an aerosol to prevent aspergillosis, which is a common serious infection in patients with leukemia or lymphoma. And so that is how AIDS has brought me from cancer back to cancer.

Thus, the prevalence of cancer analogies at Northlake is not particularly surprising. It can also be used to define risk. During a discussion of needle-stick exposures between several of the clinic doctors, Dr. Holtzman inquired about using AZT after a sexual exposure, since a number of people visiting the sexually transmitted disease clinic had asked about it. Dr. Goldstein smiled, replying, "The risk is probably a lot less than getting cancer."

Cancer also is used to construct the nature of AIDS and possible treatments. In one instance, Dr. Fields passed an article around the clinic concerning a drug already approved for use in circulation problems. The article noted that the drug has also exhibited antitumor necrosis factor properties, and since this factor contributes to wasting and fever in cancer and maybe AIDS patients, it might be useful. Dr. Fields suggested, semiseriously, starting a study on it. In the discourse presented by the article, AIDS is like cancer in its symptoms of severe weight loss and unexplained fever and thus may be treated using a drug with anticancer properties. The fact of Dr. Fields passing it around the clinic and his suggestion of a study reinforces the analogy established by the article.

There is less involvement of oncologists in AIDS in France. The Rousseau doctors treated Kaposi's sarcoma on their own, consulting oncologists only on patients with lymphoma. At Northlake, an oncologist treated all cancers in AIDS patients in a separate clinic. My French research informants had backgrounds primarily in virology or immunology. Nevertheless, in the context of interviews, cancer analogies were nearly as common as with my American informants. Sometimes the analogies are negative ones:

You know, AIDS is not like cancer. It's not a cancer. It's a tropical disease, or it's an infectious disease, so if we can find drugs to be useful, it will be very easy to show that they are effective.

There [have] to be ways, epistemological ways, of dealing with the treatment that is different from what was elaborated throughout the years for cancer. I believe cancer is not a model for AIDS in terms of the way you have to treat the patients, it's very different.

Not all French cancer analogies are negative, nor are they limited to clinicians.

But what is important is that AIDS research will open the door completely to a new way to work on viruses, especially on retroviruses. And retroviruses are certainly very important in human pathology. Many diseases that are now of unknown origin, such as lupus, for example, and even in cancer, since retroviruses are a cause of cancer in animals.

In this example, AIDS and cancer share a viral etiology. AIDS research is also constructed as leading the way in making the unknown—the origins of lupus and cancer—known.

The nature of AIDS and the practice of AIDS medicine are shaped by reference to cancer in my informants' discourse.

Many of them [oncologists] fared much better when caring for AIDS patients than some infectious disease doctors, mostly because of the nature of the specialty. Oncologists are used to caring for people with chronic, debilitating, fatal illnesses. They're also used to the idea that very toxic drugs given over a long period of time might enhance one's life, quality of life, and prolong survival. And therefore things like AZT trials, they had some familiarity with them. AZT in fact, was initially a cancer drug.

I also realized that in medical school I had quite an interest in oncology, and certainly a lot of patients we see in HIV are a lot like the oncology patients. They have a chronic disease, it's a terminal disease. . . . And it is interesting how HIV is similar in many respects to cancer.

The AIDS developed by these two narratives is like a generic type of cancer: a chronic, debilitating, painful and—unlike TB, syphilis, or hepatitis—fatal disease. It is treated by toxic drugs, even former cancer drugs, over a long period of time. AIDS medicine, like oncology, is shaped as a discipline encompassing complex treatment rather than cure. As we shall see, cancer analogies, whether emerging through discourse or practice, are at work in constructing the course of AIDS, its treatment, its doctors, its patients.

However, as is the case with all the previous analogies, there is something paradoxical about AIDS. It is close to cancer, yet not quite close enough to be understood. Just when you think you have it trapped, AIDS once again defies definition.

I think that the sum of information that has come out of these studies is to create an understanding of an illness that in many respects, to my mind, resembles what cancer is. Cancer is a disease that ultimately represents an accumulation of cells that are not helpful. And in AIDS, the bottom line is that you're dealing with an accumulation of a virus that is very harmful. The thing that happens in the progression of AIDS is that you start out with very few viruses, and you die with a lot of viruses and not much cells left. And so they're sort of conceptually paradoxical, because in the one case, cancer is the accumulation of bad cells, AIDS is the elimination of good cells and the accumulation of bad virus.

The main analogies used by my informants—hepatitis B, syphilis, tuberculosis, cancer—were all part of medical discourse when I began my research in 1987. As Treichler (1992a) and I both observe, the discourse at the Fifth International AIDS Conference centered around building AIDS as a chronic, but treatable condition, coincident with the developing lay discourse of "living with AIDS." New analogies are integral to this model of AIDS, most commonly with diabetes.

The other example I use is like diabetes, years ago. If a person was diagnosed like a juvenile onset diabetic before insulin was invented, if you developed diabetes you died of DKA [diabetic ketoacidosis] probably within a month of your onset. Then insulin came along, and those people are going to live relatively normal lives. And I truly believe that AIDS will become a similarly managed illness with certain medications.

Diabetes today, particularly insulin-dependent diabetes, is a chronic disease that requires lifelong monitoring and medical intervention. Like AIDS, it can have a depressive effect on certain aspects of the immune system. While diabetes can have devastating complications, including blindness, most diabetics live a fully able, if medicalized, life for many decades. It is this narrative of treatable and survivable AIDS that clinicians in particular are struggling to develop, as seen in these US examples.

People talk about HIV as a chronic disease. I think that's a little overoptimistic unless you're willing to count the kind of first half of infection where we were not particularly trying to intervene. It's still a very serious disease which clearly is shortening people's lives drastically, so it's not a chronic disease like diabetes. But we're more in command of it.

I have been telling patients, although I am not 100 percent convinced—that we think AIDS can be chronic disease managed just like diabetes. But I think that's the way I see it. I only hope it will come to that.

Unlike the tuberculosis analogy, the diabetes-based narrative of AIDS is often the one chosen by clinicians to be presented to patients, at least in the United States. Indeed, Northlake clinicians often used analogies with diabetes in their talk with patients, generally to reinforce the need for continuous monitoring or, as in the following interchange between Dr. Westin and a newly diagnosed HIV-positive patient, to evoke hope.

> *Patient*: You know, we've been treating cancer for forty years and people still die.
> *Dr. Westin*: I think of it like diabetes. Sixty years ago, people died after a year or so, and now they live a long time with treatment.

Using diabetes as a referent was more common among my American informants but certainly played a forceful role in French discourse as well. At one journal club meeting at Rousseau, Dr. Bernard proclaimed: "HIV infection is a chronic disease. AIDS is a complication," then went on to compare HIV disease to diabetes and chronic renal failure. Despite these assertions, AIDS is not "just like" diabetes. The analogy remains to create hope for the future.

I think AIDS is going to be a chronic disease. It's going to be treated with multiple drugs by people that specialize in the disease. I think it is going to be very much like oncology. It will be a combination between oncology and diabetes.

On the other hand, as Fee and Fox (1992, 5) observe, accepting AIDS as a chronic disease also means accepting AIDS not as an acute, time-limited epidemic but as an extended, even endemic part of human experience.

Medical discourse constructs an AIDS that is like other chronic diseases, and yet no matter what the analogy, AIDS remains a disease apart.

I would describe AIDS as certainly a chronic disease with many analogies. I already mentioned the oncology patient, diabetes patient. But I think AIDS goes beyond those chronic diseases because of the many implications of HIV infection—the social stigma of having a disease which has really resulted in hysteria among some individuals. I believe the whole contagion concerns have really been brought to the forefront. . . . It is certainly a disease with devastating complications, striking mainly a group of individuals in the prime of their life, unlike many chronic diseases you see like diabetes and cancer, which are primarily diseases of older individuals.

Unlike other chronic diseases, AIDS carries the risk of contagion, social stigma and affects primarily younger people, resulting in ambiguity and paradox.

As we have seen, medical discourse on AIDS often includes multiple analogies at work simultaneously. In fact, several techniques of construction are often used together. In a lecture to medical students, Dr. Fields made reference to hepatitis B, in terms of detecting antigen early in infection. He then stated that 50 percent of people when first infected "will have a clinical syndrome that looks for all the world like seronegative mononucleosis." He added that these people may progress to AIDS faster. He then talked about markers—p24 antigen, β2 microglobulin, neopterin—saying that as in TB and rheumatoid arthritis, a high β2 microglobulin in HIV infection suggests a worse outcome.

Within twenty minutes, Dr. Fields had constructed the diagnosis, staging, and prognosis of AIDS by bounding it with markers and through disease analogies with hepatitis, mononucleosis, tuberculosis, and rheumatoid arthritis. Medical discourse thus encompasses an extremely complex process of construction, and AIDS, with its multiple symptoms, markers, and associated syndromes, emerges as an incredibly complex disease. In fact, AIDS sometimes seems to envelope all of medicine.

A common type of reference in both the Northlake and Rousseau clinics concerned other medical problems not limited to the context of AIDS. A wide variety of these problems, particularly sinusitis and psoriasis, were constructed as being more common or more severe in AIDS patients. AIDS changes, and thus encompasses, virtually all diseases. In turn, signs and symptoms of other diseases, such as the fatigue and changed lab values seen in hypoadrenalism, are common in AIDS as well. HIV infection thus is constructed to represent and perhaps symbolize nearly the entire spectrum of biomedical conditions. HIV is all diseases, though not all diseases are HIV.

AIDS, like syphilis before it, "is internal medicine."[22] It can be any disease, as for this French clinician:

In my hospital we used to take care of any illness, so it could be cancer, immunology disease, endocrinology disease, illness with old people and infectious disease. So that's why I have to take care of AIDS people.

Or, as one American described, it can be all disease:

They get to be living encyclopedias of internal medicine, these people, these patients. In one patient, you will have everything you get to read in general medicine—endocrinology, cardiology. You have everything.

However AIDS is characterized, physicians and researchers recognize it as a symbol for a very complicated medical experience. A 1986 survey (Norton, Schwartzbaum and Wheat 1990) of 234 primary care physicians' use of metaphor in relation to AIDS revealed similar data to my own, with cancer being the most common disease analogy, although references to TB, syphilis, and rabies were also encountered. At the same time, as with my informants, many respondents referred to AIDS as being "like no other disease."[23] The findings suggest that physicians outside the AIDS field construct similar models to those of my informants, likely reflecting the larger web of discourse within the medical community as a whole.

As Black (1979) succinctly notes, "Every metaphor is the tip of a submerged model" (31). Disease analogies do not simply build a model of AIDS, to paraphrase Geertz, but a model for AIDS and AIDS treatment. Every analogy discussed here—and this list is by no means exhaustive—has implications for how AIDS is represented to patients and other members of the medical community and how AIDS is acted upon by both groups. Accordingly, the role of disease analogies features strongly in the next two chapters on natural history/staging and treatment.

NOTES

1. Patton (1985, 1990), Treichler (1987, 1992a, 1992b), Altman (1986), Crimp (1987), and Murray and Payne (1989), along with numerous others, have analyzed medical models of AIDS in terms of reproducing or reasserting the predominance of medicine/science over the discourse of marginalized peoples, and the of "self" versus "other" distinctions. I will not reproduce their work here.creation

2. The work of Peter Duesberg (1989, 1990) and others, arguing against a viral cause of AIDS, consciously breaks this identity between virus and disease, attempting to turn a "fact" back into a theory by reasserting and critiquing its origins. All the physicians and researchers that I encountered in the course of this study (not only direct informants) accepted HIV as at least a necessary factor in AIDS, demonstrating the difficulty of deconstructing facts within the medical community.

3. In recent lay discourse, there is often a distinction made between "risk groups" and "risk activities," attempting to separate people's identities from their (which may not correspond). Using a biological metaphor, however, the question, "Are your sexual partners of the same sex?" often acts, for the questioner, as a marker for that person's group—gay, IV drug user, and so on. Clinicians, as of 1993, generally use the term *risk factor*, which has a long history of use in other diseases, such as a high cholesterol and smoking being risk factors for heart disease.

4. The Front National, a right-wing French political party, advocates strict immigration control, including mandatory HIV testing of all immigrants, proclaiming immigration as the original source of AIDS in France. In contrast, American political discourse has tended to emphasize homosexuality, not immigration, as the source of AIDS (Altman 1986; Shilts 1987).

5. The wine and hor d'oeuvres served at the end of the conference, like the setting itself, was a pointed indicator of the changed status of AIDS in the French medical community as compared with 1987.

6. The transmission of HIV from a Florida dentist to several patients received extensive media coverage in the early 1990s and led to calls for mandatory testing of all health care workers in the United States.

7. See "New Concepts in AIDS Pathogenesis" (Gougeon et al. 1993), and "Pathogenesis of Human Immunodeficiency Virus Infection," (Levy 1993) for further examples of recent pathogenesis narratives.

8. *Hypoadrenalism* is defined as decreased functioning of the adrenal gland, which makes steroids controlling the body's response to stress as well as sodium and potassium balance.

9. I consider markers as directly constructing AIDS because they are seen to be a direct result of HIV, rather than a mediating opportunistic infection.

10. The 1993 CDC definition of AIDS now makes "AIDS without symptoms" theoretically possible by way of including all patients who have less than 200 CD4 cells. However, most patients with CD4 counts in this range have or soon develop some clinical symptoms related to their depressed immune function.

11. The most sensitive technique in detecting the presence of HIV is the polymerase chain reaction (PCR), which detects the virus' genetic material. While mainly a laboratory tool, it has become increasingly useful in detecting HIV infection in infants.

12. Gastric *tubage* seems unknown in the United States. None of my American informants had ever encountered it during their careers.

13. The frequent use of gallium scans as a diagnostic tool at Northlake may be a local rather than national phenomenon. My San Francisco clinical informants, for example, did not use gallium scans routinely. It can be difficult, however, to separate out national (French versus American), regional (Midwest versus West Coast), and local (Northlake versus other hospitals) differences.

14. It also demonstrates the extreme flexibility of English in creating linguistic constructs to express new interpretations, new experiences. The highly descriptive medical argot basic to American biomedicine, filled with phrases such as "an impressive X ray," "spike a fever," and "turf him to the oncology service," was curiously absent from the language used at Rousseau. Alternatively, I could have overlooked it through my lack of complete fluency in French, though missing it altogether seems unlikely.

15. Cervical cancer in women had not yet been accepted as an AIDS-related or AIDS-defining cancer.

16. Polio becomes doubly referent when one considers that one of the developers of the polio vaccine, Jonas Salk, is now working on an HIV vaccine.

17. In his analysis, Muraskin (1993) concludes that these very issues were avoided or sidestepped regarding HBV in the 1970s, leaving the gate wide open for the social turmoil over AIDS.

18. The Rousseau clinic also handled needle-stick exposures for the entire hospital, but I did not observe this procedure in action.

19. For example, syphilis can cause skin lesions and neurological problems, both of which are common with AIDS.

20. In April 1987, Jean-Marie Le Pen, head of the rightist Front National Party, appeared on a television broadcast aimed at confronting the AIDS issue. In this show, he referred to AIDS patients as *sidaiques* and recommended that they be confined to *sidatoriums*. To many French, the terminology is frighteningly similar to the *judaique* of the Nazi era (Hewitt 1987, 18).

21. Tuberculosis analogies are used almost exclusively by clinicians and epidemiologists. This is possibly due to the lack of my researcher informants' experience with *Mycobacteria,* as opposed to HBV, for example.

22. This phrase is ubiquitous in medicine and medical training, and I cannot at present attribute it to any single individual. In training, it is used to remind students of the myriad—though now seldom seen—manifestations of syphilis.

23. The lack of chronic disease metaphors is consistent with the historical period of the survey. The range of responses may also have been restricted by its written format and standardized questions.

5

The Stories of AIDS—Natural History and Staging

History—2. a continuous, systematic narrative of past events relating to a particular people, country, period, person, etc. . . . . 6. acts, ideas or events that will or can shape the future.
Webster's New Universal Unabridged Dictionary (1992, 674)

In formal medical usage, the *natural history* of a disease refers to the course of the disease within the body over time, including relevant signs and symptoms, without medical intervention. Since medical intervention in disease almost always takes place (at least in the United States and France), the term *natural history* has acquired another, informal set of meanings. It can mean the expected course of disease, based on clinical, epidemiological, and laboratory understanding, without further medical intervention. This usually is utilized when presenting treatment choices to a patient, such as, "Without the surgery, you can expect to experience increasing shortness of breath and a life span of two to five more years." More often, it is used to refer to the expected course of disease given the standard treatment of the time.

From an anthropological perspective, the natural history of a disease is narrative constructing the nature of that disease through a series of events over time within a particular setting and reaching a final conclusion, most markedly with the death or recovery of the patient.[1] Given our short experience with AIDS and the historical lack of standardized treatment, a multiplicity of natural histories have emerged over the last decade, often built around particular disease analogies. Some have fallen out of use, while others persist in lay discourse or that of medical personnel outside the field of AIDS.

To the physicians who encountered it early in the course of the epidemic, AIDS appeared as an acute, immediately life-threatening condition characterized in laboratory terms by a low number of lymphocytes and in clinical terms by one or more opportunistic infections. Dr. O'Neill recalls:

Right after that [first] case report, right after I started my fellowship, one of my colleagues had a patient admitted through the emergency room who had pneumonia [with] interstitial infiltrates—it was classic. He called me up and he said, "Hey, this guy has that strange disease they reported from Los Angeles and New York." And I said, "I don't know. I've never seen anything like that." Sure enough, that's what he had. That was our first known case of AIDS.

As the epidemic progressed, a variety of narratives emerged about the immediate antecedents of this acute condition, in part out of the practical need to recognize patients before they became hospitalized with a fatal infection. Low immunological status without symptoms and persistent, generalized lymphadenopathy (PGL) —swollen lymph nodes—in otherwise healthy gay men were tentatively linked to AIDS, as this excerpt from a pre-HIV medical textbook illustrates:

Some patients with lymph node enlargement go on to develop AIDS. It is likely that in many individuals, subclinical immunodeficiency and generalized lymph node enlargement represent manifestations of exposure to the AIDS agent. (Andreoli et al. 1986, 605)

The text goes on to conclude that AIDS itself appears uniformly fatal. The natural history of AIDS prior to the isolation and acceptance of HIV went generally as follows: a person is exposed to an agent—usually presented as infectious—and some time later may develop AIDS, a fatal condition that can present acutely as Kaposi's sarcoma, *Candida* infection, or *Pneumocystis* pneumonia. Laboratory-defined immune deficiency and lymphadenopathy may also be outcomes of this exposure.

With the discovery of HIV and continued epidemiological study, a new natural history narrative emerged, based strongly on the hepatitis B model. In hepatitis B infection, the affected person may (1) clear the infection and recover fully, (2) become a "healthy carrier" who can infect others but is not sick, (3) suffer from chronic liver disease or (4) develop the fatal outcomes of fulminant hepatitis or liver cancer. The 1986 *Surgeon General's Report on AIDS* is an excellent example of a hepatitis B–based model. The report creates three categories of responses to HIV: "No signs," "AIDS-Related Complex (ARC)," and "AIDS" (Koop 1986).

The "No signs" outcome of HIV infection is constructed as one encompassing the majority of infections and represents a healthy carrier state in which disease does not occur but the virus can be transmitted: "The majority of infected antibody positive individuals who carry the AIDS virus show no disease and may not come down with the disease for many years, if ever" (Koop 1986, 12). The ARC outcome is described as:

A condition caused by the AIDS virus in which the patient tests positive for AIDS infection, and has a specific set of clinical symptoms. However, ARC patients' symptoms are often less severe than those with the disease we call AIDS. (11)

A 1987 pamphlet put out by the New York State Department of Health notes, "Some individuals with ARC may die of their infection without ever developing full-blown AIDS" (New York Department of Health 1987, 10). ARC, a term utilized widely by lay and medical persons until about 1988, constructed an outcome that, unlike AIDS, was serious but not uniformly fatal. AIDS itself became defined formally according to the CDC criteria and was usually referred to as "frank AIDS" or "full-blown AIDS" in order to distinguish it from what were considered less serious forms of AIDS, now synonymous with HIV infection.

French medical discourse of the time is similar but not identical. In a booklet written under the auspices of the Ministry of Health and several nongovernmental organizations, distributed mainly to general practitioners, a seropositive ELISA result is explained as follows:

Presently it is considered that to be seropositive signifies only that one is a carrier of HIV. AIDS is only one of the possible forms of HIV infection. . . . Most often carriers of the virus are well (AIDES-Unaformec 1987, 22–23).

The authors add that seropositivity does indicate a risk of eventually progressing towards AIDS. Interestingly, this booklet does not utilize the term *ARC*, instead referring to major and minor symptoms. A 1986 French public education booklet, produced by the French Committee of Health Education, also does not refer to ARC but instead outlines three possible outcomes of HIV infection: asymptomatic carrier, generalized lymphadenopathy, and the manifestation of other diseases, ranging from less to more serious and potentially culminating in AIDS (Comité Français d'Education Pour la Santé 1986). Thus, although the French natural history of this period involves several discrete outcomes of HIV infection, as seen in the American narrative, the outcomes themselves are somewhat different in nature and AIDS itself presented more as part of a spectrum of HIV infection.

However, my French informants did make use of the ARC category, as seen in this excerpt from my 1987 interview with Dr. Farsi.

The second part of my explanation [to patients] is the medical consequences, what are the different possibilities: asymptomatic, the lymph nodes, ARC—what does it mean. And AIDS, what type of infection, when we talk of infection, what does it mean exactly.

This discourse, with its multiple discrete outcomes, is quite similar to that of the educational materials presented above.[2]

The 1985–1987 natural history narrative period clearly emerged out of the analogy with hepatitis B, as one American clinician made explicit in his interview:

I remember we used to call these lymphadenopathy patients to meetings, and tell them the results of what I had been learning. . . . We used to say, for example, there was always a lot of comparison between HIV and hepatitis B. I used to say not everybody that gets hepatitis B has the same outcome. Some people die of fulminant hepatic failure very quickly. Some people get sick, turn yellow, have hepatitis and then recover and are fine. Some people become infected, become chronic carriers of the virus and never even have a clinical illness. So I said, such is probably the case with this disease. And then when we knew it was caused by HIV, we used to say this is probably what HIV does. Some people will be well. Some people will become symptomatic. And some people will get a fatal illness.

As this American clinician's narrative demonstrates, analogies are not simply descriptive models. They impact how laypersons and physicians understand AIDS and how physicians subsequently treat the disease. For both clinicians and patients, the hepatitis B analogy constructed an AIDS that allowed hope.

Starting about 1987, this hepatitis–B based natural history began to be reluctantly discarded. Although AZT was available experimentally by this time, access to the drug was limited and its precise efficacy unknown, leaving many clinicians in the unsavory position of accepting the emergent natural history of HIV infection as uniformly fatal and not having any treatment for it—what one French informant referred to as "the dark days." The hepatitis B model fell to the wayside, according to informants, because it corresponded less and less with their experience, despite continued revision. As the above clinician described it:

Because as we got further down, we always increased the percentage of people that we thought were going to develop the bad illness. Then from subsequent epidemiologic studies, I think that now most people really do believe that everybody currently infected with HIV is going to die of an AIDS-related complication or an HIV-related complication unless we can do something between now and their time to forestall the destruction of their immune system. But I think we used to be a little more optimistic that different people were going to have different outcomes, and now I think most people who work in the field really feel that everybody has the same final kind of pathway. And it's too bad.

By the time of the Fifth International AIDS conference in 1989, AIDS had ceased being an acute clinical phenomenon with different outcomes and now emerged as a chronic disease process, characterized by inexorable progression to an ultimately fatal conclusion.

With increased access to antiretroviral drugs and preventative therapies against infections, new themes emerge from this chronic AIDS narrative. An example of this new natural history can be found in a 1990 public education booklet distributed by the CDC.

A positive result means antibodies to HIV were found in your blood. This means you have HIV infection. Your condition is called HIV-positive, or seropositive. You will most likely develop AIDS, but no one knows when you will get sick. Within 10 years after infection, about half of untreated people have developed AIDS. However, prompt medical care may delay the onset of AIDS and prevent some life threatening conditions. (CDC 1990, 20)

As with the hepatitis B-based model, this new AIDS allows hope, but through continued medical treatment rather than the possibility of having a "non-AIDS" outcome.

In discussions with patients, doctors at Northlake added another "moral" to this story—that during the extra time a person is surviving under AIDS-delaying treatments, more effective therapies are being developed. The theme of these stories is that AIDS is a chronic disease that is getting more and more treatable, rather than being quickly fatal. I encountered this narrative at Rousseau as well. During a routine visit, Dr. Cartier and the patient were exchanging stories of people with AIDS that they both knew—a common occurrence between clinicians and regular patients. Dr. Cartier then told a story of a patient who did not get tested because "he didn't want to know" and because his doctor had told him, "Don't bother, what can you do about it anyway?" The patient in the story becomes sick with PCP and ends up on a ventilator for three months. The theme being shared between Dr. Cartier and his patient—who is already tested and undergoing continued care, a compliant patient—is that AIDS is a treatable disease, that there are actions that doctors and patients can take to stop terrible things from happening. The shared meaning of AIDS emerges from the story in what is understood between doctor and patient.

This new natural history, AIDS as a chronic, progressive disease, also emerges from disease analogies. A common one not previously discussed is that of renal insufficiency, a condition with several possible origins, in which kidney function is diminished. Renal insufficiency generally has a slow but progressive course that, when taken with a number of accompanying sequelae, leads to "end-stage renal failure" and is eventually fatal, barring a successful transplant. In American clinics, not only in Chicago but in other cities I visited, AIDS was sometimes referred to as "end-stage HIV infection." This analogy evokes medically a sense of continuous progression over many years, with an uniform fatality not implied by diabetes analogies.

Apparent in the physician's discourse, and to the physicians themselves, is the sense that the AIDS of 1990 is not the same disease as at the beginning of the epidemic. The change in natural history narratives shapes and is shaped by this phenomenon. As Dr. Fields commented in a forum for people participating in clinical trials in the Chicago area:

AIDS is a very artificial distinction. It's how we recognized the whole problem initially, but it's part of a spectrum of disease. What we called AIDS in 1986 is not what we see today. It all gets defined as AIDS by the CDC definition, but it's not the same as it was five years ago.

In the AIDS of the early 1980s, *Pneumocystis* pneumonia meant full-blown AIDS. In the AIDS of 1990, this is not necessarily true, as emerged in a discussion during inpatient rounds at Northlake. Dr. Westin and Dr. Peters were talking about a new inpatient, and Dr. Peters remarked that she hadn't had an AIDS-defining illness. Dr. Westin asked, "Didn't she supposedly have PCP two years ago, but now her T cells are up to 800?" A little later, Dr. Westin commented: "That's something we don't address very much, that people can get a diagnosis of AIDS when they perhaps have PCP with a seroconversion illness. We know the T cells can drop, then come back up." In this construction, AIDS is made very distinct from seroconversion or even having infection with PCP. The linguistic identity between HIV, opportunistic infections and AIDS—HIV means PCP, which means AIDS—is breaking up, as "AIDS" becomes end-stage HIV infection.

Other evidence for a new AIDS comes from Rousseau, where the doctors engaged in a serious discussion about looking for toxoplasmosis before *Pneumocystis* as the cause of unexplained fever in patients. The new AIDS is marked not by presenting with PCP or Kaposi's sarcoma but toxoplasmosis (at least in France) or several minor symptoms, with an increase in Kaposi's sarcoma later rather than sooner in the course of the disease. In 1993, of course, AIDS can present entirely without symptoms (as per the new CDC definition), creating a category of patients who are considered to have severe disease without ever having been ill.

A new natural history narrative constructs not only a new AIDS but a new AIDS medicine. Disease analogies figure prominently in describing the transition from the old AIDS to the new, as seen in this French clinician's commentary.

The qualitative problem is the change in the type of manifestations. I think that we are probably in an infectious era. We are going into an oncologic era. . . . Increasing survival and use of complicated drugs will go into an oncologic era. We have to deal with cancers, things like that, and this means a lot of strain, which I see not only in the work but also in the psychological strain. Because at least from what I see from infectious disease people, they are not at all prepared for oncology. They have been trained to cure diseases, the only medical subspecialty which you can get rid of a disease. Now we are with a chronic disease, so there has to be a change in mentality.

The old AIDS here is constructed as an infectious disease with infectious, curable manifestations. The new AIDS is a chronic, incurable disease with chronic manifestations such as cancer. A different way of thinking, an "oncologic" mentality, is needed to treat and indeed cope with the new AIDS. Rothman and Edgar (1992), in their analysis of the early AZT trials, conclude that the placebo-based protocol of the early studies emerged from the infectious disease model of AIDS and the experiences of its proponents:

AIDS was a plague, an infection, the result of a viral agent, not a chronic illness of cellular origin. And those working in infectious diseases, unlike those in cancer research, generally had considerably less day-to-day contact, and less intense contact, with terminally ill patients than their counterparts in oncology.(204–205)

As in so many examples, multiple constructions emerge out of the same discourse: infectious disease, oncology, the practice of AIDS medicine, as well as AIDS itself. These are all interwoven with the evolving natural history of the disease.

Staging is an important medical concept related to natural history. Loosely, we can consider the staging of a disease as the interface between its natural history and treatment such that where a patient falls along the course of the disease determines the treatment. In practice, staging is applied almost solely to chronic diseases since most acute conditions, such as bacterial pneumonia, either resolve or result in death in a short period, days or weeks. We can also distinguish between formal staging and informal staging.

Only a relatively small number of diseases have formal, standardized staging systems, with cancers being the most prominent of these. One example is Hodgkin's lymphoma, which primarily affects lymphocytes and lymph nodes. Hodgkin's lymphoma is broken down into four stages, based on the number and location of lymph nodes involved, the involvement of nonlymphatic organs, and presence of generalized symptoms such as fever or weight loss. The prognosis and treatment are different for each stage. Staging systems for breast and colon cancer are similar, though they depend mainly on physical findings, such as the size of the tumor, rather than symptoms.

At the time of this study, two formalized staging systems had been developed for AIDS, both in the United States: the Walter Reed system and the 1987 CDC classification. The Walter Reed system was developed purposely for handling AIDS in military personnel, breaking the disease down into several discrete stages according to standardized criteria and then advocating a course of treatment for each. The CDC classification was intended as a descriptive epidemiologic tool rather than a prognostic system, but over the years, it has been utilized this latter way by public health agencies and physicians. A patient falling into the CDC Group II was usually considered to be in better shape than one falling into Group IV. The 1993 CDC classification, as discussed previously, is intended to guide treatment and even more closely resembles oncologic staging systems.

Staging systems are often used in research studies involving patients or cells from patients. This allows cross comparison between studies, since the study populations are all chosen around standard criteria. In the clinic, however, the use of formalized staging systems is extremely limited. As noted previously, reference to the CDC/WHO system was more common at Northlake than Rousseau, usually in the form of emphasizing the AIDS-defining illness. Although the concept of "AIDS-defining illness" is based on the CDC case definition, it forms part of the informal, nonstandard staging system that emerges out of the medical discourse and practice at Northlake. Similarly, a French counterpart developed at Rousseau.

Informal staging systems may be similar to each other across hospitals, regions, or even countries, but there is a significant amount of variation. Unlike formal staging systems, they do not involve named stages, often do not have standardized criteria for these stages, and emerge from daily clinical life rather than being imposed upon it. Patients also have informal staging systems, and as we shall see later, these are far from identical with those of physicians. Like formal staging systems, informal systems locate the patient along the course of the disease by a variety of criteria, which then impacts the resulting treatment. Over the years, informal staging systems for AIDS, including those at Northlake and Rousseau, seem to focus on the following factors: present signs and symptoms, present treatments, and most important, the CD4 (T4) lymphocyte count.

Recall that the most accepted pathogenesis narrative for AIDS involves the virus first entering the CD4 lymphocytes, which are then destroyed, leaving the body open to the development of cancers and infections. Research narratives on markers have further enhanced this story by concluding that the decrease in the CD4 count is the best predictor for progression to full-blow AIDS (Stein, Konvick and Vermund 1992). The importance of CD4 counts is underscored in this explanation by Dr. Peters to a Northlake patient.

HIV is a virus that infects mainly the helper or CD4 cells, a type of white blood cell responsible for fighting off infections. The helper cells are killed and decrease at a rate of about 100 a year; you start out with about 1,000. The number will fluctuate—700, then 900, then 600—but the overall trend is down. As the helper cells decrease you are more likely to get what we call an "AIDS-defining illness."

This then expands into a rough staging framework, as seen in this explanation to a new patient from another Northlake clinician:

What we do depends on how many T4 cells you have. If you have 500 or more, you don't need AZT. We'll repeat the counts every two to three months. If you go below 500, then you can start AZT; if you go below 200, you need prophylaxis to help prevent opportunistic infections. After the T cells go below 100 or 50, any kind of opportunistic infection can happen.

A similar framework is in place at Rousseau, though the details differ, with AZT and prophylaxis for infections both beginning at 200 CD4 cells. Thus, by CD4 count alone, the least-medicalized stage of HIV infection is much longer in the French clinic, and one American stage, defined by CD4 counts between 500 to 200, is nonexistent there. Still, the CD4 count is the primary staging criterion in both clinics. This is illustrated by a conversation at a Rousseau staff meeting. Dr. Martine tells a story of a young male patient, seropositive since 1985. "He has a fabulous *bilan*, 1,000 T4!" Noting that he is basically asymptomatic, she adds, "One thousand T4, that is very good for being seropositive for five years." A resident then relates, "You know Georges? He lost 200 CD4 in few months." This interchange underscores the importance of narrative in clinic discourse, with the CD4 count as the central symbol. The CD4 count is being used not merely as prognosticator but as a "health meter." A patient's level of health at both Northlake and Rousseau is often not judged by signs/symptoms such as fever or cough, or the patient's own designation of feeling sick versus healthy, but by the CD4 count.

There are some distinctions between the French and American use of CD4 counts in staging discourse. At Rousseau, the actual number was mentioned less often, and a descriptive term such as *good immunity* or *good immune labs* was substituted, lending a continuous rather than discrete quality to the staging. Additionally, the prognosticative value of the CD4 count was sometimes questioned, a rare occurrence at Northlake. The Rousseau clinicians sometimes spoke of this in terms of there being fewer labs in France that do reliable CD4 counts. As Dr. Bernard exclaimed during one such discussion, "If you want to make your patient happy, get your lymphocyte typing at this one lab here in Paris. Everyone gets 1,500 T4!"

However, French stories of patients with low CD4 counts who were doing well were not uncommon. After observing a consultation, I mentioned the patient's dropping CD4 count. The doctor expressed uncertainty about the value of the CD4 count, then launched into a story: "I had a patient who had a T4 of eight two years ago. He's alive and has nothing [no problems]. He's working, drinking, smoking, going to the gym." In this narrative, not only does this patient with an incredibly low CD4 count not have AIDS, but he is living a full, hard-driving French life: working, drinking, smoking.[3] However, stories such as these generally act as exceptions that prove the rule of the importance of CD4 counts.

The CD4 count, while necessary to informal staging, is not sufficient. Two other elements contribute, those of symptoms and treatments. At Rousseau, if a patient had persistent symptoms, such as oral candidiasis, at a CD4 count above 200, AZT would then be started despite not meeting the CD4 criterion. The following is a Northlake example, with its characteristic emphasis on AIDS-defining illness. One clinician presented a new inpatient—"with no prior AIDS-defining illness." The patient, who had a relatively high CD4 count, had developed a fever and cough over the last five days and now showed a low oxygen level in his blood. Dr. Peters remarked that the patient could be considered (1) asymptomatic or (2) acting "like ARC" with wasting or more minor symptoms or finally (3) having AIDS with a high CD4 count, which he states is unlikely but possible. The patient is thus being staged according to his present symptoms, which may or may not be associated with HIV infection, his past symptoms, and his CD4 count. Note the reference to "ARC," which is used here as a shorthand for an intermediate stage of HIV infection.

Staging discourse often includes reference to present treatments, as in another Northlake example where the patient was described as being "asymptomatic HIV, on Bactrim, AZT, with a T cell count of eighty-two."[4] Symptoms, present treatments, and CD4 counts thus determine the stage of HIV infection. The stages, except sometimes for full-blown AIDS itself, are not named in any consistent fashion but are signified by the descriptive shorthand seen in the above example.

As the patient becomes sicker, with lower CD4 counts, the count takes on less importance in assessing the patient's status. As one Rousseau clinician responded to a patient asking about his low CD4 count, "It is difficult to explain. Ten or 50 T4, there is no difference. Fifty or 500 is different, but not 10 or 50." At Northlake, when a patient with CD4 counts under 100 or after a noted AIDS-defining illness would ask for repeated counts, the doctors would reply that how someone is feeling is more important than numbers at this point. In talking about a patient carrying a CDC AIDS designation, Northlake doctors would sometimes omit the CD4 count altogether and focus solely on signs, symptoms, and treatments.

In these informal staging systems, the most severe stage, AIDS, is defined generally along the criteria of CD4 count, symptoms, and treatments, particularly at Rousseau. When I asked one doctor if he used the term *ARC*, he replied, "No, it's too artificial. If a person has infections and is taking Bactrim and other drugs, I would classify that as AIDS." During a staff meeting, a resident asked whether a patient on prophylaxis for PCP can be considered to have AIDS. Dr. Farsi replied, "The biological reality, in a patient with zero CD4, on primary prophylaxis for *Pneumocystis* is that he has AIDS. Epidemiologically, it doesn't count as a case of AIDS until he actually gets the infection." The 1993 CDC definition formally incorporates, and thus legitimizes, this interpretation.

At Northlake, as at Rousseau, patients with low CD4 counts and symptoms were generally ascribed to the same treatment category as those with similar labs and symptoms who carried the actual CDC AIDS diagnosis. However, identifying whether a patient has had an AIDS-defining illness was a significant element in Northlake discourse, with no equivalent counterpart at Rousseau. The term was ubiquitous in daily talk around the clinic, both between doctors and patients and among doctors themselves. The development of CDC-defined AIDS was thus marked, in discourse if not always in practice, as a separate stage from patients who were symptomatic with low CD4 counts. For example, a physician described a new inpatient by stating, "He has a low helper count but no AIDS-defining illness."

One contextual force driving this discourse is the US health care system. A patient is definitively eligible for disability (and thus Medicaid coverage) and other benefits only if he carries the CDC-defined AIDS diagnosis. Occasionally, people with severe symptomatic disease but not AIDS are accepted for disability as well (El-Sadr et al. 1994). At Northlake, patients without CDC-defined AIDS often waited months for coverage in the course of "proving" their disability. The Northlake clinicians were usually aware of patients' insurance and financial status, since it could affect a patient's treatment if appropriate action were not taken when needed. Thus, public policy helps to perpetuate American physicians' use of the "AIDS-defining illness" and constructs three categories or stages of HIV infections, of which CDC-defined AIDS is the most severe and considered automatically disabling.[5]

This benefits-based meaning for the AIDS-defining illness emerges out of doctor-patient discourse as well. For example, during a visit with an patient hospitalized with an opportunistic infection, Dr. O'Neill inquired, "Have you had any so-called AIDS defining illnesses before this?" The patient replied, "Just thrush twice." Discussion then ensued about whether the patient had applied for disability yet. Dr O'Neill ended by stating that once you have an AIDS-defining illness, the disability application "will sail right through."

Another contextual influence concerns clinical trials. Many clinical trials for experimental medications are limited to patients carrying the CDC AIDS diagnosis. Thus, the AIDS diagnosis controls access to a number of new treatments. Patton (1990, 52) notes that persons with AIDS participate in clinical trials due to "smart shopping" for treatments as much as an altruistic desire to further medical knowledge. I would add that Northlake physicians often acted as "smart shoppers" as well, keeping an eye out for the experimental "bargain" for their patients. At Northlake, patients or clinicians would mention a possible experimental drug, only to review the patient's history and discover he does not carry the requisite AIDS diagnosis, leading the doctor to comment, "Well, I guess you're just too healthy." Additionally, one way for patients to receive medications for free was to enroll in a clinical trial. In fact, when a patient's insurance or other financial resources ran out, the Northlake staff would scramble, looking for an appropriate trial so that the patient could continue treatment. The role of many clinical trials at Northlake, and perhaps at other American clinics, emerges not only as a means of advancing scientific understanding of AIDS and its treatment but as a way to provide adequate health care for increasingly impoverished patients. The French socialized health care system, by contrast, would not tend to reinforce an AIDS-defining illness discourse.

However, these immediate, contextually mediated meanings are not enough to explain the power and prevalence of this terminology at Northlake. It was frequently utilized in cases where patient benefits and clinical research were not an issue, and more often than not, discussion that focused on the AIDS-defining illness did not include any mention of such benefits. For example, the team was going to see an inpatient with *Cryptococcus* in his blood, his first opportunistic infection. Dr. Westin asked Dr. Peters, "Have you told him that he now has AIDS? It's a very difficult threshold for patients." We went in, and Dr. Peters explained to the patient that his treatment would not change except for the addition of one drug to his daily medications, but that "we now call this AIDS instead of being HIV positive." The patient asked, "Did my immune system get weaker?" Dr. Peters replied, "Not necessarily. You were at an increased risk of getting an infection before." It is the nurse who commented that we, the HIV team, didn't see this as any different, just that the CDC needed to know for epidemiological purposes.

This incident is illustrative of the focus on information sharing in the American doctor-patient relationship, which will be addressed in a later section. It also brings up an interesting question, with ethical implications: If this AIDS diagnosis truly makes no difference, why tell the patient in the absence of any inquiries? The answer is that, for Northlake physicians, it *does* make a difference, not so much in the treatment aspect of staging but in the placement of the patient along the natural history of the disease. For the Northlake physicians, the patient is now in a new, distinct stage of the disease as the result of a discrete event, the AIDS-defining illness. It perhaps marks an important difference in the character of American staging of AIDS as evidenced by Northlake, compared to the French. With its greater emphasis on the actual numbers of the CD4 counts, and its separating out of at least one stage by a single event, the American system more closely resembles the discrete, standardized stages seen with cancer. The new definition of AIDS does not necessarily change the model, only the event defining the stage known as "AIDS." Further detailed research at other US clinics would be helpful in clarifying this aspect of American models of AIDS.

The French system is somewhat more continuous, with fewer and more descriptively oriented boundaries—"good immunity" versus "bad immune tests." "Being on AZT," in the discourse of the Rousseau clinic, is often used in place of "less than 200 CD4 cells," as is primary prophylaxis for PCP. "He taking Bactrim for secondary prophylaxis" or "He's on Malocide because of toxoplasmosis" means that the patient has had at least one episode of opportunistic infection, identifying a more serious stage of the disease. The French system tends to be descriptive rather than quantitative, constructing a more fluid AIDS, though there is considerable overlap with American models.

Informal staging systems based on CD4 counts, symptoms, and treatments are not limited to Chicago and Paris. A San Francisco clinician emphasized the importance of the CD4 count in determining the stage of the disease:

I'm much more interested in how long somebody with 500 helper cells survives, or how long does somebody with 200 helper cells survive now, because that's a much firmer, more defined way to pin down where the person is in their disease, rather than just what they happen to have had or not had.

As in the Chicago examples, the emphasis here is on a "more defined" way to stage a patient, generally through the quantitation of the CD4 count.

The informal staging systems are flexible. I suspect that there is some variation between institutions and, definitely, between regions. At one San Francisco clinic I visited, AZT was often begun at above 500 CD4 cells, placing the "asymptomatic but in need of treatment" stage earlier than in Chicago. However, in a 1988 medical text on managing AIDS, a San Francisco physician outlined the important questions for staging[6] a patient:

1. Is the individual symptomatic or asymptomatic?
2. What is the extent of the immunologic compromise?
3. Is there sufficient evidence from preliminary studies to make a definitional diagnosis of AIDS?
4. If not, what is the risk of progression to disease?
5. Given the stage of disease, is the individual eligible for any traditional or experimental therapy? (Hollander 1988, 107)

Question 1 asks for symptoms, question 2 for CD4 count, and question 3 asks if there is an AID-defining illness, putting this 1988 San Francisco staging system well in line with the one that emerges out of daily medical discourse at Northlake. Thus, the basic components of the informal staging system I saw in Chicago—CD4 count, symptoms, treatments—seem to hold true across the United States, and, to a lesser extent, across the Atlantic as well.

By no means is this informal staging system static. It is reshaped every day in every medical encounter, retaining much ambiguity along the way. As we saw in a previous encounter, a Northlake doctor had difficulty deciding whether a patient was in the asymptomatic, "ARC-like," or AIDS stage. Ongoing discussion about whether to institute PCP prophylaxis based on absolute CD4 counts or as a percentage of total lymphocytes occurred at both clinics. The Northlake physicians, in fact, went "percentage crazy" one day, reassessing all the day's patients after discovering that a few patients who were above 200 CD4 cells had developed PCP. Another Northlake discussion concerned continuing to look at CD4 counts regularly even when a patient drops below 100, after a study suggested that a drop below 50 indicated low survival past a few months. Recently, a French commission has recommended beginning primary toxoplasmosis prophylaxis at CD4 counts below 100, and *Mycobacterium avium-intracellulare* (MAC) prophylaxis below 50 (Mayaud 1993a). Thus, the exact criteria for each stage remain ambiguous, evolving on a near-daily basis, much like the whole of AIDS.

NOTES

1. In French, not unexpectedly, *histoire* can mean both "history" and "story."

2. I suspect that "ARC" found its way into French medical discourse through the American medical literature—the syntax is incorrect for a French acronym—and popular usage. Rousseau clinicians used the term rarely during my 1990 visit.

3. I did encounter American stories of this type, though less frequently. "Low CD4" stories, utilizing the discourse of both patients and physicians, have appeared in the American lay press. One such article, which initially appeared in a gay paper, *The Advocate*, was later reprinted in a medical journal (Gallagher 1994).

4. Dr. Daniel Buff (1994) observed that physicians can and often do describe the entire medical history of an AIDS patient using only abbreviations. His poem "An Abbreviated Life" recognizes our avoidance of the person behind the acronyms.

5. The 1993 CDC classification expands the number of people meeting the criteria for AIDS and so theoretically increases the number of people eligible for disability benefits. It is impossible to tell whether the CDC changed its definition in part due to these socioeconomic pressures. However, the CDC notes: "The CDC's AIDS surveillance case definition was not developed to determine whether statutory or other legal requirements for entitlement to Federal disability or other benefits are met" (CDC 1992a, 8). The article goes on to state that the new definition does not alter the Social Security criteria for evaluating claims and that agencies should develop their own criteria dependent on needs, not the CDC case definition.

6. The term *staging* was specifically used in this text and frequently by American informants as well. While my French informants did occasionally use the word *stage*, as in "a more advanced stage of HIV infection," I could not discover a consistent French equivalent to the American words *staging* or *staging system*.

6

Treatment

We have already seen how treatments play an important role in constructing AIDS by designating its boundaries. The types of drugs, past and present, used to treat AIDS also construct the nature of the disease for the medical community.

In the early part of the epidemic, a wide variety of treatments emerged. Among the earliest drugs used, particularly before the isolation of HIV, were immune modulators, a diverse class of medications sharing the common property of affecting the proliferation of immune cells (Grmek 1990). One seemingly paradoxical drug, an immune suppressant known as cyclosporin, was used briefly around 1985 by a group of French clinicians, but was quickly abandoned. The use of this drug constructed a model of AIDS based on an autoimmune mechanism, whereby the body develops an immune response to some of its own cells. Although cyclosporin has been discredited, two of my informants presented models of pathogenesis that contained elements of an autoimmune narrative, while scientific articles on the topic continue to be published (Gougeon et al. 1993; Katz 1993). Additionally, there has been an increased use of steroids, which also act as immune suppressants and are used in autoimmune diseases such as lupus. In the context of AIDS, steroids are used alone to treat aphthous ulcers—non-specific inflammation—in the mouth and esophagus and as an adjunct in treating PCP. Thus, AIDS retains some of its paradoxical autoimmune nature even today.

More common immune modulators that have been used in AIDS are immune stimulants. These include interleukin-2 and alpha-interferon, both immune stimulants found naturally in the human body. DTC, commercially known as Imuthiol, is a synthetic compound with immune modulating properties. It was widely used as an experimental drug in parts of Europe, particularly in France, and continues to be used at the Rousseau clinic on a limited basis. The application of these drugs constructs AIDS as primarily the result of a deficit in the immune system. These drugs, and the narrative they helped build, fell out of use due to (1) increasingly accepted research narratives that these drugs were not effective and (2) the isolation of HIV and the emergence of the model of AIDS as a viral infection.

Immune modulators have not disappeared however, and remain a strong part of medical practice and discourse on AIDS. Alpha interferon is now used to treat Kaposi's sarcoma, and Imuthiol remains in use in Paris for those patients that seem to have responded, as well as being the subject of renewed interest worldwide for use in combination with AZT. Another immune stimulant, GM-CSF (granulocyte macrophage colony stimulating factor), is used as an adjunct therapy to maintain the number of white blood cells (WBCs), especially neutrophils, while administering marrow-toxic drugs to treat cancer or CMV retinitis. Many informants, as seen in the following French and American excerpts, mentioned immune modulators when talking about future AIDS treatments, usually as an addition to antiviral drugs.

It will be different at each stage of the disease. Because very early asymptomatics might need only combined antiviral treatment, then more advanced into the disease, it might be important for combined antivirals plus immunomodulators. And at the late stages of disease, we are going to need antivirals plus bone marrow transplants.

I think that as we begin to find agents that may work at different places in the virus' life cycle, that we will be combining various antiretroviral agents. Hopefully we might find some immune modulator that could build back a little bit of the immune system that's been destroyed by the virus, and I think that probably patients will be taking prophylaxes for all of the different opportunistic infections.

However, a number of the Americans were quite skeptical of immune modulators:

Immunotherapy is and has been a therapy looking for a condition or disease. I think we don't understand enough about the immune system right now to be able to even pretend that we're manipulating it in any more than a grossly empirical way.

This is a disease that I'm not worried about immunomodulators. A patient with leukemia doesn't need immunomodulators for his bone marrow to recover. Once the disease is eradicated, the immune system reconstitutes itself. What we need are better antivirals of a very different sort than we have now.

The latter comment constructs a model of AIDS as being the effect of HIV on the body—a unicausal narrative extremely common in biomedicine. This approach dates back to the development of the germ theory of disease and proliferating with the bacteriology discoveries of the later nineteenth century (Starr 1982). In discourse on AIDS, however, there is a distinguishable split between the American and French emphasis on the role of HIV. There is no doubt that the majority of French clinicians and researchers see HIV as necessary. On the other hand, unlike many of my American informants, their discourse suggests that attacking HIV alone is not sufficient, as was seen in the French researcher's suggestion of immune modulators and bone marrow transplants.[1] As the head of the Rousseau clinic cautioned, "We know also that we cannot expect of antiretroviral therapy something like a restoration of the immune system. We can only expect diminution of the viral load."

Why this French focus on an immunological approach to AIDS treatment when its viral etiology is well accepted? This may be due to the French concept of *terrain*, a body's overall ability to ward off disease, of which the immune system is an important part. As Payer (1988) notes:

Many diseases result from a combination of some type of outside insult and the body's reaction to that insult. While English and American doctors tend to focus on the insult, the French and the Germans focus on the reaction, and are more likely to try to find ways to modify the reaction as well as fight off the insult. (1988, 61)

Terrain is a concept that is fundamental to French biomedicine—and perhaps fundamental to French constructions of AIDS. For example, the topic of pathogenesis came up in a Rousseau staff meeting. Dr. Bernard pointed out that some people become rapidly sick with HIV, while others stay healthy a long time, expressing it as a compatibility between the individual's immune system and the virus. He concluded, "And there must be an immune response, because it [AIDS] is a slow disease. Otherwise, it would be like in infants, who don't have developed immune systems."[2] The immune response, as well as the virus, is integral to these French clinicians' construction of AIDS, with a subsequent treatment discourse and practice that includes immune modulation and vaccine therapy.

In both French and American discourse, the virus is still central to AIDS. After HIV was isolated, experimental antiviral medications proliferated, including HPA-23, a compound with activity against certain animal retroviruses, and acyclovir, used to treat herpes. AZT, the medication in widest use today, was developed in the United States as a cancer drug. That it has antiviral activity is likely no accident, since the Federal War on Cancer initially put most of its funding toward finding a viral cause for cancer (Payer 1988).

Payer suggests that for American physicians viral causes are often attributed to unknown or poorly understood conditions, such as cancer and now AIDS. Viruses, and by extension antiviral drugs, stand for the external origins of disease in American biomedical discourse.[3] All the antiretroviral drugs now commonly used in AIDS—AZT, DDI, DDC—were developed in the United States. Although DDI and DDC were developed explicitly for use in AIDS, they are chemical cousins to AZT, utilizing the same mode of action that was once thought to be effective against cancer.

The dominant analogy of cancer in the United States extends into how AZT is used by medical communities. At Northlake and a number of US clinics, AZT is started when the patient's CD4 count drops below 500. In the San Francisco area, it is sometimes begun even earlier. The discourse surrounding this practice is thematically very clear: the sooner treatment is begun, the better.

Personally, I will often suggest starting AZT before that [500 CD4]. And that's my personal philosophy based on nothing but intuition. I want to give people the option of taking AZT earlier. I mean, I would be on AZT if I was HIV infected regardless of what my T cell count was.

During a lecture at Northlake, Dr. Fields recounted the story of the first AZT studies and the decision to examine the early use of AZT in people with few symptoms and a 200 to 800 CD4 count. He concluded:

With TB, if you take someone whose skin test converts, you give them INH [trademark for *isoni*cotine *h*ydrazine for the preparation of isoniazid] and they don't get TB. In contrast to this, in people with cavitary TB, you need three drugs because the bug load is so high. It's much easier to treat early infection than late infection. So the same type of thinking was applied to HIV.

As discussed below, the French do not use purified protein derivative (PPD) testing and INH prophylaxis in treating tuberculosis and, analogously, use AZT at lower CD4 counts. Tuberculosis thus resurfaces as an important analogy for both discourse and practice in both countries.

The "aggressive" approach to treatment is pervasive throughout American biomedicine. Even the word itself is ubiquitous in talk among American clinicians, as in "Let's treat this aggressively." The whole process of staging cancer often functions to determine how aggressive the physician can or must be in treating. In Hodgkin's lymphoma, staging determines whether radiation or the more aggressive chemotherapy will be used. In breast cancer, radical mastectomy was, until the last ten years or so, the treatment of choice for *early* stage treatment, with the goal of cure through early, extensive surgical intervention. More recently, adjunct chemotherapy is being recommended for breast cancer even without evidence of metastases (Hacker and Moore 1992, 450). The more strictly defined staging and the early use of AZT in the American approach to AIDS emerge from and sustain the analogy between cancer and AIDS.

The French discourse on AZT is equally revealing. The institution of AZT treatment when a patient reaches 200 CD4 cells is not limited to Rousseau but was the recommendation of the national panel on AIDS treatment. Looking at a major American clinical trial of AZT, the panel concluded: "It is advisable to remark that the mean length of follow-up in this trial was only one year, that the effects of treatment in the long term are unknown and that the data on in-vitro and in-vivo resistance are very fragmentary" (Dormont et al. 1990, 9).[4] The concern over long-term toxicity of the drug was expressed by a number of my French informants:

It's [AZT] a chronic treatment, so its long-term side effects are also important for all the drugs we use in the future.

To create such very long trials, many months or years, you don't know about the toxicity of the drugs. And I think that the American position to say we have to give AZT to all people who are seropositive under 500 CD4 lymphocytes is *fou* [crazy]. And very good to give money to the laboratory.

French objections to early use of AZT also concern efficacy. Both Northlake and Rousseau physicians utilized clinical research data to support their positions. In separate presentations to both medical students and patients involved in clinical trials, Dr. Fields stressed that AZT prolongs the period before development of full-blown AIDS and seems to extend life span somewhat. On the other hand, in a presentation to Rousseau clinicians, Dr. Bernard emphasized that CD4 levels in all patients return to baseline between six months and one year of initiation of AZT. In a staff meeting, Dr. Bernard poked fun at the American interpretation of AZT's effectiveness:

In the United States, there is a study of over 3,000 patients, compiling statistics on changes in T4 with AZT. So there are increases of 10 percent, 20 percent. A patient can have 10 percent increase going from 10 to 11 [T4 cells]!

Besides presenting an observed French skepticism of American reliance on statistics, it again focuses on the status of the immune system, represented by the CD4 count, as the appropriate indicator of the drug's effectiveness. The Americans, on the other hand, emphasize the delay of clinical manifestations of the virus's activity as the best indicator. The preliminary results of the French-British Concorde study indicated no delay in clinical progression of disease over a three-year span despite early use of AZT (Aboulker and Swart 1993). Debate over the interpretation of Concorde and similar studies continues the narrative contest over AZT, highlighting the impact of cultural constructions of disease-body interaction on the scientific enterprise.

French medical discourse on the use of AZT often revolves around the issue of resistance. As seen in the French panel's recommendation, concern over the development of resistance is one of the primary reasons that AZT therapy is begun later than in the United States. This reasoning was reiterated in a guidebook for French physicians:

In effect, the spontaneous evolution of patients having a CD4 level between 200 and 5,000 carries a weak risk of complications (on the order of five percent a year); this is opposed to the risk of cumulative undesirable effects in the time of AZT, as well as the appearance of resistant viral strains, perhaps in association with clinical resistance of which the frequency equally increases over time. (Rozenbaum 1990, 46)

In informal conservation with my French informants, this concern with resistance was expressed not only as increasing resistance within an individual patient over time but as the development of resistant strains *within the population.* This discourse on resistance in AIDS mirrors French discourse on resistance of tuberculosis.

We don't treat contact people with isoniazid because we suppose that the vaccination is more or less sufficient. It is a bet. And also that isoniazid alone may provoke resistance. And if you are looking at the rate of resistance in United States and in France, I think that perhaps we are right. You have a very big increase in resistance in United States, I think. And as the primary prophylaxis in tuberculosis is proposed [in the United States] in AIDS patients, I'm afraid that it may have some trouble.

This contrasts strongly with Dr. Field's narrative on TB and AIDS, which centered on the effectiveness of early intervention rather than the issue of resistance.

My American informants spoke of resistance as well, and though they all agreed it needed to be studied, most concluded it was not a major problem. Dr. Fields, during his presentation on the ACTG meetings, noted:

An individual that has AIDS or ARC is more likely to develop resistance in six to nine months, independent of dose. In contrast to that, individuals who were in 019 [a clinical trial] who were asymptomatic have isolates out to three years that are still sensitive to AZT. . . . The correlation of clinical failure with resistance doesn't exist, which is fascinating.

Another Chicago physician addressed the issue of resistance at a forum for patients in clinical trials. He defined resistance as the "failure of therapy" and cited tuberculosis as "the best example of resistance in treating a chronic disease over a long period of time." Turning to HIV, he remarked that there is a low load of virus early in the infection: "It doesn't break the laws of biology. When you get infection with HIV, your immune system responds to that infection." He stressed that the more virus around in the body, the better the chance of developing a resistant strain. Thus, since AZT works to reduce viral load, early use of AZT would delay development of resistance. The emphasis here, as in all resistance discourse I encountered in the United States, is on developing resistance to AZT in the individual patient, not resistant strains emerging within the population.[5]

The French model of resistance, as seen in their approach to tuberculosis, is that the longer you expose a large number of people with an infectious agent to a single drug, the more likely it is that a resistant strain of the agent will evolve. The French would be horrified at the suggestion of one American physician to give all IV drug users—who have a high incidence of tuberculosis—isoniazid as prophylaxis, whether or not they have a positive skin test for TB exposure. Thus, the caution of my French informants regarding early use of AZT is more comprehensible, given their approach to tuberculosis and resistance issues, their concern over toxicity, and the fundamental concept of *terrain*. Why give a potentially toxic drug when the patient's *terrain* is relatively healthy, only to risk the development of resistant strains? This argument is compounded by the time lag in getting new antiviral drugs from the United States into France; once you have lost efficacy with AZT, backup treatments such as DDC are difficult to come by.

The American argument is centered around basic American biomedical values of aggressiveness and the benefit gained for the individual patient. As Dr. Peters commented, "I'd rather have AZT when I'm healthier." The Rousseau physicians saw the American approach to TB and AIDS as naively aggressive and socially irresponsible, while the Northlake doctors viewed the French approach as unscientific and harmful to the patient. Payer (1988) notes that this has historically been the view between the two biomedicines as well.

Despite the variations in discourse and practice regarding AZT, both my American and French informants rely on the drug heavily in daily practice and envision the combination of several antiretroviral medications as the treatment of the future.

Some of my San Francisco informants remarked that combination antiviral therapy was already in use, either through doctors or patients acting independently.[6] One noted, "I am already seeing my patients combining AZT and DDC when they fall below 500 helper T cells."

Combination therapy, usually referred to as combination "chemotherapy" as in cancer treatment, is supported discursively by three main narratives. First, that combining antivirals would allow a lower dose of each and thus decrease the toxicity for the patient, as seen in the comments of an American clinician and French researcher.

The current rage is combination therapy, which it was for in oncology. We have some drugs that are unacceptable with toxicity, so it is rational to put more than one antiviral together.

Now it's more like cancer. It took twenty, thirty years to develop drugs that were at the beginning more efficient, usually toxic, and by working on combinations and some modification of the chemistry of the drugs, tried to reduce the side effects, it was possible to achieve some success in the treatment of cancer. So I'm afraid it's going to be the same for AIDS.

Second, combining different drugs, particularly those with different mechanisms of action, would increase effectiveness, as described by an American clinician.

I think it's going to be a combination chemotherapy like in cancer, and I think that the nucleoside analogs like AZT, and DDI, and FLT [fluorothymidine] will be the cornerstone, the lynchpin for the foreseeable future, with other drugs such as the interferons, perhaps protease inhibitors or gene active agents as additives and synergistic combinations—that is, looking at ways of attacking different parts of the host cell–virus interaction.

Finally, as the following French epidemiologist and American clinician remarked, combining drugs would impede or alleviate the development of resistance: "I think that we will have better drugs than AZT. But I suspect that they will still need to be used in combination with drugs, for example, AZT, to prevent resistance."

As one can see, some narratives emerge out of analogies with cancer treatment, while others are associated with tuberculosis. While both models are present in both countries, the analogy with cancer chemotherapy seems somewhat more predominant in the United States.[7] However, the analogy between cancer and AIDS is reinforced in both French and American practice by the use of antibiotic and antifungal drugs as prophylaxis against opportunistic infections.

The concept of giving medication to prevent rather than treat infections has a long history in biomedicine. Outside of the American use of isoniazid to prevent TB, most long-term prophylaxis occurs in response to some sort of immune-compromised state, most prominently to patients on cancer chemotherapy or transplant recipients on immunosuppressant medications to fight organ rejection. For example, fluconazole, an antifungal drug, was developed in Europe as both treatment and prophylaxis for infections in cancer chemotherapy patients and now has worldwide application in AIDS. While *Pneumocystis* pneumonia had been known in immune-compromised patients before AIDS, the idea of prophylaxing against it, first against secondary recurrence and later against even the initial infection, seems to have developed entirely within the context of the AIDS epidemic. Many of my informants give PCP prophylaxis at least as much credit as AZT in increasing the quality and quantity of life for people infected with HIV.

Prophylaxis against the myriad opportunistic infections in AIDS, primary and secondary, has mushroomed: herpes recurrence, atypical *Mycobacteria,* candidiasis, and toxoplasmosis. In the context of AIDS, prophylaxis generally means that patients stay on the medications indefinitely rather than the limited time frame seen in cancer chemotherapy. Some of the preventive therapies are relatively standardized, such as aerosolized pentamidine or Bactrim for PCP, while others vary from hospital to hospital, region to region, or country to country. The Rousseau doctors used a different combination of drugs against atypical *Mycobacteria* than the Northlake doctors, while until recently, San Francisco informants focused on aerosolized pentamidine for PCP and East Coast informants seem to have relied more on Bactrim. While my exposure to clinical practice outside of Chicago was necessarily limited, these type of data suggest three levels of biomedical culture: local, regional, and national/societal.[8]

Much public attention has been focused not on the immediate treatment of AIDS but on the possibility of a preventative vaccine. In the daily life of an AIDS clinic, vaccines are rarely the subject of discourse except when brought up by patients or in the media. What discourse there is, is highly fragmented, with little uniformity over the possibility of ever developing a vaccine, its potential efficacy, or the best immunological basis for its action. Most of the clinicians were extremely pessimistic about there being any vaccine in the foreseeable future. Not surprisingly, those informants who are involved in vaccine research, both French and Americans, were the most optimistic. There is extensive disagreement over whether the vaccine should be based on cell-mediated immunity, which is seen at work in encounters with poison ivy, or humoral immunity, as used in measles vaccines. One American researcher suggested that stimulating antibodies against HIV could even enhance rather than inhibit its action. There seems to be no larger pattern for which people espouse which narrative, other than perhaps institutional affiliation.

The same is also true of a discourse on vaccine as therapy for HIV-infected people, either to prevent or improve symptomatic disease. This use of vaccine has historical precedent in present-day treatment of rabies, which, like AIDS, has a slow onset of disease following infection, as well as in the nineteenth-century treatment for TB and syphilis. As we have seen, all of these diseases are used as strong analogies for AIDS. A positive discourse on vaccine as therapy seems more common among my French informants, and it was this type of vaccine that was developed by French immunologist Daniel Zagury and a team of Zairian physicians in 1986, when Zagury inoculated himself to prove the vaccine safety and immune-provoking response (Grmek 1990). Though Zagury's well-publicized act was decried in both France and the United States, his vaccine model itself was not heavily criticized in France, where several other researchers were working on similar projects. This idea of vaccine as immunotherapy fits in well with the French emphasis on immune modulation and the role of *terrain*.

Still, the discourse among my French and American informants was heavily divided even on vaccine therapy, including on how they should be made, how they should be used, and if they would be effective. Overall, this proliferation of vaccine narratives is strikingly similar to that seen earlier in the epidemic for causes of AIDS. This discourse, like that surrounding etiology, is another step in the construction of the nature of AIDS. Here, too, I suspect that a full narrative contest will ensue over time, ending in the adoption of an authoritative vaccine narrative—that is, a fact—by most of the medical community.

My informants often recalled the initial variability of AIDS treatment, commenting on the proliferation of therapeutic approaches in and out of the biomedical community.

I think a lot of things have changed since 1986 or '87 in that in the mid-80s there was sort of a mad scramble for access to the "treatment de jour" whatever it was. . . . It's really not access that's inhibiting progress against this disease. It's the nature of the foe. It is the virus that is outwitting us.

I think that earlier on in the epidemic when knowledge of illness manifestation disease and treatment were not nearly as standardized, or effective interventions hadn't been delineated as clearly, I think that you had more of a physician-specific and patient-specific approach treatment of illness. Those were the years when alternative health became a cottage industry for illness, treating the HIV infection, and I think that is not the case as much anymore.

As noted by the above clinicians, this "mad scramble" has narrowed somewhat over time, approaching but not achieving the point of "standardization" across all biomedicines. As of 1994, most treatment plans included the use of an antiretroviral, usually AZT, linked to the patient's CD4 count, as well as prophylaxis against opportunistic infections chosen from among certain known medications, such as Bactrim. I am using *standardization* for AIDS drug therapy as Koenig (1988) does in her discussion of "routinization" of a technological treatment. The standardization of at least some parts of AIDS, such as staging and treatment, enables clinicians to talk and act without a complete reconstruction of AIDS at every step. As Koenig suggests, standardization provides a counter to the chaos inherent in illness, a chaos particularly characteristic of the paradoxical, fast-changing AIDS.

The increasing standardization of AIDS emerges clearly from my informants' discourse, as does a sense of the increasing comfort in regard to treating patients:

We're less shooting in the dark. We have often more options when something doesn't work—there's something else to try. And we have much more of a feeling that you know where you are at a particular point. . . . Decisions have become very standardized, at least in this country [United States]. The point at which AZT should be introduced is standardized. There are a couple of quite standard approaches to PCP. There are a couple of quite standard approaches to toxoplasmosis and to KS, for that matter.

There are treatments available, antiretroviral drugs available, and PCP prophylaxis, and the different symptoms and signs of HIV infection are much more easily known and treatable. Most of the things are treatable, like rash and different pneumonias that people get and that sort of thing, so you learn to anticipate a treatment much easier. And so primary care's become routinized, which is—I like that—if you could see things in a certain way and automatically react.

However, though certain aspects of AIDS treatment have become more routine, it is still anything but standardized, either in the United States or France, as seen respectively below.

As we reduce the uncertainty and management diversity at some decision points, we get more aggressive about other, often later, decision points. So, there are areas of gross lack of standardization, particularly the management of people on AZT whose CD4 counts continue to fall.

Eventually, I think we will see more standardization, and I think right now it's fairly standard because we have so few options. I would expect that in the future as the number of options increase for the treatment of HIV, it will get less standard. People right now are doing everything from not treating to treating with immediate combinations of AZT and DDC even in asymptomatics. I think that spectrum of approaches reflects the kind of awareness of the doc and patient, and aggressiveness of the doc and patient will for quite a while result in quite an array of different approaches.[9]

As far as AZT is concerned, it is not exactly very uniform. But this is an international problem—nobody has the answer. Maybe treatments are getting a bit more uniform, but still, for instance, as far as Kaposi's is concerned, I still see sometimes odd types, for instance, prescribing interferon in very high doses in a patient who has five T4 cells and everybody knows it won't work.

AIDS treatment is constituted not only by continued diversity in discourse and practice but by daily innovation and improvisation as well. I use *innovation* to refer to use of new drugs, or old drugs in new ways, in a number of patients outside of formal clinical trials. *Improvisation* refers to treatment approaches developed "off the cuff" in relation to a particular patient's situation. The development of aerosolized pentamidine as prophylaxis for PCP, rather than the intravenous version, was an AIDS innovation in response to the troublesome toxicity of the drug when used intravenously.

We discussed, wrestled, with the idea of giving it as an aerosol for a long time. Resisted because everybody knows that the aerosol route is not very good for treating pneumonia. In fact, the same is true of pentamidine—it's not very good at treating pneumonia. It can be quite good at preventing it.

I encountered innovation at Rousseau on day one, when I observed the doctors prescribing thalidomide, a drug that has been banned or restricted worldwide due to its deforming effects on the developing fetus. According to Dr. Bernard, the drug was initially developed for its antiinflammatory properties. Since AIDS patients often develop severe, resistant oral aphthous ulcers, "canker sores," he theorized that thalidomide might be helpful. According to the Rousseau clinicians, several patients have benefited by the unusual treatment, and the innovation has become a part of the Rousseau repertoire.[10]

Improvisation was also common at Rousseau. The following case, again based on the use of thalidomide, is illustrative of the improvisation process. A patient had long-standing perianal lesions, initially thought to be due to either CMV or resistant herpes, and, after failing more conventional therapy with acyclovir and ganciclovir, was treated with foscarnet, an experimental drug at the time. The lesions did not improve after two weeks of treatment. Dr. Farsi then speculated that patients often will have noninfected aphthous ulcers of the mouth and esophagus—why not of anus and rectum? He suggested that maybe a trial of thalidomide would be in order. Thus, faced with a puzzling and painful aspect of AIDS, Dr. Farsi improvises, basing his approach on an extension of a previously developed innovation.

At Northlake, innovation was vital to daily practice. The paradoxical use of steroids to treat a variety of AIDS-related problems was one such creative approach. During inpatient rounds one day, we noticed that three of the patients were on prednisone, a steroid, leading Dr. Westin to comment, "I think maybe patients are suffering from prednisone deficiency." AIDS in this way is constructed as prednisone deficiency or thalidomide deficiency or AZT deficiency: AIDS is lack of appropriate treatment.

Another Northlake innovation was the use of an antibiotic, erythromycin, to treat delayed stomach emptying and subsequent persistent vomiting. This condition, known as *gastroparesis*, is seen in long-standing diabetics with neural complications and was diagnosed in several Northlake patients with neurologic symptoms.[11] The antibiotic often causes diarrhea due to faster gastrointestinal mobility when used normally, so Northlake clinicians theorized that it might counter the slow gastric mobility in their patients. A published report on its use in diabetics was cited to support the novel application of an old drug. Still another innovation involved an antiinflammatory drug used in arthritis. Dr. Westin theorized since that the drug inhibits a chemical in the body that can also speed up intestinal mobility as well as cause pain and swelling, the same drug might be useful in treating a patient's diarrhea. The drug was improvised for use in one patient initially, then spread as an innovative response in treating several other patients. In all these cases of innovation, doctors are constructing how AIDS acts on the body and acting on those constructions.

Innovation and improvisation seem to be a common denominator for those involved in AIDS medicine, more so than for other diseases. As one San Francisco informant astutely describes:

People are much more willing with AIDS to invent a therapy and just give it than I think characterizes other diseases. . . . But certainly in heart disease, say, I know that we didn't just do things—make up combinations of therapy without clinical trials telling us to do it.

The informant then gave the use of combination antivirals as an example, noting that this was illegal outside of clinical trials.[12]

The only other point I was going to make about combinations is that in fact there is no legal way to proscribe combinations now. So 60 percent of high AIDS treaters who are doing this are not only willing to invent therapies involving modestly toxic agents that we don't have a huge amount of experience with, but they're willing to somewhat misrepresent what they are doing to the people who are providing the drugs.

It is this reliance on innovation and improvisation on the part of many AIDS clinicians that distinguishes AIDS from other diseases, and AIDS medicine from other medicines.

Thus, at the same time that medical discourse and practice are striving to build a uniform, standardized AIDS, my informants recognize and rely on off-the-cuff constructions of the same disease to order their experience. The improvised nature of AIDS medicine emerges through discourse, as in the following Northlake examples from rounds:

> *Nurse*: If he can't tolerate that [amount], then we'll just have to get creative.
> *Dr. Westin*: That's what it's all about. Improvise. We make it up as we go along.

In another instance, Dr. Westin, Dr. Peters, and a resident are discussing a patient's PCP treatment. Dr. Westin cites a study about dosing, then comments to the resident: "We're making this up [as we go along]. It's the Dr. Peters plan. It's a well-tolerated dose, it just costs a fortune. But hey, we're a high-powered medical center [laughs]."

These examples are very similar to the comments of physicians in Koenig's (1988) article regarding the experimental phase of a new technology: "Dr. Parker kept repeating throughout that he didn't know what he was doing" (474). I heard the same phrase often at Northlake, particularly when the clinicians were at a loss regarding an increasingly sick patient. Unlike the case of Koenig's experimental technology, AIDS treatment is an ongoing experimental process. It is not limited to one room or one piece of equipment but is virtually everywhere: in the clinic exam rooms, in the clinic office, in the X-ray room, on the inpatient floors. The focus of all this improvisation is not a piece of equipment or a procedure but a disease, a nonmaterial construct of discourse and practice. The procedure in Koenig's article eventually becomes routinized, part of ordinary medicine. While medical discourse on AIDS and its treatment strives for this, and achieves it to a limited extent, there is a sense among both the medical community and the lay public that we will never "know what we are doing." One French researcher compared the development of AIDS treatment to that of organ transplants:

So, in transplantation, kidney transplantation, heart transplantation, a lot of progress has been made without any progress in the immunology of transplantation. When transplantation began forty years ago, the immunologists said, "It won't work because from what we know it cannot work." And in 1990, a lot of people are living with their transplants, and ask a transplant immunologist and he will tell you, "I don't know why."

NOTES

1. Bone marrow is the site of blood cell generation, including cells of the immune system. Bone marrow transplants are thus an immunological, rather than antiviral, approach to AIDS.
2. Dr. Bernard also postulated an immunological etiology for Kaposi's sarcoma. At a staff meeting, he remarked that several patients had developed KS lesions on sites of prior trauma on their body: A patient who had had vein stripping on the legs got lesions on the legs; a patient who had had lung damage as a result of inhaling a drug developed pulmonary lesions. He concluded, "I think that stimulation of the immune system has a role in the development of KS." Dr. Bernard's model of KS thus fits in well with the French *terrain* based construction of disease.
3. Obviously, a "viral discourse" exists in France as well, but it is not as common. When HIV-asymptomatic patients at Rousseau became ill with symptoms such as fatigue or a stuffy nose, doctors were more likely to attribute their symptoms to sheer lack of rest or sinusitis than to the "viral syndromes" commonly diagnosed in the United States.
4. A similar panel was convened in 1993 to update these recommendations, and citing the Concorde study, the panel again recommended initiating AZT at CD4 counts of less than 200, rapid drop of CD4 counts below 500, or with signs/symptoms related to immunodeficiency (Mayaud 1993b).
5. The American focus again is on the action of the virus and the benefits of swift intervention: Early treatment is more effective and provokes less resistance because there is less virus.
6. Buyer's clubs, in which subscribers can gain access to large quantities of prescription and certain experimental medications, have become popular among the HIV/AIDS community. This allows people to decide to attempt various treatments without enrolling in trials or waiting for Food and Drug Administration approval.
7. The use of drugs developed to stimulate appetite in cancer patients, such as Megace, at Northlake (and not Rousseau) supports this, though this may vary regionally between the Midwest and the West Coast as well.
8. Another point of note on the national level was a difference in antibiotics used to treat the "non-AIDS" infections. French physicians used a variety of antibiotics I had never encountered in the United States, such as fusidic acid and josamycin. In contrast, the cephalosporin class of

antibiotics, a mainstay of American physicians, was almost never used. When I mentioned this to my Rousseau informants, I was given a variety of explanations including cost, less stringent clinical trials for new drugs, and protectionism toward French drug companies such that hospital pharmacies will tend to stock French antibiotics over others. I suspect all of these explanations are valid—cephalosporins are both American and costly—combined with, perhaps, a historically based penchant in French biomedicine for pharmaceutical research in the area of bacterial infections.

9. This and the previous excerpt are from American physicians, marked by the use of *aggressive*.

10. More recently, a US research team has been studying the inhibitory effects of Thalidomide on tumor necrosis factor and HIV (Makonkawkeyoon et al. 1993).

11. Similar to many of the other Northlake "HIV-opathies," I never heard this diagnosis discussed at Rousseau.

12. Combination antiretroviral therapy, such as with AZT and DDC, has since been approved for use under limited conditions.

7

Paradoxes and Patients' Stories

> The second point is that as a disease of the immune system—not merely as a disease, as an infection of the very cells which the body uses to defend itself from infection, it is the ultimate scientific paradox. It really is to me one of the most intellectually challenging subjects that I can think of. It's the ultimate Trojan Horse.
>
> Washington, D.C. clinician/researcher

THE AMBIGUITY OF AIDS

Why does AIDS fascinate us, after more than a decade? For my informants, American and French, AIDS is still a new disease, suffused with mystery and challenge.

I'm sort of a person that likes to be intellectually challenged. . . . So, starting right out in the beginning, and being a pioneer in understanding a new disease, has been incredibly challenging, very exciting, very frustrating, very sad.

Personally, sometimes I feel like I'm on an adventure. We have discovered a new disease. . . . The etiology of the disease has come very quickly. In the history of medicine, no one has an opportunity like that.

For those informants who have been involved with AIDS since early in the epidemic, AIDS was initially defined by this sense of discovery, of touching the unknown, an experience unlike any of their previous encounters with disease.[1]

It was very interesting initially to be sort of standing right there. And in fact, to be able yourself and with your twenty-six-year-old peers to say this is obviously a new disease, not have to be told by somebody else.

The thing that was the most interesting was the amazing array of diseases, and the fact that during the first part of the epidemic, every time we walked into a patient's room, we learned about a new disease. Everything we saw was new.

For many of the clinician informants, especially the Americans, AIDS is the ultimate challenge—multidisciplinary, ever-changing.

With HIV, there are so many things going on—the patient, the virology, the evolving epidemiology—I mean, there are so many things going on at once with this disease that it really just sort of keeps you interested. You cannot blink your eyes without missing something actually fairly important.

For the researchers, HIV is the ultimate puzzle, marvelous and mysterious. As one US researcher explained, "It is, I think, probably next to the living cell, probably the most marvelous critter around."

I would argue that AIDS retains its newness, its challenge, its power and danger, from the ambiguity inherent in the medical experience of AIDS. As we have seen, AIDS is extremely difficult to categorize because it can affect every organ system in the body, crossing the boundaries of several scientific and clinical disciplines including virology, immunology, infectious disease, and oncology.

At that time, I knew I wanted to get involved with what emerged as the AIDS story. The trouble is that at that time there wasn't really a clear-cut delineation of where this particular thing ought to be studied. Was it cancer? Was it epidemiology? Was it immunology? What was it?"

It [AIDS] is a compelling thing to work on, mostly because it's an extremely important public health problem, and also because it is new. It requires a variety of different approaches to deal with it. In other words, there is one aspect of the problem, its molecular biology and basic science, to understand the pathogenesis to develop therapies and a vaccine. Another part is to continue to try to understand the individual and population factors that contribute to transmission and spread, survival, epidemiology. The third is the whole public health prevention and control efforts, which span health education, health promotion techniques. . . . And so it has multidisciplinary interests and hence it's an interesting problem that's also very important.

AIDS not only crosses disciplines; it crosses disease boundaries; AIDS is like and yet unlike every other disease. As described earlier, my informants construct a disease that is analogous with syphilis, TB, and cancer and yet is paradoxical with each in some fundamental way. Thus, medical discourse on both sides of the Atlantic strives, on the one hand, to create an AIDS that is just like any other disease caused by a virus that is just like any other virus. As one informant stressed, "AIDS is a virus which really doesn't break the rule of infectious diseases." Yet, on the other hand, medical discourse also constructs an AIDS that is unique, both in its cause and manifestations.

The virus is interesting because it is so complex and appears to be tricky and unique in many of its ways of intervening with cell function and postimmune function. . . . From a disease point of view, and from being an infectious disease specialist, obviously the infections we have seen have been different and unique and unusual.

The nature of AIDS that emerges out of the medical discourse is inherently ambiguous, even paradoxical. Unlike cancer and most chronic conditions, AIDS is also an infectious disease, breaking the medical model of an infectious disease as an acute, usually curable condition. Neither a cancer nor an infectious disease, but containing elements of both, AIDS is thus conceptually more powerful, more dangerous. Like the abominations of Leviticus discussed by Mary Douglas (1966), "There is no order in them" (56). This might account for some of the historical reluctance of established clinicians and researchers to become involved with AIDS, and for the relatively young and eclectic mix of specialists presently working with the disease.[2]

The ambiguous nature of AIDS emerges through the daily life of the clinic, as we saw in the necessary innovation and improvisation used in diagnosis/treatment. Treatments for AIDS, like the disease itself, often fall outside the boundaries of standard medical practice. During inpatient rounds at Northlake, Dr. Westin decided to send a patient home despite his continued unexplained fever. Dr. Westin shook his head and commented, "I used to be bothered by sending these patients home with an unidentified source of fever, but now it's the norm." What goes against all standard medical practice becomes routine in AIDS.

The concept of AIDS medicine being different from regular medicine in turn gets passed on to residents in their encounters with clinic doctors and patients. For example, after seeing another inpatient with puzzling fever and respiratory symptoms, a Northlake resident commented: "We're getting a bunch of patients that we don't know what's going on, all these weird pulmonary things." Dr. Westin responded, "This is normal for us." The resident added, "It's very frustrating. I remember when I was a junior medical student, I used to be so mad when I would draw all these cultures and they would come back negative. Finally, I realized that this was normal." The resident here is using discourse to incorporate AIDS into normal medical experience. What is "weird" in standard medicine is normal in AIDS, to the point that AIDS medicine becomes an inversion of "regular" medicine.

While at work in the clinic, I would be called upon to diagnose patients, just as I would during any of my medical school rotations. As I had been taught, I would list the differential diagnoses, that is, the various possible disease explanations for the patient's problems. After about two months at the Paris clinic, I realized that most of the diagnoses I was listing were not likely to be appropriate explanations in the context of AIDS, though they would be acceptable in almost any other medical milieu. There is a common medical dictum in the United States, often used as a moral to some clinical narrative: "If you hear hoofbeats, think horses, not zebras." With AIDS, the reverse is the case. It is always PCP and never common bacterial pneumonia that we think about when we encounter a patient's symptoms. In the medicine of AIDS, one must think of zebras because they are more common than horses. It is a world turned upside down, and perhaps that is why many doctors still avoid treating AIDS patients—not for fear of contagion but for fear of zebras.

In many cultural contexts, inversions express power and danger and are often part of rites of passage. Turner (1969), for example, discusses the installation of a new chief among the Ndembu, which involves the incoming chief performing menial tasks. Brazilian Carnaval also involves inversion, people dressing and behaving opposite to their usual social roles, and, as DaMatta (1984) states, it is "an extraordinary moment" where the ideal is "that everyone can do everything" (234). Both of these examples are bounded by time. The installation of the chief and Carnaval have definitive beginnings and endings, constraining their power to a particular time and place. AIDS, however, is always inverted, always ambiguous, though medical discourse may sometimes strive to contain it through standardization. Thus, AIDS is medically dangerous, not merely through the possibility of contagion and death but to the entire order of the medical world.

A humorous example concerns a sign I noticed posted on a P2 laboratory door in Paris. A P2 lab is one in which whole virus is utilized, and special precautions, including double doors, gloves, mask, and a change of lab coats, are required. The sign read: "Controlled entry—katana, nunchaku, shuriken, kimono, gloves, mask obligatory." The martial arts additions to the notice had been made by a doctoral student interested in karate. AIDS here is constructed as a highly dangerous opponent, to be fought with all the weapons and regalia essential to combat.[3]

The ways of AIDS are mysterious, even magical. When describing the case of a patient who had stopped taking AZT, a Rousseau clinician began, "His T4 count went up, due to electromagnetism or something." At Northlake, a resident, Dr. Holtzman, and myself were discussing the common increase of eosinophils, a type of white cell, in AIDS patients:

> *Dr. Holtzman*: We don't know if that's due to occult parasites or whatever.
> *Jamie*: I read a study saying that it doesn't appear to have any consistent cause they could find.
> *Dr. Holtzman*: It must be *Fahrfurgnugen* [the German word used in advertising the experience of driving a Volkswagen].

The sheer strangeness of AIDS rattles the foundations of French and American biomedicine, as seen in these comments by two respective clinicians.

My medical practice has changed because I find that when you're working with AIDS patients, you are always on the defensive. You're never sure that things are going well. The slightest fever, the slightest diarrhea, the slightest problem, you always think that you've got something new coming up—a new opportunistic infection, or things like that. So you don't feel safe with things. The second thing is that you always have to think in a multietiological basis, and that goes against our basic medical training. You always think about different germs, about different etiologies.

The law of economy of diagnosis is completely confounded by the advent of HIV. One unifying diagnosis is not something you usually find with HIV. Often time there are many.

AIDS thus not only defies the usual nature of infectious and chronic diseases, but it also defies a basic dictum of medicine. As the first (French) clinician stated, "You never feel safe."

At Northlake, discussion of a patient's rapid decline sparked the following interchange between three of the clinic doctors.

> *Dr. Westin*: I don't understand this disease. Some people come in looking horrible, and the next day they're doing fine. Other people come in, and the next day they're dead. We pat ourselves on the back when people get out of the hospital, but I'm not sure that we're really doing anything.
>
> *Dr. Landry*: The nice ones die and the nasty ones you can't get rid of.
>
> *Dr. Westin*: Look at Bob Smith [patient who died recently]. He just went down the tubes.
>
> *Dr. Landry*: It's just when their natural resilience wears out.
>
> *Dr. Norman*: There are people with T cells in the single digits who do fine for two, three years.
>
> *Dr. Landry*: There are inscrutable factors here impossible to assay. [*Mild laughter by the group*]

The frustration of these doctors is palpable, for, trained in the world of regular medicine, they now practice in a world of ambiguity, paradox, and death, regulated by "inscrutable factors." That they do this out of choice testifies to their own distinctiveness. As we shall see in the next chapter, it is part of what makes them "AIDS doctors."

The uncertainty and ambiguity that is AIDS provides fertile ground for the proliferation of multiple voices, among the lay public and even within the medical community itself.

I think the most difficult [concept] is the one that is an inherent paradox, which is it's hard to get HIV, but it's easy to get HIV. It's not easily communicable and yet people get it very easily, and everybody's at risk. That is, for the layperson, such an inherent paradox, that it's almost always set up as a contradictory point of view. And you end up with a lot of professionals taking sides on that one.

Given the incredible variety of discourse about AIDS, some of it vicious, much of it confusing, it is not surprising that the discourse of medicine is consciously directed at providing an effective structure for the AIDS experience, particularly on the issue of transmission.

Many of my informants encounter lay discourse on AIDS on a regular basis, not only from patients but from friends, government officials, and media representatives. These clinicians and researchers have had, to some extent, the role of "AIDS educator" thrust upon them and, as such, are sensitive to lay narratives that directly challenge the authoritative narrative of the medical community.

They [the French general public] talk about AIDS, but not well. The press is very badly informed. The people don't know anything. People who came to give blood had strange ideas about transmission; every day I hear that one can get AIDS from the needle, from the blood bag.

The preceding narrative constructs the lay public as afraid, confused, and uninformed. It also comments on the existence of unauthorized stories, which illustrate and are, to the medical professional, responsible for this public confusion.[4] From the perspective of my informants, these stories create fear and yet flourish in spite of education campaigns. Bernard Paillard, a sociologist studying these stories, recounted one narrative about young men running through the Paris Métro, pricking women with contaminated needles and giving them AIDS (personal communication, 1987). As discussed previously, the French medical community felt the same need in 1990 as in 1987 to construct a unified discourse on transmission to present to the lay public. Elsford (1987) observes that anxiety among a group of medical students over transmission via drinking glasses and cutlery never disappeared, despite intensive AIDS education.

Why do these unauthorized stories persist? Many of my informants, as in the above example, blame the press for inaccurate and sensationalized reporting on AIDS. The heart of the matter lies deeper, however. There is no story that remains uncontested; that is the nature of dialogue. Discourse on AIDS, I have found, is inherently dramatic, incomplete, and uncertain because it attempts to make coherent a terrifying and equally uncertain experience. The burden of this work has, to a large extent, fallen on the medical community. Physicians and researchers, French and American, utilize a variety of powerful discursive tools in their search to make sense of AIDS, to write the authoritative story. AIDS is cancer, AIDS is HIV, which is HBV, only different. AIDS is homosexuals, drug-users and Africans, toxoplasmosis, Kaposi's, and wasting. AIDS is a puzzle, an opportunity, an adventure. Their efforts to generate a uniform discourse are not directly aimed at suppressing alternate voices but at building an AIDS that is knowable, as free from uncertainty as humanly possible. Because ambiguity can never be eliminated, particularly from a phenomenon as anomalous as AIDS, alternate stories continue to flourish and compete with the dominant medical narrative.

Though their work and their language are grounded in science, my informants often used non medical metaphors to give meaning to AIDS. One French physician compared it to a stock market crash. Other analogies were blunt, even brutal: "AIDS is Berlin in 1945—destroyed, leveled, bombed out with almost nothing alive." Yet in the midst of the harsh experience that is AIDS, there is also poetry. When I asked one French informant, a general practitioner, "What is AIDS?" his answer encapsulated the sorrow of this disease.

What is AIDS? It's a very bad image, maybe, but it's something. You know, when you were a little boy, you make a castle in the sand on the beach. And with the tides, the water is going up. If you make castle so the waves are going up, once a wave will destroy a bit of your castle, so you make it again. And then again, and then there is a big wave and everything is vanished.

PATIENT VERSUS PHYSICIAN MODELS

> AIDS is *une source de merdement*. I think the patient will describe it as,
> "Doctor, you can say it's a source of diagnosis." Fantastic. For the patient,
> I think it's a source of problems.
>
> Resident at Rousseau

> I don't want any medical people touching me, only people that have read
> James Joyce.
>
> Patient at Rousseau

Though the focus of this study is on the medical community, it is impossible to talk about medical discourse without talking about patient discourse. The two impact each other on a daily basis in the clinic, and at times can be so interwoven that one may hardly distinguish them. Clinicians must at least minimally hear the patient's story in order to create their own, while patients must integrate something of the doctor's story into their own illness narrative in order for the medical encounter to be meaningful. Yet the two discourses are fundamentally and irreconcilably different, even when patients and their doctors are of the same class, gender, age, ethnicity, and sexual orientation, as indicated in studies by Gullick (1985) and Cassell (1976). Kathryn Hunter (1991), in her work on the narrative structure of biomedicine, concludes, "Physicians and patients, by virtue of their roles in the illness encounter, are always engaged in the narrative construction of different realities, telling different stories about what is nominally the same malady. This is the irreducible substrate of communication in medicine" (140).

At the same time, patients' stories are not identical with other lay narratives, due to three important factors. First, patients, unlike the rest of the lay public, actually experience the illness. Second, as part of their illness, patients often encounter other patients and share their stories, a phenomenon I observed at both clinics and often commented on by the physicians. Finally, patients encounter medical discourse on a more personal, frequent, and regular basis than do the rest of the lay public. All of these factors are exemplified, even exaggerated in AIDS, so that the patient's discourse is at the same time like and unlike that of the physician.

At both the Rousseau and Northlake clinics, there was little conflict between doctors and patients over HIV as the basic cause of AIDS, though there would be occasional discussion over cofactors. A more usual narrative contest between doctor and patient occurred over the nature of AIDS as a chronic, treatable disease versus a more rapid, fatal one. I witnessed one such contest at Rousseau, between Dr. Farsi and an American patient. Dr. Farsi began by lecturing the patient about his tendency to travel on business and vacation every other week, such as a newly planned visit to Australia. The doctor argued that this made it difficult to keep track of his care, including chemotherapy for KS. Dr. Farsi then added that it would be different if he were going to the United States to enroll in a therapeutic trial, because there would be a doctor who would have a copy of his charts and could follow his care. The patient then raised the point of vacation and travel being good for his emotional health. Dr. Farsi countered with the concept of priorities and that someone with his level of KS needs consistent treatment and follow-up, adding that if he is going to Australia because "you think you might never get to see it otherwise, well that is something understandable." "But," he concluded, "the kangaroos can wait."

In the above encounter, the physician is constructing a model of AIDS as a treatable chronic illness that requires constant monitoring, rather than an imminently fatal disease—"the kangaroos can wait." The lecture seems similar to those given diabetics who refuse to eat meals at consistent times or who do not check their blood sugars regularly. In both cases, the patient is not behaving acceptably as a chronically ill person. By contrast, the patient is constructing AIDS here as a fatal illness in which the jaunt to Australia is more therapeutic than medical intervention. Dr. Farsi displays some understanding that the patient may still see himself as "dying." As Dr. Bernard commented during one staff meeting, "The problem with AIDS today is that people think there are no treatments because we haven't got a cure." The ambiguous nature of AIDS feeds the narrative contest between the emerging authoritative medical discourse of a chronic, treatable disease and an alternative lay narrative of an incurable, fatal disease.

This doctor-patient difference over the nature of AIDS also emerges through the use of different disease analogies. In a Northlake encounter between Dr. Westin and a new patient, the patient commented that she had thought she only had a year or so until she got AIDS. Dr. Westin explained that he wanted to recheck her CD4 count to decide about using AZT, but if she needed it, it will prolong her life and decrease her chance of infections. The patient responded, "You know, we've been treating cancer for forty years and people still die." Dr. Westin countered, "I think of it like diabetes. Sixty years ago, people died after a year or so, and now they live a long time with treatment." The patient here again constructs HIV infection as a more or less rapidly fatal condition and utilizes a cancer analogy. The clinician, on the other hand, models AIDS to himself and his patient as a chronic, treatable disease, using diabetes as the reference point.

In committing themselves to continuous and sometimes unpleasant treatment, patients are at least partially incorporating the medical narrative into their own model of AIDS. A few refuse to medicalize their condition, as I discovered during one patient's visit at Northlake. The patient's CD4 count had dropped below 500 at the last check. With the patient present, Dr. Westin explained mildly, "He doesn't take AZT, even though it's clearly indicated." Dr. Westin again broached the subject of taking AZT, and the patient replied that he might talk about it sometime but probably would never take it, and the same of prophylaxis against PCP. The patient then asked to repeat the CD4 count, not to start any therapy but to decide if he wanted to move up his October vacation. He remarked to me, "People say, 'You have AIDS? What do you take?' I say, 'Vacations.'" Dr. Westin, while he does not agree with his patient's approach, respects the patient's wishes readily. He admits that the patient is doing well with his strategy and seems to bring up AZT only to let the patient know that the topic is open for discussion at any time.

Like the American patient at Rousseau, this Northlake patient's narrative presents patient decisions concerning emotional well-being as being equally or more important than medical intervention, a discourse that I noticed less among French patients, who give over more control of their care to the physician. This encounter also focuses attention on CD4 counts and AZT as important markers, but with different meanings for physicians and patients.

As we have seen in clinicians' discourse, CD4 counts are extremely important in gauging the progression of disease. To the physician, not all CD4 counts are equally significant, with 500 marking the start of AZT for Americans, 200 marking AZT for the French and PCP prophylaxis for both, and under 100 as indicating poor prognosis and less need to do further counts. For patients, all CD4 counts appear to be equally significant. To the amusement and frustration of Rousseau and Northlake doctors, patients frequently ask for repeated counts, rejoicing at any increase and despairing at any decrease, no matter how small. Stories about this phenomenon were common at Rousseau staff meetings, as in the following example: "I have a patient who is very happy now. His T4 went from three to thirteen—a fourfold increase!" The irony is evident in constructing the difference between what is meaningful for doctors and what is meaningful for patients.

The Rousseau clinicians also discuss strategies for handling this dissonance. One doctor tells a story of an encounter with a patient: "I said, 'You have three T4. He said, '300?' 'No, three.' And he started to cry." A resident added that you have to hide these things. The doctor replied, "I say, 'It [the CD4 count] is 'stable.' Perhaps it's stable at six, but. . . " The strategy is to switch the focus of the discourse from the number to the stability over time. This technique is also seen at Northlake, again more common in talking with patients with low CD4 counts. In meeting with one such patient, Dr. Landry summed up by saying the patient is doing well. The patient replied, "Well, as long as the count remains stable." Landry then contributed, "Don't focus on the T cell count. T cell counts are ballpark figures which we use to initiate therapy and later to judge the response. For you now, T cells counts aren't really appropriate for looking at how you're doing."

The initiation of AZT therapy is a significant marker for clinicians and patients, though its meaning is fraught with ambivalence among both groups. Historically, it has defined the patient as now being "sick," as opposed to a "healthy carrier," since in the past AZT was begun only when the patient was quite ill. Now AZT is begun when the patient feels perfectly well, and incongruity between the medical disease and the patient illness emerges in force. As one Rousseau clinician explained:

Maybe in 1986, '87, in the mind of the patient and also the mind of the doctors, there was a difference in the border between sick people who had treatment and people not yet sick who had no treatment. Now, we say that we don't wait for the period of sickness to give treatment, and we know when we saw people that it's necessary. . . . People who approach the period where they could be sick should have a treatment. In the relationship with the patient, it's sometimes difficult to explain to people that they must take it, even though they are in good physical form, they don't feel any symptoms, they have no fever, no diarrhea, they have no weakness, and accept the idea to take pills every day.

For the physicians, the person taking AZT is now someone who "could be sick," while for the patient, the taking of the pills constructs them as someone who *is* sick. At the same time, the beginning of AZT therapy marks the first time that the doctor and patient can "do something" against the disease, rather than simply to sit back and monitor the situation. This meaning seems especially prevalent among San Francisco patients, and to a lesser extent their clinicians, since my San Francisco informants report their patients as taking AZT and combination therapy at higher and higher CD4 levels. One Rousseau informant presented this interpretation as having been more common when AZT was first available, but not anymore:

In '87, every patient spoke about "when will I take AZT?". . . In retrospect, it's not the same discourse. Now when you speak with a patient and you propose AZT, it's not the sign of hope, because the disease is more advanced. Three years ago, when you proposed it, it was at least a drug for the problem. Now, it's completely different. Now it is DDI. . . the DDI takes the place of AZT for three years, but we know now that a patient knows too that DDI will not resolve the problems. This is an important thing. When we spoke about AZT three years ago, it's not the same message.

Over time, the meaning of AZT has changed for both patients and physicians. Once a symbol of hope, now it is for patients a daily reminder of their sickness. As one Northlake patient explained to Dr. Westin, she has gone through a grieving process at three times: when she was first diagnosed as being HIV-positive, when she began taking AZT, and when she had her first opportunistic infection indicating full-blown AIDS. This is an example of a patient staging system, informed by, but not identical to, that of the clinicians. An encounter between a Rousseau resident and a patient again illustrates this distinction. The resident told the patient he has a mild oral candidiasis infection. The patient responded, "This doesn't have anything to do with the HIV?" The resident answers, "But, yes. It is the same stage as the lymph nodes [lymphadenopathy]. It is not an opportunistic infection, no." For this patient, illness associated with HIV means AIDS. In other words, he is constructing a system similar to that of clinicians earlier in the epidemic: If you're symptomatic, you're sick, while if you have no symptoms, you are a "healthy carrier." The resident is utilizing the more recent view of HIV as a continuum of disease. No one is ever "not sick"; one is simply more or less suffering effects of the disease. The two constructs of AIDS are quite different and serve their respective speakers better than they serve their intended audience. That is, the continuum of disease narrative tends to support constant medical intervention in AIDS, while the sick/not sick construct of the patient gives authority to the doctor only when the person is experiencing illness.

As is the case with high blood pressure (Kleinman 1988), this particular dissonance between medical and patient narratives generates issues of *compliance*—the biomedical term for patients not carrying out the medically prescribed therapy. Both Northlake and Rousseau doctors talked of patients who altered the dosage or stopped taking medications altogether, usually sparked when the patient had become increasingly sick and expressing a sense of frustration on the part of the physician. However, as was the case of the Northlake patient who refused AZT, my clinician informants also told "noncompliance" stories in which the patient is respected or even admired for outsmarting them.

During one inpatient rounds at Northlake, we visited a patient who has had CDC-defined AIDS since 1982, an almost unheard of survival time. Dr. O'Neill then told the story of how the patient was initially diagnosed with *Pneumocystis*, survived, and then would not come in for follow-up:

We all thought he would die. This was the time when people weren't living six months. . . . He survived AZT [the initial high dose trials] and decided not to take it, saying, "You guys don't know shit." And he was right. He lived in spite of us.

This story serves to remind the clinicians about the unpredictability of AIDS, as well as constructing a moral of "When you don't know shit," the patient may well know more than you.

The clinicians' staging system is a way of ordering their experience of the disease, of constructing a medical model of AIDS and a model for treating it. The patient's staging system, too, is a way of ordering experience, but it is the experience of the illness. The meanings developed in the clinician's staging system may not hold much value for the patient. Another inpatient encounter at Northlake illustrates this point. In the clinic office, Dr. Peters described to me his visit with an inpatient who had recently been diagnosed with his first opportunistic infection. The patient then explained that his fevers are not from infection but are caused by AZT clogging his pores so the body heat cannot get out, making him unable to regulate his temperature. He also added that his fever spikes are due to too many blankets. Dr. Peters replied to the patient, "Sir, you're not a reptile," explaining that humans do not need to rely on ambient temperature to regulate body heat.

This is an excellent example of a narrative told by one doctor, Peters, to another, myself, in order to illustrate "wrong" lay interpretations, as well as showing negotiation between doctor and patient about how the human body works. There is a collision here between the authoritative narrative of the patient's sickness—an opportunistic infection—and the alternative narrative of AZT clogging the pores. The patient has great stake in not having infection because then, in the alternative model, he wouldn't have "AIDS." In the alternative narrative, AIDS is something distinct from being seropositive or ARC, while in the new medical narrative, they are all basically a spectrum of the same disease—everyone is sick. The clinician, on the other hand, has a great stake in staging the patient appropriate to his system, because to accept the patient's narrative is to disrupt the medical meaning of AIDS. It would leave the physician unable to act as a physician and perhaps open the way for professional and legal recriminations. Alternative narratives are not simply a threat to medical power but a threat to the meaning of the medical experience.

At Northlake, the discordance between the two staging systems often emerged through the common use of the term *ARC* by patients. As noted previously, *ARC* was rarely used by clinicians as of 1990 but had been an important component of earlier medical models of AIDS. The term and some of its meanings seem to have been integrated into patient constructions, persisting in the face of a different medical terminology. A new Northlake patient exclaimed, "What do I tell my family? I can't tell them I have AIDS." Dr. Westin replied, "You don't have AIDS." After the physical exam, the patient asked, "Am I ARC or AIDS or what?" Dr. Westin answered:

You're at the stage that used to be called ARC. We don't use that term any more because it's vague, really meaningless. There's no real term for the stage you're in, other than saying you're HIV-positive and that you're having some symptoms related to that. You don't have AIDS. That stage requires some additional symptoms, like unusual infections or those spots on the skin.

The patient here is concerned with what to tell her family, and ARC perhaps presents an acceptable alternative to AIDS. Additionally, ARC gives a name to the patient's condition, which, in the clinician's responding discourse, remains ambiguous.

As is the case with transmission, my clinician informants try to present a unified discourse to counter the persistence of "misinformed" lay narratives, seen in the following two encounters about ARC.

Patient: Would you say I have ARC?
Dr. Westin: We don't use that term anymore because it's kind of nebulous. There's AIDS, which you definitely don't have, symptomatic HIV infection, which you don't seem to have and asymptomatic HIV, which is where I think you are.

Patient: I was told by somebody I didn't even have AIDS— I had 'AIDS-related complex,' which sounds a lot better. I don't even feel sick.
Dr. Peters: It's a matter of semantics. I think if you don't feel sick, you don't have to think of yourself that way. You have a disease that we can help treat.

Northlake clinicians find the persistent use of *ARC* by severely ill patients especially ironic, a situation in which the discrepancy between the medical interpretation and the patient's interpretation is the greatest. For example, during inpatient rounds, Dr. Westin, Dr. Holtzman, and the social worker were discussing a particular patient. Dr. Westin commented, "Last week he looked like he was going to die, so we pulled back on the treatments. And now he's looking so much better. So much for our therapies." A little later, the social worker brought up the home situation: "He never uses the word *AIDS*. He tells everyone that he has ARC." Dr. Westin shot back, "Yeah, full-blown ARC."

As noted before, ARC is not a significant element in either clinician or patient discourse at Rousseau. Yet there is still an interpretive gulf between French patients and physicians, most often concerning the meanings of patient's symptoms. Recall that for physicians AIDS is an inversion of the usual medical dictum of diagnosing the common before the exotic. The ambiguous nature of AIDS leads to a problem for clinicians in distinguishing what is important from what is trivial; thus, nearly everything becomes related to HIV infection. As Dr. Farsi commented during one staff discussion, "It's very difficult to tell the difference between the little problems that everyone gets and the big problems. We often panic." For the clinician, not diagnosing and treating an opportunistic infection early enough means a more seriously ill or even dying patient. For the patient, diagnosing an opportunistic infection means a more medicalized life, repeated unpleasant tests, and a redefinition of self as a person sick with AIDS rather than "like everyone else."

This conflict in meaning was illustrated during one of the few encounters with an inpatient at Rousseau. A clinic patient had been admitted for fever and shortness of breath but was refusing bronchoscopy, the standard diagnostic test for *Pneumocystis*. The test itself is invasive and unpleasant, since it involves inserting a tube through the mouth into the air passages in the lung. I went with a clinic resident to talk with the patient. He first spoke about a previous bad experience with the test, then added that his cough is just a cold, a normal bronchitis. He commented, "Why is it that whenever I get a cough, everybody panics? Why is it that because I have AIDS, I can't have a cold like everyone else?" The resident responded:

It's true you can have a cold like everyone, but your immunity is not like everybody's. You have had a fever that we can't explain. When you are in the hospital and we can't find anything, we have to decide what to do. What if you go home now and have a fever tomorrow?

I witnessed similar conflicts at Northlake. Negotiation between doctor and patient usually bridges the gap, though never erases it. In the above case, the patient eventually agreed to the test as long as he received an antianxiety drug beforehand.

In conclusion, patients' and physicians' constructions of AIDS may be quite different, and negotiation between the two is a significant part of daily life at the clinic. Clinician informants would approach this dissonance, as in the case of *ARC*, by presenting a relatively uniform medical narrative to the patient and entering into negotiation when needed to proceed with an action. Patient discourse on AIDS appears marked by its close encounters with medical discourse, seen in the emphasis on CD4 counts and the use of older medical terminology such as ARC. Though the words themselves may be similar, they have emerged from the patient's discourse with significantly different meanings, meanings that order the experience of patients and sometimes disorder the experience of clinicians. One may wonder how doctors and patients manage to talk meaningfully with each other at all.

Yet with AIDS, the meanings between doctors and patients may overlap considerably, as seen in the example of AZT. In a number of situations, my informants readily acknowledged their lack of certainty to patients, enabling them to share the ambiguity of the AIDS experience. As Sharf (1990) concludes, doctors and patients are coauthors of a negotiated story of disease and illness, and in order to be effective, neither one can have their initial tale unchanged by the encounter. AIDS doctors and AIDS patients are thus an integral part of each other's lives, as near to each other as they are separate from one another. Each encounter is a learning process, part of the evolving doctor-patient relationship.

CONCLUSION

AIDS is not a singular object to be discovered and then described. There is not one AIDS but many AIDS, and they change over time, emerging from medical discourse and practice through a complex process of construction. Physicians and researchers use a variety of discursive techniques to give meaning to AIDS, such as naming and the delineation of boundaries via risk groups, symptoms, and treatments. Analogies with known diseases—hepatitis B, tuberculosis, cancer, diabetes—are another powerful and pervasive tool for constructing the nature of AIDS. They play a role in shaping the natural history of the disease, as well as its staging and treatment. There are differences in these constructions and their associated practices between countries, regions, and institutions, as well as differences between doctors and patients. As we have seen, medical discourse on AIDS is not "simply" a matter of semantics. There would have been no research or treatment for AIDS had it not been constructed as a disease apart from other diseases. Treatment practices both shape and are shaped by constructions of AIDS in a continuous feedback loop. Thus, medical discourse on AIDS can literally be a matter of life and death. Yet such discourse is hardly uniform. It is fluid, situational, multivocal. Evolving narratives of AIDS compete in both oral and written forums as the medical community strives to build a uniform discourse to present to each other, to patients, to the lay public, with the latter groups creating their own narratives in turn.

The proliferation of discourses is fed by the inherent ambiguity of AIDS. No matter how we name, enclose, or analogize, AIDS slips free of its constraints. There is always an element of paradox about any AIDS constructed by medicine. It is like and unlike every other disease, fascinating and frustrating. The very practice of AIDS medicine is an inversion of usual medical practice, with the exotic becoming commonplace. The ambiguity of AIDS, while dangerous, is also powerful. It allows innovation and improvisation to flourish; opens up new ways of speaking about disease, medicine, and the human body; and acknowledges the limitations of medical knowledge. As has been hinted at Part II, medical discourse never only constructs AIDS, but simultaneously produces a host of meanings for other experiences. AIDS is both constructed and constructive, a medium for other discourse and, as such, is the topic of Part III.

NOTES

1. Koenig and Cooke (1989, 76) report a similar response among a group of San Francisco residents treating AIDS patients, particularly early on in the epidemic.

2. Homophobia, the lack of financial remuneration and the stigma attached to AIDS play important roles as well (Zuger 1991).

3. Obversely, science here is constructed, via AIDS, as the provision and correct use of these weapons. One might even conclude that science is the weapon itself.

4. One might also consider the anti-HIV narratives of Duesberg and others to be unauthorized narratives, considered by the rest of the medical community to be even more dangerous because of their professional origin (Fujimura and Chou 1994).

Part III

AIDS AS CONSTRUCTOR

8

AIDS Bodies, AIDS Patients

AIDS has generated a phenomenon which goes so far beyond the actual
scope of clinical illness which it causes—political, social, religious, ethical,
moral—that it's not only changed the shape of medicine, but it's changed
the face of society as well.

Dr. Campbell, Chicago clinician

INTRODUCTION

In the previous part, we saw how AIDS is constructed through medical discourse, yet
in nearly all examples, other constructions were being made simultaneously and
inseparably from those of AIDS: the nature of medical practice, health care systems,
the roles of doctors and patients. AIDS is not unique in this regard, as Brandt (1985)
demonstrates in his historical analysis of venereal disease: "In fact, venereal disease,
as a social construct, provided a means of organizing and explaining many of the
social dilemmas which Progressivism sought to address" (9). AIDS is at the same
time constructed and constructive, and my separation of its two roles in medical
discourse is purely artificial, an analytical convenience for myself and my audience.
As exemplified by Dr. Campbell's statement above, my informants recognize the
constructive power of AIDS, using it as a medium for talking about, and thus
refashioning, a wide variety of medical and social experiences. Some of the objects
of this discourse are intimately linked to AIDS, such as the nature of AIDS patients
and their bodies. Other issues are broader in scope: health care systems, the doctor-
patient relationship, the practice of medicine, the scientific enterprise. Finally, there
is the question of identity—national and professional—in which AIDS serves to
shape self, society, and the interaction between them.

BUILDING THE AIDS BODY

Patients and their bodies are essential elements of the medical community's experience with AIDS and, as such, are often the subject of discourse. Generally, this discourse falls into two categories, those constructing the body of the patient and those constructing the nature of the patient as a person. As often as not, discourse encompasses both categories simultaneously. A theme of medical discourse from the earliest days of the epidemic is, "Who is an AIDS patient?" From the historical context of the epidemic alone, we can see that the answer to this question changes over time and place. In the United States in 1981, it was gay men, while in France in 1982, it was gay men and African immigrants. As one San Francisco physician explained: "Obviously, the association between presenting with AIDS and being gay is breaking down. But for us for years, anybody who presented with an AIDS complication was gay or bisexual."

While the concept of the "Four H's"—heroin addicts, Haitians, homosexuals and hemophiliacs—has fallen into disrepute, it has left its trace on subsequent discourse about patients. It provides a framework for talking about different groups of people who are heavily affected by AIDS using criteria of ethnicity, sexuality, chemical dependency, and economic status.

We're seeing gradually a change in the sort of profile of an AIDS patient. Whereas in the early '80s the stereotypic patient would have been a white gay male, who was probably middle class and lived in a big city. The stereotypic AIDS patient in the '90s is probably going to be a black or hispanic heterosexual man or woman, living in the inner cities, in one way or another tied in with drug use, either IV drug use or crack use.

Changing the patient changes the disease and how clinicians approach it. Among my informants, the possible exception to this lies in male-female distinctions. There was surprisingly little discourse at either clinic distinguishing women patients, either in terms of their female bodies or in terms of their characteristics as patients. I suspect that this may change as a greater percentage of women develop AIDS and enter the daily life of the clinic. However, as Treichler (1987), Patton (1990), and others have observed, medical discourse does construct the bodies of gay men, hemophiliacs, drug users, and various ethnic groups as being different in the context of AIDS.

Even outside of AIDS, physicians distinguish gay male bodies by way of increased incidence of certain infections. This seems to be a transatlantic phenomenon, observed at Rousseau and Northlake. During a Rousseau staff meeting, a discussion of a patient's intractable diarrhea led one clinician to mention the high incidence of certain gastrointestinal infections among gay men. Another doctor commented, "It's a good test for homosexuality." The first doctor agreed: "Yes, if I test for [*Entamoeba*] *histolytica*, and [names two others], I can say he is homosexual." This exchange was light hearted in nature, and no one seemed to intend it as a serious screening test for homosexuality, but it nevertheless distinguishes the gay male body.

I encountered a similar discourse at Northlake. Dr. O'Neill saw a new patient who denied any drug use or sexual activity with other men. The doctor found anal warts, often caused by a sexually transmitted virus, on physical exam and later told me, "So much for not knowing how he got it." In broader terms, physicians will speak of "tests" for sexual activity—pregnancy tests, tests for sexually transmitted diseases such as gonorrhea. With homosexuality, however, physicians often fail to distinguish between the identity and the behavior.

My informants also construct the gay body as having AIDS differently than other bodies. This is usually expressed in terms of the higher incidence of Kaposi's sarcoma and cytomegalovirus among gay patients. During a Rousseau discussion of a possibly sexually transmitted infectious agent for KS, Dr. Bernard noted that in his experience the only female patients who develop KS were infected with HIV through intercourse with a bisexual partner.

My informants' constructions of the gay body as different, susceptible to different ailments in and outside of AIDS, emerges largely out of the daily demands of their clinical practice. If the patient is a gay male, the AIDS clinician will take extra care to look for signs of Kaposi's or manifestations of cytomegalovirus, just as a physician in general practice will watch closely for signs of hypertension in African-American men. The trick, of course, is not to ignore the possibility of Kaposi's in heterosexual people or to incorrectly ascribe the gay patient's diarrhea to infection rather than some other cause. What surprised me is not that my informants distinguished the gay male body as different but how rarely they did so. Rather, the gay body emerged as the norm against which other patients' bodies were measured. At Northlake, the wife of a hemophiliac patient asked if the course of AIDS was different in hemophiliacs, and Dr. Westin replied, "Well, hemophiliacs don't tend to get some of the infections that others like gay men get, such as Kaposi's sarcoma and CMV."

Hemophiliacs are a significant part of the patient population at Northlake, but the hemophiliac body seems defined largely outside of its relation to AIDS. The interaction between hemophiliacs and the medical community has had a long history prior to AIDS, and I suspect that medical discourse about hemophilia and the hemophiliac body will be comparatively less impacted by AIDS. Similarly, my informants generally talked about the intravenous drug user's (IVDU) body in relation to the gay body. One exception is the construction of all IV drug users as being infected with HIV. At one Rousseau journal meeting, a resident presented an article from Spanish researchers looking for prognostic markers of AIDS in drug users and mentioned that study used a control group of drug users that test HIV-negative. Dr. Bernard quipped, "There still are some?" My informants generally distinguish IV drug users in reference not to their bodies but to their behavior as patients, as will be discussed later.

The bodies of AIDS patients are distinguished by ethnicity as well as sexuality. At Northlake, the African-American body in AIDS is distinguished by an increased incidence of kidney problems associated with HIV, "HIV nephropathy." In a presentation on HIV nephropathy, Dr. Westin noted that "the key epidemiological point" is that the condition is more common in African-American patients, citing a high incidence in New York and Miami clinics in contrast to San Francisco, "where patients tend to be white and homosexual."[1] Dr. Westin presented the standard case of severe HIV nephropathy as being "a black patient with heavy dense kidneys on echo [sonogram] who is rapidly progressing." When another physician asked about other factors, such as family history of kidney disease, Dr. Westin replied that a genetic factor may be at work since African-Americans in general have higher rates of kidney disease.

The African-American body that emerges from the discourse of the Northlake doctors is distinguished by one or two different responses to AIDS but is ultimately the same as every other body in terms of its response to treatment. During a presentation on the AIDS Clinical Trials Groups meetings, discussion centered on a recent Veterans Administration (VA) study (Hamilton et al. 1992) comparing the use of AZT early and late in the course of HIV infection among white, African-American, and Hispanic populations. This study was interpreted by my informants as suggesting that African-Americans and Hispanics do not benefit from early AZT treatment, a conclusion with which they strongly disagreed. Dr. O'Neill remarked, "Now everyone knows that being black or Hispanic doesn't change the way a drug works," adding that the outcome in the VA study was a "statistical fluke."

While the discourse at Northlake characterized mainly African-Americans, the talk of Rousseau physicians covered a wider range of ethnicities, though the focus was primarily on Africans. The senior physicians would remind the residents to look for an additional set of unusual infections among African patients, such as leishmaniasis, a parasitic infection transmitted by sandflies. On the other hand, the reminder was often extended to well-traveled European patients, so perhaps this discourse is less a construction of the African body and more a construction of Africa itself. Because of the proximity of Africa and the presence of African immigrant patients, Rousseau clinicians would occasionally discuss the differing definitions of AIDS in Europe and Africa. As Dr. Lefevre reminded the residents, "Except in Africa, diarrhea is not in the definition of AIDS." Africa and African bodies are important enough to Rousseau physicians to be subjects of discourse (unlike the situation at Northlake) yet are constructed as the exception, special cases requiring special knowledge.

Rousseau physicians encounter patients from a wide variety of nationalities, covering all continents except Australia. Americans are the most common foreign patients, and their bodies are distinguished in discourse as well. Like African bodies, American bodies require some measure of special knowledge, particularly regarding tuberculosis, and this knowledge is passed on by senior physicians to residents, as in the following example.

The US doesn't use it [tuberculosis vaccine]. The BCG is very French, French-African. The US has less incidence of TB. If you get an American patient, which isn't too unlikely, or a patient born in the US, you must do the skin test to look for possible exposure to TB.

As often as bodies of AIDS patients are subdivided into various distinct groups—African, American, hemophiliac—they also emerge in discourse as a single entity, made distinct not from each other but from the bodies of non-AIDS patients. As we have seen, this is usually expressed in terms of tolerance for debilitating conditions, such as recurrent severe infections and neutropenia. Often AIDS patients are contrasted with cancer patients, as seen in this remark by Dr. Holtzman to a hospital resident: "AIDS patients tolerate their neutropenia pretty well. With chemo [cancer chemotherapy] patients, they generally have GI ulcers, and that's why we make sure we cover gram negatives [type of bacteria]." Ultimately, daily clinical practice revolves around the interaction between the physician and an individual body. Each patient's body emerges from the discourse as distinctive, requiring special knowledge and special care. For example, Dr. O'Neill remarked to a patient recently started on DDC (an experimental antiretroviral): "You're looking a lot better. DDC is your drug." Each patient's body has "its" drug, and the physician's task is to find that drug. As one Rousseau resident told a patient concerning treatment for KS, "The treatment for all patients is different." In the daily life of the clinic, it is this theme that predominates over any other, emerging out of every formal case presentation or quick hallway conference. As Kathryn Hunter (1991) aptly describes, "The single patient provides the text that medicine must read and make sense of and explain" (45).

FASHIONING THE AIDS PATIENT

The distinction I have made between discourse about patients' bodies and about patients is artificial. As we have seen, my informants do not talk about African bodies; they talk about African patients. However, there are two distinct constructions occurring in medical discourse about patients, one focusing on the physicians' experience with a patient's biology and another focusing on their experience with the patient as a patient, a person behaving within a specific social relationship. Charles Bosk and Joel Fraser (1991), in their discussion of the impact of AIDS on medical practice, describe a hierarchy in the status of AIDS patients, with hemophiliacs and recipients of transfusions having higher status than gay men or, at the bottom, IV drug users. Bosk and Fraser present the lower status of gay men as being due to their activism, unacceptable to the physicians, and their extensive social network, which allows less "heroics" for residents. IV drug users, according to Bosk and Fraser, are perceived as problem patients due to being "guilty" victims, having brought the disease on by their own unacceptable behavior, as well as a fear of contagion on the part of residents.

My experience at Rousseau and Northlake supports the construction by physicians of a patient "caste" system but not the specifics as presented by Bosk and

Fraser. In discourse at both clinics, gay men are not marked, unlike hemophiliacs (at Northlake only) and, more markedly, IV drug users. During informal case presentations, for example, the patient's sexuality is not mentioned as part of the opening identifiers. A gay male patient would be introduced as "a twenty-seven-year-old white male," with any reference to his sexual orientation either absent or presented as part of the patient's social background. In contrast, IV drug use is almost always mentioned in the opening introduction—"a twenty-seven-year-old white male with a history of IV drug use." Ethnicity has been a part of the initial identification of the patient in the case presentation long before the AIDS epidemic and does not seem to play a large role in the status of the patient among AIDS physicians. At Northlake, one of the doctors would prepare a daily list of all the inpatients on the clinic's service, with a quick summary of each patient's history and present ailment. Hemophilia and IV drug use were always noted, but sexual orientation was not. In my experience, gayness emerges as the norm rather than the devaluation proposed by Bosk and Fraser.

That the gay patient is the norm at Rousseau and Northlake does not mean that gay patients are not characterized in discourse. For the most part, gay men are constructed as educated people with strong financial resources who take an active part in their health care.

My clinical practice is biased in that the majority of the patients I have been personally responsible for have been gay men who are highly educated, who are very interested in the disease and know everything that there is to know really, so it is more a discussion among equals than the usual doctor-patient relationship where you are having to bring people up to a level of understanding.

I think that we in San Francisco benefit from having a very highly educated gay male community. Because of all the newsletters and all the seminars and all the support groups, I think that people are really quite sophisticated.

This construction of the gay patient is so pervasive that my clinician informants would express genuine surprise at encountering a gay patient that knew little about AIDS and its treatment. After seeing one such patient, a Northlake doctor commented, "You'd think a gay man in 1991 would know something about HIV, but this guy doesn't have a clue."

Among the senior Rousseau physicians, the *toxicomane*, the drug user, is more often the center of attention than the gay patient. Except in truly exceptional cases—a very flamboyant personality, for example—gay patients are taken as the norm at Rousseau, with other types of patients distinguished in relationship to them.

However, the Rousseau residents would occasionally discuss the nature of gay patients informally. A lunchtime conversation among the residents followed this path. One resident remarked, "Their lovers are really nice, but the mothers . . . [makes a face]." Another agreed, "The mothers are hell." They then described encounters with several patients' mothers and concluded that the mothers tend to cling tightly to the patient, trying to oversee and question everything about their care. The discussion moved on to talk of the gay patient themselves, alternating between jokes about the ease of doing rectal exams to expressions of difficulty relating to the more flamboyant patients and, ultimately, admiration for the close relationships often seen between patients and their lovers. One resident remarked, "It's very touching to see them," while another added, "They are couples, really." In this way, the residents fashion the gay patient, whom they have rarely knowingly encountered prior to the AIDS clinic, in a way that brings meaning to their experience.

Bosk and Fraser, as discussed above, suggest that the activism of gay patients lends itself to a devaluation on the part of physicians. However, gay activism in France and the United States are two different phenomena, carrying different meanings for both patients and physicians. The gay community, which has played such a large role not only in politicizing but in providing practical responses to the epidemic in the United States, only relatively recently has adopted those functions in France. Due in part to greater tolerance, if not acceptance, of homosexuality in French society, the gay community is more fragmented, and some would question whether one could even speak of a "gay community" in France, at least in the US sense of the term. Thus, when the AIDS epidemic took root in France, there were few existing support structures available for gay men (Pollak 1988).[2]

French support groups such as AIDES tend to stay out of the political arena directly and focus instead on providing legal assistance, housing, education, and emotional support. While these groups may petition clinics for office space or the government for added help with such issues, they are rarely, if ever, involved in demonstrations or protest activities directed either at the government or at the medical community. This contrasts strikingly with American groups such as ACT UP (AIDS Coalition to Unleash Power), which utilize confrontation tactics at medical conferences and government hearings. Thus, as one of my informants put it, activism in France is "gentle," though stronger for AIDS than for other health care issues. Additionally, French patients seem to be less equal partners with their physicians than American patients.

In contrast to Bosk and Fraser, I would contend that American patient activism is constructed ambivalently, not negatively, by my informants, often emerging as a positive element of working with gay patients. Not uncommonly, an article brought in by a Northlake patient would rate serious discussion among the physicians. Activism in the form of patients taking an active, informed role in treatment is generally received favorably, even when the patient disagrees with the physician, as was seen with the Northlake patient who refused AZT in favor of vacations.

The interested, educated, high-status gay patient is often contrasted with the undeniably low-status IV drug user, both in France and the United States:

Here you have mainly homosexuals and usually upper-class social economic classes. So it's much different from the IV drug addicts that we can have in north Paris or suburbs of Paris, where it's certainly more difficult to explain and to be understood by the patients.

The dichotomy of the AIDS population is sort of interesting. The gay population just tends to be a good population of the people to work with. They are very overall cooperative, and interested in learning, and interested in doing what you want them to do in order to take care of themselves. The other extreme obviously is the IV drug abuser population which is incredibly frustrating.

Bosk and Fraser suggest that IV drug–using patients are devalued because of a moral judgment on the part of physicians, constructing them as "guilty" victims. While I do not disagree that moral judgments may play a role, this theme rarely emerged from my informants' discourse, either in the interview or in the clinic setting. What did emerge was the construction of IV drug–using patients as frustrating, time-consuming, disinterested, and noncompliant, evoking a sense of powerlessness among their physicians.

At Rousseau, IVDU patients were consistently identified in the talk of senior physicians, residents, and nursing staff. During a statistics-related conversation between myself, a nurse, and Dr. Farsi, the latter unhappily mentioned that four patients had come into the emergency room last night with AIDS-related problems and that they wished to be followed at the clinic. He then added, "And by chance, all four are drug users." Recalling that the director had officially closed the clinic to new patients, the theme of the story becomes clear: Not only are we going to have still more patients and thus more work, but the additional patients are drug users, requiring additional attention. Drug users are marked in discourse in part to alert staff to a potentially "difficult" patient.

An encounter between an IVDU patient and the Rousseau staff illustrates this construction in action. The patient, a young man, was initially seen by one of the residents. Because he keeps his clinic appointments intermittently, more time is required to review his history and present symptoms. He did not leave the clinic at the end of the consultation but remained all day, stopping every physician, including myself, with a variety of medical and nonmedical demands. Each physician, in turn, spent several minutes responding to the patient. By the end of the day, Dr. Farsi almost physically pushed him out the door, as staff complained that they were being prevented from seeing other patients. After one confrontation between this patient and a resident, another resident commented, "It's just like a drug user." The resident quickly added that she knows it is not appropriate for her to say such a thing, but her frustration was evident. The resident's remark constructs the nature of the IVDU patient as being disruptive to the functioning of the clinic. Because the clinic is structured around the norm of the participatory, educated gay patient, the relatively small percentage of IVDU patients stand out as a chaotic element and thus are marked in discourse and practice.

The sense of powerlessness and frustration is evident in the discourse of Northlake physicians as well. Some treatments for opportunistic infections require intravenous drug therapy over several weeks, and a long-term "central" line is usually placed into a large blood vessel for this purpose. IVDU patients will sometimes inject their drugs into this line, resulting in potentially fatal infection or, depending on the dose, sudden death. This presents a dilemma for clinic doctors. Without the line, the patient may die, and with the line, the patient may die as well. As happened during rounds on one such patient, the patient was instructed "not to abuse the line" or otherwise risk a fatal infection.

Another patient presented a similar dilemma. This man had pancreatitis, a painful condition usually relieved by narcotic pain medication and giving food through an IV line rather than by mouth. The patient in question, hospitalized on and off for several months, had abused all his pain medication and continued to eat, even sneaking down into the cafeteria while in the hospital. After much discussion, Dr. O'Neill decided that the patient must be given something for his pain but limited the prescription to one week at a time. Again, the sense of frustration and helplessness is evident, as it seemed that no matter what we as physicians did to treat the patient's pancreatitis, he was likely to die, given his present behavior. As Dr. O'Neill remarked to the social worker, "Sometimes you have to give up."

Unquestionably, in the physician-constructed status hierarchy of AIDS patients, IVDU patients are at the bottom of the pyramid. After an emotion-filled consultation with a new patient, a young woman, a Northlake clinician remarked, "It's so hard [emotionally] with mothers. I mean, if it was some grizzled old drug user . . . " Yet I would suggest that this status is as much due to how they are constructed as patients as due to preassigned "guilt" for their infection with HIV. My Northlake and Rousseau informants may tend to detach themselves from many of these patients because of a sense of being unable to prevent, or at least delay, their deaths.

Not all of my informants constructed IVDU patients in this way. One prominent example is a New York physician who, unlike the Northlake and Rousseau physicians, sees a large number of IVDU patients.

Surprisingly, I think that the assumption is that drug addicts are stupid and don't want to know about their health and won't understand, and that's completely wrong. There are stupid ones who don't understand, but there are stupid people who don't understand in all walks of life. And in fact, I think some of the drug addicts, once they get to know about HIV, exceed some other groups of people in terms of what they want to learn about themselves.

Additionally, IVDU patients may escape their low status among clinicians and even cease to be marked as drug users, as I discovered during a conversation at Rousseau. Two residents and two nurses were sharing horror stories about particular IVDU patients, each demonstrating the difficult, disruptive nature of these patients. One resident brought up the name of a patient not previously mentioned. A nurse responded that this patient was not like the others at all and was immediately characterized as cooperative, never coming to the clinic high, keeping all her appointments. Though I had encountered this patient previously, no one had ever identified her as a drug user. Thus, though she used intravenous drugs, this patient was not marked in discourse because she did not fit the definition of an IVDU patient in terms of the meanings constructed by the Rousseau staff.

Hemophiliac patients at Northlake were generally seen by one physician, a hemophilia specialist, for all outpatient visits. The other clinic physicians encountered them usually as inpatients, and talk about the nature of hemophiliac patients as patients tended to be minimal. Unlike Bosk and Fraser, I observed no status or lack of status associated with hemophiliac patients at either clinic. At Northlake, ethnicity-centered discourse was also minimal. More common were remarks about public aid or poor, uninsured patients, who seemed to be coming to the clinic in increasing numbers. Poor, uninsured patients require more work on the part of these physicians, in terms of finding a way to provide them with medication, for example. However, as will be seen later, this discourse tended to be more constructive of the health care system rather than the nature of the patients themselves.

I encountered a similar discourse at Rousseau, not about French poor, who are covered by Securité Sociale, but about uninsured foreigners, usually Africans and Americans. As is the case at Northlake, discourse about *les irreguliers* tended to emphasize the nature of the French health care system rather than the patients themselves. Compared with Northlake, however, there was more ethnicity-centered discourse overall, perhaps due to the relatively larger numbers of foreign-born patients. During a staff meeting, Dr. Farsi told the case story of a man, his pregnant wife, and child, all seropositive and/or symptomatic, from Zaire. He commented, "It's typical. He comes in for a consultation and has zero T4." The African patient is constructed as one who has received little care, in worse condition than other patients, and presenting increased medical and social problems for the medical community.

The discourse of my French informants constructs American patients as well, though the reference is usually to American patients in the United States, rather than American patients at Rousseau. One example involves a discussion between Dr. Bernard and a mixed group of French and American media representatives. They began talking about the clinic and the AIDS epidemic, and one person asked Dr. Bernard about differences he sees between the United States and France. Bernard replied:

Both French and American patients are educated [about their disease], but they are very different. Patients here aren't as aggressive against medical institutions as they are in the US. For example, there was this patient that Jamie saw today, with a big allergy to a drug. In the US, the patient might sue over this, but here, no.

He then commented on differences in clinical trials: "In the US, it's almost impossible to do clinical trials because the patients take everything anyway. . . . In the US, as soon as a new drug comes out, everybody is taking it, so it's difficult to evaluate them." This discourse, part of a generalized discussion contrasting France and the United States, is as constructive of Americans as a group as it is of American patients. Bernard is not talking about Americans as patients, such as those he encounters regularly in the clinic, but patients as Americans, enamored of lawsuits and the latest fads, in contrast with the cooperative French. As will be discussed later, this type of discourse serves to construct French identity more than it serves to give meaning to encounters with American patients.

Medical discourse also constructs AIDS patients as a unified group, to be distinguished from other types of patients, usually those with cancer.

These [AIDS] people are activists, and you tend to hear the activists much more than you hear the pacifist who's laying at home with cancer or something else.

I think what it is going to do socially, though, is hopefully drag this country into some kind of compassionate, rational health care delivery system. The AIDS patients being so vocal, they just don't lie back and take it like the cancer patients or the diabetics who have suffered for years.

As seen in the above examples, both by American clinicians, my American informants tend to construct AIDS patients as activists, particularly in reference to the inequities of the US health care system. Sometimes clinicians interpreted patients' dissatisfaction as being directed at them:

First, you have the unusual circumstance of a lot of angry people, who are angry in the same way that cancer patients are angry with their doctor. So people who are trying to do something good get dumped on. And this is perhaps on a larger scale than many other diseases. It may have to do with the fact that we're dealing with an epidemic—where cancer patients have been not as organized in the past. Maybe the constituencies that are involved in HIV infection are much more vocal and had sort of a civil rights agenda to begin with.

This last example evokes the ambivalence I observed in the American medical community toward patient activism, an uneasiness in mixing politics with medicine. The construction of the AIDS patient as a political activist is absent from French discourse, at least in reference to French patients. As I was told on several occasions, French AIDS patients do not demonstrate in the street, unlike Americans. This difference in discourse likely stems in part from the differences in the health care systems, as well as the historical lack of organized activity on the part of the French gay community. In addition, I would suggest that the contrasting natures of the French and American doctor-patient relationships, to be discussed later, contribute substantially to the difference in discourse.

French and American medical discourse about AIDS patients do share one fundamental construction, that of more active participation in the treatment process than other patients, with increased interaction among the patients themselves. As one American clinical researcher remarked:

In the early days the aerosol word [aerosol prophylaxis for PCP] quickly spread, and we had patients coming here for their pentamidine from as far away as Toronto and Washington, DC, but that quickly became available throughout the country. Cancer patients are, their motivations are very different. Word spreads in different ways through that group of patients, and most patients with leukemia start chemotherapy very shortly after their disease is diagnosed and the word *prophylaxis* is a word that they've never thought of except as condoms.

One of the Rousseau residents described communication between AIDS patients in a similar fashion:

Most of them understand [AIDS] quite well, and even they are talking together, because of the population. Most are homosexual; they are talking together much more and are learning many facts. They have different points of view, and I think that's why they know much more than people who have got cancer; they [cancer patients] won't discuss with another one at the hospital. Because it's taboo, you know. . . . They [AIDS patients] see the evolution of the treatment, and they are very interested in their disease and their treatment and about the news.

From the physician's point of view, and perhaps from the patients' as well, AIDS patients form a community in which they learn from and support one another, enabling a rapid sharing of experiences and information. At both Rousseau and Northlake, patients would greet each other and discuss their condition and treatments. With each clinic following approximately 2,000 patients, one gets a sense of being in a small town, where everyone, for better or worse, is an integral part of everyone else's lives. My informants incorporate the idea of an AIDS patient community into their practice. When a Rousseau patient was beginning aerosol prophylaxis, the physician instructed him in how to do the treatment properly, then asked if he knew what to do from watching other patients.

My informants, French and American, recognize that the community of AIDS patients is often as divided as it is cohesive. One Rousseau nurse remarked that the variation in patient population in Paris AIDS clinics is partly due to an informal peer network, suggesting that gay men tell their friends about Rousseau, while African immigrants pass the word about other hospitals, and drug users still another. The construction of the AIDS patient information network is here broken down along transmission group lines.

I encountered a similar discourse at Northlake. After meeting with an IVDU patient who had dropped out of a "mostly gay" support group, Dr. Westin informed me that it is still difficult for heterosexuals and people of color to find a support group; "The support system is still set up to serve primarily white gay males." He then talked about divisions in the "HIV community," with gays resenting newcomers, since gay men themselves established most of the support systems. The discourse of physicians may well contribute toward supporting this division. Their construction of AIDS patients in general as highly participatory activists, especially in the United States, bears striking resemblance to their discourse about gay patients specifically, further evidence of the gay patient being the unmarked standard for all AIDS patients.

Despite my informants' acknowledgments of the divisions among AIDS patients, Dr. Westin's use of the term *HIV community* is significant. The term was extremely common among my American informants, a model of and a model for the interaction of AIDS patients with each other. In the representations of my informants, AIDS patients form a unified community that experiences some divisions, rather than sharply divided groups that occasionally come together. As we have seen, though my

French informants lacked a common word for this community, it nevertheless emerges from their discourse in the form of a learning or communication network.

The HIV community also emerges as an ideal for both French and American physicians. In the United States, this network often takes the form of patient-clinic forums and community-based research (in contrast to research done in academic medical centers). In France, the establishment of a few large, relatively unified support organizations and the avoidance of political affiliations contribute to the development of community. Many French professional and social organizations are formed along political lines, including physician associations. This often leads to ineffective lobbying efforts vis-à-vis a strong central government and infighting between groups that share nominally similar goals (Wilsford 1991). Thus, keeping an organization apolitical is a significant feat, requiring an unusual amount of solidarity. As one French clinician involved in AIDS education remarked:

If you want to help people who are sick, you cannot help these kind of people who are of one political color and not other people. We don't want that. We want to help everybody—black, white, Catholic, Jewish, gay, straight. Everyone, and we don't want to ruin the beginning, you understand.

As we shall see later, physicians in both countries construct their own roles in the HIV community.

In conclusion, patients and patient bodies are an integral part of medical discourse on AIDS. While a status hierarchy is certainly present, it emerges predominantly out of discourse on the nature of gay men, hemophiliacs, and IV drug users as patients, rather than preassigned "guilt" in contracting HIV. Gay men emerge as the norm, in terms both of their bodies and their behavior as patients, with other patient groups being constructed in reference to them. Ethnicity appears to be less important in regard to the issue of status, though it serves a variety of other purposes in my informants' discourse, such as distinguishing manifestations of AIDS and constructing national identity. Finally, the concept of an HIV community emerges from discourse on patients, ultimately emphasizing the distinctiveness of AIDS patients from other patients, and their unifying social relationships as experienced in the daily life of the clinic.

THE DOCTOR-PATIENT RELATIONSHIP

In redefining patients, my clinician informants also redefine the doctor-patient relationship. While the interactions between physicians and patients have been the subject of discourse by both clinicians and social scientists well before AIDS (Cassell 1976; Hahn 1985), AIDS acts to highlight its intricacies and serve as a context for refashioning this complex relationship. My American informants developed central themes of information sharing and empowerment, while the French emphasized the value of trust.

Much of the American discourse on the doctor-patient relationship appears as an extension of discourse on the stereotypical AIDS patient. Since AIDS patients are constructed as educated and actively involved in their care, the relationship emerges as more of a partnership, based on shared powers of decision.

I have a very sophisticated patient population—they can read; they are intelligent. I say, "Here, read these two things, and you can do whatever you want to do."

I think really the major difference between now and 1986 was the incorporation of the patient voice and the AIDS advocate voice into decision making and designing clinical trials and determining what the priorities are and should be for doing studies. I don't know any disease where there is that much of an integration of the patient into the decision-making process.

AIDS thus changes the nature of the doctor-patient relationship, reapportioning decision-making powers more evenly between the two parties. This discourse of empowerment is more prominent among the San Francisco informants and is presented as a regional accomplishment.[3]

I think that San Francisco early on understood the importance of empowering patients to assume a lot of the responsibility for their own care. Giving the patients the opportunity to take risks. . . . Patients coming and saying, "I know the studies aren't in. I want to take this drug. I understand it may kill me, but I'm going to die anyway." I think most of us would say, "Great, we understand that. Here is what we see as the risk there, and here are what we see as the rewards." But not say to the patient, "If you are going to make a decision like that, I as a Western medicine provider will not care for you." Which was sort of the model of before the AIDS epidemic. So, I think we have come a long way in patient empowerment in realizing medicine can only provide part of the answer to this thing, and that patients need to be allowed to make their own decisions.

Even when the patient's decision is contrary to the clinician's advice, my informants tended to respect the patient's decision. I observed this on several occasions at Northlake, again, the most striking example involving the patient who decided to take vacations instead of AZT. Another common practice is for patients to increase their dose of Bactrim, a drug for PCP prophylaxis and treatment, when they start feeling sick. The physicians would not reprimand patients but, depending on the results of the exam, would often suggest an additional drug or a return to the lower dose. This is not to suggest that such conflicts are not problematic for American clinicians:

The third kind of patient is somebody who is smart and can't comprehend an intelligent, rational discussion about drugs and how we arrive at our decisions to use what drug and what not to use, what would be dangerous or unknown or foolish or whatever. . . . They don't want to take a drug that I know will help them, or they want to take a whole pile of drugs that I don't think is going to help them at all and possibly is going to complicate things. . . . Basically, it's their decision—it's their life.

The doctor-patient partnership emerges from the discourse as a challenge for the physician, in terms of both accepting patient decisions and keeping pace with patients' increasing understanding of the disease.

There's a more sophisticated group of patients with AIDS than any other disease that I have ever known, and I think that has helped enormously. . . . It has helped physicians realize that they can't just say, "Well, we don't know too much, and this is the best that I can do, or go talk to somebody else." It's really challenged the physicians to stay up-to-date.

As the above excerpt suggests, empowerment is achieved through information, particularly biomedical information. At Northlake, I observed that patients initially become hyperaware of any changes in their body. As time goes on, patients learn to translate their experiences into medical categories of meaning, learning which of their experiences are "relevant" to HIV disease. This learning is never complete—patients do not "become doctors" in the interpretation of AIDS, though they may at times approach it: "Some of my patients—I know you have heard this a thousand times—know much more than I do. For them it's a full time job."

AIDS emerges from the discourse as unusual, if not unique, in the level of patient information and empowerment it promotes. This refashioning corresponds to Koenig's (1988) analysis of the doctor-patient relationship in the setting of experimental therapy:

Patients play a role in creating the "standard therapy" meaning of TPE [therapeutic plasma exchange] as it develops in individual treatment units. In highly experimental settings, patients are much more likely to be treated as partners in the research endeavor rather than as passive recipients of treatment. (47)

AIDS, being an "experimental disease" involving experimental therapies, allows a redistribution of information and power between doctors and patients, something that is not only accepted but valued.

There are a lot of textbooks over there that say AIDS on them, but I still think that you cannot take down a textbook, open it up, and get the answers to everything. So I still think almost essentially everything we do in this disease falls into an investigational/research category. And I don't know all the answers, so I am very willing to have patients teach me by doing their own experimentation.

The question becomes, If and when AIDS ceases to be experimental, will the relationship between patient and practitioner become less of a partnership, closing off access to medical meanings? Or, as most of my informants suggest, has a new model of and for this interaction emerged out of the AIDS experience?

The discourse of my French informants shares some basic similarities with that of the Americans, namely, that AIDS changes the doctor-patient relationship and that patients take a more active role in their treatment. For the French, however, AIDS provides a medium for constructing the traditional values of the relationship in a new way. The theme in this discourse is not empowerment but trust.

Most of patients are aware of their disease, what are their risks. It's not like in cancer, when especially in France, people used to lie to patients, to say, "It's nothing, it's not a cancer." But with AIDS, I think it's impossible because . . . most people that come here with AIDS have seen it before. . . . So it's something new, too, because the relationship with doctor and the patient can be different than before, because people are aware. And I think it's important not to lie because when you lie to people, they will never accept treatment if they don't trust you.

Whereas talk of decision making lies at the core of the American discourse, truth telling emerges as the central issue for the French.

Is it difficult to tell the truth to a patient? That, I believe that is equally for me a big lesson, because I learned to tell the truth. And, before this, I did not have this attitude at all. . . . I believe a lot in this relationship, in trust and in explanation. I explain a lot, I always spend a lot of time in speaking with patients. Thus, I believe one can say a big part of the truth. That's a big lesson for me, a big change since the taking in charge of HIV-seropositive people.

Information sharing is valued not in and of itself but as an aspect of telling the truth, which in turn is important as a means of creating a relationship based on trust. Trust is not a new value in the French doctor-patient relationship. Rather, AIDS allows this value to be played out in a new way. The amount of information shared, the level of truth told, is dependent on the desires of the patient: "If he is truly AIDS [not simply HIV-positive], and he asks me, 'What am I?' it depends. If he doesn't want to know that he has AIDS, I say that he is HIV plus, in a serious stage."

The Rousseau physicians generally offered new information not affecting treatment, such as a change in prognosis, only at the request of the patient. To do otherwise would place an emotional burden on the patient without necessarily improving the doctor-patient relationship.

I tell them [seropositive patients] I'm not a fortune teller, I have no crystal ball. If the biological and clinical results are good, I tell them they can sleep easy for the next six months. If there is pathology in the results, I try to judge their psychological state. If he is suicidal, I don't tell.

I never use the word *AIDS*. I say, "You don't have AIDS," and that's the only reference I'm using for AIDS. . . . I say, "You have *Pneumocystis*." I let them do their own connections—I don't give it to them.

This may also be a more generally European approach. In reviewing the 1993 CDC definition, for example, the European Centre for the Epidemiologic Surveillance of AIDS remarked on the unfavorable psychological consequences of having asymptomatic seropositive persons seeing themselves now labeled as having AIDS (Bouvier-Colle, Jougla, and Schwoebel 1993).

In the American discourse, in contrast, information is constructed as a source of empowerment, and physicians must present information in order for patients to participate in decision making. The following encounter at Northlake illustrates this difference.

During rounds, we visited a patient with his first opportunistic infection. Before entering the room, Dr. Westin asked Dr. Peters: "Have you told him that he now has AIDS? It's a very difficult threshold for patients." Dr. Peters then spent several minutes explaining to the patient that he now has CDC-defined AIDS. Afterward, Dr. Westin commented, "Despite your eloquent speech, that's [having AIDS] got to prey on his mind." Despite the acknowledged burden to the patient, the American clinician nonetheless presents the information. I never observed this type of encounter at Rousseau, and it would be unlikely to take place in any French medical context. Unless the course of treatment were being changed significantly, a French physician would wait until the patient asked if they had developed AIDS or were getting worse. Information sharing, in the French context, is only valuable if it promotes the foundation of trust between doctor and patient. There is overlap, as always. American clinicians assess the receptivity of patients to information and try their best to offer hope: "I tend to be vague often with the response unless they really press me to numbers [mortality statistics], and some people do want to know numbers."

The French clinicians, like the Americans, represent AIDS patients as taking a more active role in their care than other patients. In the French discourse, this refers to patients requesting information more frequently, or asking about experimental therapies they have heard about through the media.

I think people there [in the day hospital], their relationships with patients are much better, because they are not in bed waiting for someone, totally passive. And I think it's a very good way to make people take care of themselves.

Maybe the most difficult will be to deal with the new treatments, and what is said in the media. The patients we see here are well aware of the new advances which very often have no clinical significance. . . . And they ask many questions about why don't we try this new treatment or this new viral medicine. And that's quite difficult to deal with that. Maybe the most difficult is to convince the patients that many of the treatments which are sometimes proposed by physicians, or not physicians, are not good for them.

French clinicians, like their American counterparts, find active patient involvement a double-edged sword. In the French case, the physician still retains much of the decision-making power. The challenge for the French, seen in the above example, lies in convincing patients that they may be making a poor decision rather than accepting those patients' poor decisions.

An encounter between a resident and an inpatient at Rousseau illustrates the difference in decision making. The patient had refused bronchoscopy to diagnose possible *Pneumocystis*, asking why he cannot be treated for PCP without the test. The resident explained that the treatment can be too toxic to do without proof. After convincing the patient to undergo the test, the resident commented to me that many doctors don't explain things to their patients, who would be satisfied if you talk with them a few minutes. She added that AIDS patients ask more questions than other patients, who create their own problems by not asking anything, instead waiting passively for explanations. An active patient, in the French interpretation, solicits information that will allow him to expand his trust in the doctor's capabilities and intentions, not necessarily taking on more decision-making power.

He [the patient] knows, he reads the papers, he reads the books. This is the first time, for example, in the history of medicine where we saw patients who know more than their doctors. This is true. I think all of us are in very good relationship with the patients because . . . if there is no sympathetic relationship, they don't come again.

A Rousseau encounter with an American patient exemplifies this difference. Several of the clinicians and I were discussing the patient, who was present behind a partition about ten feet away. We reviewed the lab results and the recommendations of the specialist. The resident mentioned one drug specifically, and the patient, a disembodied voice at this point, called out, "No, he said another drug besides Voltaren, too!" We laughed and Dr. Farsi commented, "The patient is joining in on the consultation!" During the rest of the discussion, the patient continued to add commentary from his bed and later negotiated a delay of treatment so that he could travel on vacation. This American patient contrasts with many of the French patients who do very little direct negotiation over treatment and who never "chime in" on discussions between the clinic physicians. As one of the Rousseau clinicians stated:

Yes, there are differences in the relation between physicians and patients, which is more simple in France than in the States. . . . But I think the regulation is different, and generally speaking, the confidence, I think, is stronger in France than in the States. It's quite rare to have a discussion about the treatment or the way you work with a patient here. If the patient disagrees with his physician, he will just go and see another physician. He will not go in front of the law.

For the French, the level of confidence that the patient can place in the doctor is empowerment, not information. As Dr. Bernard observed:

At the beginning, the patients were very well informed about the treatment, all the aspects of the disease, until, I will say, '88, '89. They wanted to know everything. And I feel there is a retreat from that. Because they realize that the amount of information is so big that it's very difficult for them to manage. And also for the oldest patients, I think that they realize that it's impossible to manage by themselves, these kind of things. So I think they are looking for a more traditional kind of relationship—"You are doing the technical job, and I'm a patient."

A notable difference in French and American interactions with patients involves organized patient activism in the form of support groups or lobbying efforts. One of my French informants constructed this as a fundamental cultural difference:

For example, in a sickness like AIDS which has no good treatment, in France, I think the response against the *l'angoisse*, the anguish, is to look for a small group, with friends, relationships, family. In the United States we see, many times, more big groups with a very large component of spirituality, which we don't see here. And this kind of response depends on the mentality of people in each country.

Outside of references to the International AIDS Conferences, French clinicians rarely speak of encounters with patient activist groups. Regular conflicts with such groups are seen as a particularly American experience, one not to be envied: "The activists are much less activist than in the States, that's true. And that's true for all the medical field, not only for HIV. . . . And the activist groups are very gentle in France, so that's easier."

American clinicians usually encounter activists at clinical research meetings or community forums, and their discourse on patient activism evokes a strong sense of ambivalence. An encounter between a Northlake physician and a long-standing patient provides an excellent example. The patient asked the physician about the recent AIDS Clinical Trials Groups Meetings, which the doctor had attended. The physician provided an overview, then observed:

The activists were out in full force, asking their usual dumb questions. Earlier on, they used to ask better questions. . . . Now they must have a broader range of people. The investigators are getting pretty tired of it. Here they are, bending over backwards, trying to help, especially since things have gotten more flexible.

As will be seen in the discourse of research scientists, this discourse carries a nostalgia for the "old days" of AIDS, as well as sense of a personal insult. The doctor then told the story of an argument at one session between white lesbian activists and African-American straight women activists. The lesbians argued that studies looking at the use of AZT in pregnancy should be made into studies on all women. The African-American women then told the white lesbians that they weren't the ones having babies and they didn't get AIDS anyway, so they should stay out of the discussion. The doctor told the story in a highly animated style, mimicking the name-calling between the two groups. He ended by saying:

Tim Rogers [the NIH session leader] knows when to take a stand. He's not wishy-washy. He stood up and supported the black women's position, and the rest of us are sitting here saying, "Yeah, another usual meeting."

This narrative constructs what has become "usual" at AIDS meetings and defines the ambivalent relationship between activists and clinical researchers. Rather than attempt to silence both activist groups, the leader of the meetings recognizes their discourse as important by participating. At the same time, the other medical participants emerge from the story as frustrated, perhaps by their impotence in the face of the activists' conflict. After this story, the doctor noted that some clinical researchers have received death threats and violence to their property. The patient

replied that there are some "loonies" but that most of the gay community is serious
and cooperative. The doctor agreed, concluding, "Overall, I think the impact of the
activists has been positive. Research studies have become a lot more flexible, and that
was a good thing."

Patient activism emerges from this discourse as a force for both constructive
change and disruptive conflict. The most striking part of this doctor's narrative is not
how it constructs activists but that it is shared with a patient rather than another
physician. It suggests a sense of community between doctors and patients, an unusual
fluidity in the boundaries between the two groups. Northlake physicians, for example,
would routinely express their uncertainty to patients about prognosis or treatment
options, rather than simply relate a set of known facts. One such discussion took
place between Dr. Westin and a patient who was intolerant to several antiviral
medications.

> *Patient*: Well, let me ask you. How long would you expect me to live, given no
> T cells, positive antigen and no antiviral?
>
> *Dr. Westin*: You've already gone past the average, with or without AZT, so we're
> in uncharted waters here. I know that's the type of information you need to
> make an informed decision, but I just don't know.

Dr. Westin directly acknowledges the patient's desire for information and his own
inability to provide that information. At this point, the patient and the physician are
exploring the outer limits of the human body, like *Star Trek* explorers, together
boldly going where no one has gone before.

The sense of shared experience, along with the active involvement of patients,
seems to encourage more intimate and informal relationships between doctors and
patients in both the French and American contexts. Two French examples follow.

Maybe the human relation is different here. It is much more friendly, much less strict, less
academic than in another hospital. . . . The way of speaking to the patients, and when I say the
way of speaking, it's not only from the physicians, also the nurses. The nurses are very friendly
with the patients here. All the team is much more friendly with the patients. It's more familiar.

When I saw you the first time, in 1987, the patients I saw, the oldest patients, I knew them for
several months. Now, certain patients, I've known them for three years, four years, several years.
So because of this, with certain patients I have another, closer relationship. And secondly, now
I see patients dying that I have known for a long time. . . . The relationship is *forcément*
different. Even with the new patients, because they know the disease better, because some of
them have a friend who is dead. So, with the new patients, the patient and I have the same
history.

At Northlake, Dr. O'Neill mentioned that a lot of the "old-timers" and "veterans"
come to see him on one particular day of the week, since he has treated them for years
and they do not feel comfortable with anyone else. Patients would sometimes bring
the Northlake staff candy, and long-standing patients were generally on a first-name

basis with at least one of the clinic physicians. At Rousseau, not a day passed without a patient bringing flowers or candy to the clinic, in addition to the abundance of gifts for the nurses around Christmas. Nearly all physicians and patients addressed each other by first name. The ambiance at both clinics was one of warmth, a particular closeness between physicians and patients that I have yet to encounter in other medical settings.

The intimacy of doctor-patient relationships in AIDS may also emerge from their potent experiences with death and dying. When I arrived at the Rousseau clinic, I expected to be confronted with death on a daily basis. To my surprise, not only was death an uncommon event, but the majority of patients did not even seem to be dying.[4] Even at Northlake, I was startled at how little my prior visions of a death as an omnipresent force coincided with the actual clinical experience of AIDS. Doctors and patients spend more time talking about AIDS and life than they do about death. Nevertheless, death has become an integral part of the experience of AIDS—a shared and regulated process at Northlake, a private matter between doctor and patient at Rousseau.[5] Issues of resuscitation, palliative care, and physician-assisted suicide are confronted regularly, though not routinely, in the world of AIDS. In one form or another, death becomes integrated into the physician's experience of AIDS. Physicians participate in the suffering of patients, the grief of their families. None of us are apart from death.

Physician-patient interactions in the clinics occasionally border on the strange. At Northlake, a patient of mine asked to see Dr. Westin as well. When Dr. Westin came in, the patient brought out a fabric sample and tape measure and announced that he would like to make Dr. Westin a pair of pants. After a discussion about style and color, the patient had the doctor take off his coat and began taking measurements. When the patient measured the inseam, he told Dr. Westin, "This might be a little uncomfortable. Just stand up straight and cough"—a parody of the standard hernia exam on men. By the end of the encounter, all of us were laughing. The intimacy of the doctor-patient relationship in the context of AIDS opens it up to inversions such as this, creating a place for the strange in clinic life.

AIDS appears to bridge, to some extent, the cultural gap between doctors and patients. The HIV community described earlier includes, at times, clinicians and researchers as well as patients and activists. In Chicago, I attended a regularly held forum for physicians, researchers, and patients, particularly those in clinical trials. The medical participants presented new information from the ACTG meetings, but most of the time was spent in a discussion of clinical issues. I was struck by the repeated use of "we" in the physicians' discourse, such as "how we should approach the problem of AZT resistance." Again, it suggests a sense of community between patients and physicians. Though the power to speak was unequally distributed—the physicians did all the presenting—patients and physicians questioned each other, struggling together to create meaning for these experiences. Through their close and complex relationships, AIDS doctors and patients may well share more meanings with each other than with those uninvolved with AIDS.

My last day at Northlake, I handled the visit of a new clinic patient. Although he met with Dr. Westin afterward, I felt somehow responsible for him. After an hour or so talking about his concerns and learning about his body, we had formed a bond. He was newly diagnosed with HIV, and in doing a history and physical, we had walked through the threshold together into the HIV community, person with HIV and physician of HIV. You do not let go easily of that, and I suspect it is the hallmark of the singular relationship between doctor and patient in the world of AIDS.

NOTES

1. Not only is the African-American body constructed in this discourse, so are New York, Miami, and San Francisco.

2. Over time, however, a large number of associations have evolved, based to some extent on US models, such as Gay Men's Health Crisis in New York. The oldest and largest of these organizations, Associations AIDES, was started in 1984 in Paris and now has a number of other regional offices. Like many of the US organizations today, they are not limited to gay men but provide services for all persons with HIV infection.

3. See J. Feldman (1993) for further discussion of regional differences and the San Francisco model of care.

4. This may, in part, be due to the absence of inpatient rounds.

5. There are notable differences in French and American approaches to death and dying, including issues of palliative care and physician-assisted suicide. For a detailed assessment, see J. Feldman (1993).

9

Health Care and Medical Practice

AIDS may actually tip the whole thing over. Somebody may wake up and say, "What are we doing?"

Chicago clinician, on the US health care system

HEALTH CARE SYSTEMS

The AIDS epidemic has an enormous impact on any health care system, necessitating funding and personnel for research, treatment, prevention, and support services. The US Public Health Service estimated the direct cost of care for AIDS patients in 1991 to be between $8 and $16 billion (Velimirovic 1987). The average lifetime medical cost for a person with AIDS has been estimated as high as $147,000 (Ozawa, Auslander, and Slonim-Neva 1993).[1] My clinical informants, particularly Americans, confront this issue daily in their practice, and it is the subject of much discourse. The American discourse is amazingly uniform. Nearly all, regardless of region or institutional affiliation, spoke of AIDS as a spotlight, exposing tremendous weaknesses in the health care system, particularly in regard to the poor and minorities.

The main problem is that AIDS is adding a burden onto an overburdened, collapsing, chaotic, horrible medical system. . . . The bureaucracy is astounded and the medical system is slowly responsive because it's already overburdened by a population that's incredibly underserved and medically horribly sick.

I think this epidemic provides a spotlight on most of what I view to be significant weaknesses in this country's system of health care. In general, the way it deals with underrepresented, underprivileged, nonaffluent people.

There is less uniformity about whether the system will actually change in response to AIDS or simply increase existing disparities. In all cases, AIDS is constructed as the force that can either save the system or break it.

It's all tied up into the whole problem of how we manage health care in this country in general. I am assuming that the trends in the last two to five years will continue, and we are regressing back to a two-tier system of health care due to the economic pressures of the system. Clearly, that's a disaster for managing HIV infection in this country.

I think it provides an opportunity for some innovation, and at the very least, it's providing stress on the system in general, that the system might not be able to stand up against. It's been possible to kind of brush a lot of the weaknesses in the health care system under the carpet. It may not be possible now.

I think what it is going to do socially, though, is hopefully drag this country into some kind of compassionate, rational health care delivery system. This whole idea of basically crisis intervention, and only the workers are insured, and then only if you work for a company with more than twenty-five people.

Since private insurance lies at the core of the US health care system, it is not surprising that it lies at the core of health care discourse, as seen in the last example. Insurance issues are an integral part of the Northlake physicians' experience with AIDS. As noted previously, the medical team that follows each patient is composed of an attending physician, a clinical nurse manager, and a social worker. When a patient's case is discussed among the team, the doctor often turns to the social worker for an "OK" of treatment, in the sense of, "Can we do this? Will the insurance cover it?" Patients are continually asking about insurance, and a major concern of both doctors and patients is that the patient will be canceled or refused insurance if the HIV infection is discovered. For example, a new patient to the clinic explained that he was first diagnosed as HIV positive in 1985 but never received any follow-up since he had been trying to get insurance first. In such cases, the HIV infection would be considered a "preexisting condition" and often would not be covered.

Occasionally, a patient's insurance status affects treatment decisions. A patient of mine had been on a drug for preventing a fungal infection but then developed a recurrence. I suggested he go on a different antifungal, more powerful and more expensive. Dr. O'Neill, however, decided to keep him on the original drug. Later, he mentioned to me that the patient had no insurance or public aid, implying that the patient would have had no way to pay for a more expensive drug. In a staff meeting, Dr. Westin asked the psychiatrist, "If a hypothetical patient with documented HIV dementia came in, where would he be hospitalized?" The psychiatrist answered, "The Institute of Psychiatry says that if it's a demonstrated organic cause, it's a medical problem." He then cited a case where the patient had no insurance and was refused admission to the Institute. "If he'd had good-paying insurance, who knows?"

Throughout the day, Northlake physicians would be called upon to cope with insurance questions, usually filling out forms or talking with company representatives about a patient's coverage. Rarely would such interaction pass by without some expression of frustration on the part of the physician, particularly when the insurance company or the hospital (which absorbs costs not covered by insurance, including uninsured patients)[2] would question the need for hospitalization, a regular occurrence known as "utilization review." For example, Dr. O'Neill was called during rounds about whether a new inpatient needed to be in the hospital. Dr. O'Neill exploded afterward:

He's one of the sickest patients on the service! They don't mind and I don't mind if they call. It's just that there isn't any code[3] they can understand, like "gallbladder, five days" or "normal labor and delivery, three days." They look at this AIDS stuff and it's . . . [screws up his face].

Utilization reviewers, generally nurses, emerge from the discourse as particularly ignorant concerning AIDS. As Dr. O'Neill remarked in clinic, "I get calls from all these utilization review nurses about our patients. They don't know anything about AIDS, and I'm educating them over the phone." The Northlake physicians resent the time spent handling insurance issues, and their discourse evokes a sense of powerlessness. Insurance companies, in turn, are constructed as dominating and disinterested in patient care.

I actually have a nurse that spends hours every day dealing with all these health care agencies. And agencies will say, "Well, this guy has full Blue Cross coverage, but we don't cover anything that is injected as an outpatient." Okay, so what does that mean? Well, that means that if you get the patient to the hospital every day or have him come to your office and inject him yourself, then it will be paid for, even though it costs more. . . . We have two full-time social workers. We shouldn't even need a social worker. Or we should need maybe at the most a part-time social worker to orchestrate what is needed. We know what is needed; we just can't get it. So we have to juggle fifteen different agencies and whatever. It's a huge wasted effort.

Horror stories about insurance encounters abound, expressing themes of powerlessness, fragmentation, and waste. Dr. O'Neill's narrative below is one example.

Everybody is limiting care, whether you have insurance or you don't. You want to admit the patient to the hospital, and they are on public aid. One of the first questions they get, "What are the four things that you are doing in the hospital that you cannot do as an outpatient?" Well, the patient is comatose. Second, I think he needs to be intubated. [And then they ask,] "Isn't there a fourth?" . . . One guy—I didn't know what was going on with the patient—was very ill. I was afraid he would collapse in the street. How do you document that? I mean, that's a clinical decision. I've treated thousands of AIDS patients, and how do I know that guy was going to collapse? . . . They wouldn't approve the admission because the insurance company wanted me to try it at home. And I said, "Look, where are you?" He said, "What?" I said, "Where are you, physically speaking, where is your body?" I said, "I am hiring a limousine. I'm paying for it myself. I am sending the patient over to you, and you can take care of him, because I can't take care of him like this. You can have him. I mean, I can't do it. I'll pay for it." And he said, "Well, okay, I will give you three days." I don't think they get the concept here.

While loss of autonomous control forms a part of this discourse, what emerges from these stories is not simply physicians resenting having to share power. Rather, it is the sense of powerlessness, of having to struggle against a powerful and fragmented commercial bureaucracy in order to provide care for their patients and to actively practice their identity as physicians.

Government programs, and the lack of them, provoke similar discourse. A staff meeting discussion turned to the increasing number of clinic patients coming from the public county hospital, usually on public aid or with no coverage at all. One physician remarks, "There's definitely a lot of pressure from the hospital not to see public aid patients. I've gotten a lot of letters [from the administration] about it." This concern is due to lack of government reimbursement for many public aid patients. One nurse commented that the problem is not just new patients coming in on aid but that patients now live longer, often lose their insurance, and end up on public aid. She added, "And next year it'll be worse." At another meeting, the staff was discussing an inpatient newly diagnosed with lymphoma. The social worker brought up the problem of paying for his chemotherapy and other drugs with Medicaid. Dr. Westin said, exasperated, "So this guy wants chemo but can't afford it? What are we supposed to say about that?"

Public aid thus emerges as only a marginal financial improvement over having no insurance, while requiring as much time and effort on the part of the physician as private insurance. In another example, an incoming public aid patient sparked a discussion between a Northlake physician and the psychologist on the hospital staff about not having enough money to hire more staff. The physician remarked, angrily, "He needs care, he needs to be hooked up with studies, and I'm the only one to do it." This type of resentment toward disenfranchised patients was less evident at Rousseau, where the focus was usually on the sheer number of patients rather than their financial status.

The flaws in the health care system are constructed as a social or political problem, not a medical one: "The AIDS epidemic has been a force—the government has to do something about access to health care, because it's just getting out of hand." Thus, for the American clinician informants, time spent on the financial access problems of their patients is constructed as taking away time and effort from "real" medical problems. Additionally, access issues emerge as the purview of social workers, not physicians. My clinician informants present themselves as having neither the training nor the desire to do this type of work.

Despite the challenge to their identity as physicians, Northlake doctors have developed a number of creative practices to subvert access barriers for their patients. AIDS patients with non-AIDS-related problems may be admitted under the HIV service to get around utilization review. For example, a patient with urinary retention and HIV was admitted, and the resident asked Dr. O'Neill about his immune status. Dr. O'Neill commented that the patient really has a urology problem, adding: "Urology didn't want to admit him because they knew it wouldn't pass the utilization review. With me [HIV service], you get AIDS, KS, et cetera. I mean, I sign more death certificates than the oncologists." Dr. O'Neill is using the reputation of AIDS as a complicated and fatal disease—note the cancer reference—to obtain hospital-based treatment for his patient and thus subvert utilization review.

Constant creative trickery goes on in the clinic as well. One technique involves claiming a more serious diagnosis on billing sheets in order to get adequate reimbursement from insurance companies or particularly public aid. As with the hospitalization case, this is made easier by the general confusion over the staging of AIDS and the limited diagnostic categories provided by the hospital's billing department. Another important practice involves creative diagnosing and payment to keep insurance companies from knowing a patient is HIV-positive for as long as possible. For example, the physician will record a diagnosis of "pneumonia" rather than "*Pneumocystis* pneumonia" on the insurance form.

Finally, one of the common means of funding patient care is through clinical research. Northlake physicians will regularly suggest such studies to patients as means to provide medications and follow-up care. In fact, the practice was so common the physicians had to be reminded at staff meetings that not all studies cover doctor visits as well as the study drug. Still, the staff agreed that enrolling patients in studies was a valuable way of decreasing their financial burden. Northlake physicians would sometimes go to great lengths to insure that needy patients met the study criteria. For example, a study on weight loss, which paid for the patient's labwork, required a 10 percent loss to qualify. One patient weighed in initially two pounds short, so the doctor had the patient strip down to undershorts and get on a "better" scale to officially qualify for study, even though all other weights I had seen for this study were done with the patient wearing clothes.

Physicians express pride in their other, less subversive, ways of coping with the problems of access to the latest treatments. For example, Dr. Fields emphasized the increasing availability of clinical trials to all patients:

There is an attempt here to organize and to integrate clinical research into the health care system that is available to HIV-infected people. That's relatively recent and was not true five years ago, and I think it may have every chance of being successful. For instance, in the renewal, we are proposing to establish subunits at the county hospital.

A San Francisco physician focused on community cooperation between public and private sectors:

I think, more than anything else, it is the sense that working together as a community we've tried to encourage. I think that extends to really not a great deal of competition between private and public sectors here. We respect the fact that people with private insurance certainly can and usually do choose to go to private practitioners that in turn don't accept patients that don't have that level of reimbursement, and yet it works out pretty well, I think.

Despite talk of local successes, most of my informants called for the development of some type of national health care to insure access for all their patients and relieve themselves of administrative tasks.

And somehow or other a national health system, however embryonic, has got to be considered in this country.

It [AIDS] has challenged all of our medical system. The crisis that we are facing now, with the controversy about national health insurance versus a national health service plan and the Canadian model, is at least in part related to AIDS and what glaring deficits we have seen. It was present before AIDS, but it's dramatic, and all the more dramatic and highlighted when there are 39 million Americans who have no third-party payment and have to go to the public sector. You can see the way the public sector is getting crushed now by the additional burden of AIDS and HIV disease.

Many of my informant use unflattering comparisons with European health care systems to highlight the inequities and burdensome fragmentation of the American situation.

It has to be a government responsibility, at least half of it, and governments don't want to have anything new in this disease. . . . We have a bigger problem here because we don't have any national health insurance system. And so when we want early intervention here, often we have to go out and get money for the whole thing. In Europe, where most people are covered with insurance, the actual care of the individual is taken care of, and all you have to do is add on the part of notification and the counseling issues, which take a little bit of money, but those are really marginal compared to the major stuff of getting people medical care and drug treatment, AZT and that stuff.

In Italy, for example, where the greatest proportion of AIDS patients are among drug users, they just decided that AZT looks like it works, so we will give all of the drug addicts AZT. That was just basically the government deciding what they were going to do. Here, each state has twelve different ways to try to get the people who don't qualify for Medicaid and see if you can get them AIDS related, and meanwhile there are people who fall through the cracks.

On the other hand, because they [European countries] all have basically socialized medicine or at least guaranteed health care, once the drugs are approved, they don't worry about costs, cost efficiency, who is getting admitted, who is not getting admitted. All of that is just gone from their lives, or it is just never in their lives. I was just in Greece giving an update on new drugs and experimental agents, and half the drugs I talked about had already been released there. They had many patients on these drugs, and there was absolutely no problem getting them. . . . It was kind of sobering to see a country that has got just a fraction of the gross national product that we do has an annual per capita income of about half of what ours is and they don't talk about rationing health care. They talk about who needs this, who needs that. . . . It made me more embarrassed—the American coming from this very confusing, silly system where I just spend so much time justifying a certain medication, a certain admission to the hospital.

Whereas American medical discourse about the health care system evokes themes of powerlessness, fragmentation, and embarrassment, French discourse about their system is comparatively benign. For one Rousseau physician, AIDS highlights the advantages rather than the problems in the French system, even while recognizing the financial stress it places on that system.

It's true that it is a big security, the Securité Sociale, for such a disease, which is a chronic infection, which lasts a long time, which can perhaps necessitate heavy care, very expensive treatments. It is true that all this is taken in charge by the collectivity. And this is a truly remarkable element. Me, I was very critical of the Securité Sociale. I am a lot less today. . . . But, I think that our system is an excellent system for resolving this type of problem. It costs quite a bit, collectively speaking, but I believe that all those people would not be at all taken care of.

Just as the Americans compared their system to those of Europe, my French informants used comparisons with the United States to underscore themes of fairness. During her presentation on the San Francisco model of care, the Rousseau head nurse talked about the financial problems of American patients in general, citing several US studies about patients needing money to obtain care. She emphasized the high cost of insurance for the chronically ill in the United States, as well as the need for HIV-positive Americans to hide their status from insurance agencies. She summarized by saying, "Nothing is free in the US, even attention." Another Rousseau physician, involved with a lay support organization, made a similar comparison.

The third thing is the social aspect. And in this third aspect, there is a very big difference. In France, for example, there is a system of social protection which is *obligatoire*. It's the law. It's legal. In the United States, the companies are private, and it's impossible to ignore the difference of this protection when people are really sick.

As was the case with the Americans, access to health care is considered a social rather than a medical issue and, for my French informants, distinguishes French identity, French values. The above physician underscored his point with a story about visiting AIDS assistance organizations in the United States.

I didn't work in the United States, but I went there many times, in many parts of the United States, on the West Coast and the East Coast. And during my last travel in November of '89, I spoke with a lot of associations and groups who take care of people who are sick, without work—that means without money, without house or apartment, without anything. . . . We know also this kind of situation sometimes, but it's very, very rare, and I think that the problems we are up against are not the same.

French physicians do share a few problems with their American counterparts in regard to access. A small but significant percentage of patients are covered by private insurance, rather than Securité Sociale, and experience problems similar to American patients in retaining coverage. French physicians, in turn, resort to similar subversive practices to get around these difficulties.

For the moment, medically, I admit to you that I cheat. I cheat to the maximum that I can do it. I don't make lies, but I "forget" to tell certain things [laughs]. . . . Oh, for example, someone has insurance and he gets a pulmonary *Pneumocystis* and I'm asked for the diagnosis. I answer that he has a "pneumopathy." One must not make false documents, but on the other hand, I am effectively persuaded if one marks "pneumopathy A," one marks "P. *Pneumocystis*," and one marks "*P. carinii*," no one pays attention to the fact that this *Pneumocystis* is thus an AIDS [laughs].

Another issue commonly brought out in discourse is that of "marginal" patients, people not covered by any type of insurance. In the United States, this refers to about 40 million people and, as seen previously, is often expanded to include all public aid patients as well. In France, the population of marginals is considerably smaller, encompassing mainly immigrants or visitors from other countries, usually Africa. For example, during a staff meeting, Dr. Farsi mentioned a patient from Zaire who was living "among *les squats*," homeless squatters. She had lymphoma of brain and liver, and Farsi suggested the only question is whether she would stay here or go home to Zaire to die among her family. At another staff meeting, a similar patient provoked discussion on where she should be treated. Dr. Bernard commented that sending her back to Africa would be "brutal," but there was nothing else to be done, adding, "It's not a medical problem; it's a social one." I encountered an analogous incident at Northlake concerning a Mexican patient in the country illegally. Despite the physicians' attempts to circumvent obstacles to his care, he was sent back to Mexico. At Rousseau, Americans are sometimes marginal patients but often emerge in discourse as marginals in their own country:

I think that many times patients in the States have no money for treatment. But the patients of the States we see here in Europe are quite rich, or they have insurance, and so on. I think they have no problems and we never see the poor ones.

French physicians construct their health care system as being fair to patients but problematic for the medical community. One issue concerns the central allocation of money for AIDS care. Rousseau staff were regularly preparing charts and statistics to prove the need for additional funding to the administrative board for public hospitals. One resident related a story about an encounter between Dr. Bernard and an administrator on a recent television program. The administrator had remarked, "Oh, there is enough money [now]," and Bernard had replied angrily, "How much is spent for one Exocet [missile]?"

Another major theme of French informants was that of employment, for both physicians and clinical research assistants.

The problem is to find first the money to have people, and secondly to find people. I imagine if the salary would be sufficient, it would be easier to find people. . . . So even we have difficulties to get grants to pay people. You know, in France when you are working in the public field, they're employed for life. So a number of positions don't fill, because everybody is afraid that if they grant the position, it's for life. So positions are not created. It's very hard. We need people to see patients, we need people to do clinical trials. It's quite impossible actually to employ people.

The health care system is thus constructed as static in regard to personnel, with a few powerful people entrenched in tenured positions. French patients may have access to care, but French physicians do not have access to positions.

A related and more common topic of discourse among the Rousseau physicians is the monolithic French bureaucracy.

I don't know how it is in US, but in France the bureaucracy is very heavy. And the bureaucracy has not changed. You know, between the decision and the realization, you may have two or three years. On the administrative point of view, nothing changes in France. For the [research] protocols, it's also the same. The bureaucracy has taken charge of the protocols, and it's very hard to make it more efficient. I don't know exactly, but, for example, in the US, the ACTG groups have done much more than we have done in France.

We had filed a demand for a retrovirology laboratory, which was financed. And the source was there, and it was refused, on purely administrative grounds. Nothing structural, nothing important, but purely for administrative procedure—that's all. . . . I have the impression that despite the fact that there are a lot of people who have a high quality of education and good technical knowledge of their job, but they're sort of—sometimes you wonder if they're not on another planet.

The health care system that emerges from French discourse is powerful, static, and politically motivated, compared to the American constructions of a fragmented, economically motivated system.[4]

Overall, the French spoke less about their health care system than the Americans. While the French expressed concern about the impact of AIDS on the system, unlike the majority of American informants, they did not construct AIDS as a vehicle for the potential breakdown/overhaul of the entire system. The fit between French culture and the health care system appears strong, as underscored by the nature of the discourse. The intensity of American medical discourse on health care, however, points to this issue as involving a fundamental social value, and AIDS as a medium for reexamining this value.

THE PRACTICE OF MEDICINE

> AIDS has changed medicine in the same way bubonic plague changed
> medicine in the Middle Ages, or the flu epidemic, or polio epidemic, or
> tuberculosis. It brings out some of its quirks.
>
> Chicago clinician

Physicians have likely talked about the practice of medicine since its earliest beginnings. Robert Hahn (1985, 64) refers to this type of discourse as "meta-medical," being about how medicine is or should be done. My informants' discourse is shot through with such meta-medical talk, much of it not specific to AIDS. Nevertheless, my informants use AIDS to explore significant changes in their everyday experience of medical practice, such as the interaction between medical specialties, the role of primary care, and the sense of both personal danger and professional commitment. The boundaries between "medical" and "social" problems are refashioned through discourse, while medicine itself is resituated in a historical context.

Interactions between medical specialties can profoundly impact clinical practice (Helman 1985), while physician discourse about the specialties serves to shape their acknowledged areas of competence, or "turf" (DelVecchio-Good 1985). In the context of AIDS, physicians redefine the nature of the specialties and their practitioners, setting their boundaries in relation to the epidemic. Both French and American informants, many not trained in oncology themselves, often spoke about the field of oncology, contributing another element in the analogies between cancer and AIDS.

It's surprising that oncologists don't work on AIDS. . . . They don't have the same spirit, they are more resigned, more fatalistic. . . . These patients are dying of infectious disease and we [infectious disease specialists] feel "they can't be dying of an infectious disease." We have more fight, we treat the infectious disease, whereas cancer people say, "We can't do anything."

This French excerpt constructs the nature of oncologists and the speaker's own specialty, infectious disease (ID), at the same time. Oncology here is constructed as a field based on acceptance of dying, while infectious disease emerges as its fundamental opposite. Because AIDS is both chronic and fatal, the practice of infectious disease, at least in regard to AIDS, is becoming, or should become, more like oncology. As one French clinician noted, "Now we are with a chronic disease, so there has to be a change in mentality." This theme is shared by my American informants as well.

Many of them [oncologists] fared much better when caring for AIDS patients than some infectious disease doctors, mostly because of the nature of the specialty. Oncologists are used to caring for people with chronic, debilitating, fatal illnesses. They're also used to the idea that very toxic drugs given over a long period of time might enhance one's quality of life and prolong survival. . . . Infectious disease doctors, on the other hand, are usually consultants to other physicians on transient problems, often in life-threatening cases, but usually they would last for a few weeks at the most and you go on to something else. So the mentality of the oncologist was particularly good.

Many of my informants were trained in infectious disease and their discourse, particularly among Americans, represents AIDS as a major agent of change in their field.

Taking care of a relatively young patient population who has a horribly fatal disease, debilitating in many regards, changes a lot of the development of infectious disease as such a premier subspecialty. ID used to be—it was like a cushy-cushy subspecialty that if you wanted to do a fellowship and play golf or something then you did ID. . . . It has really become a very hard, interesting subspecialty. It's almost become an AIDS subspecialty rather than true infectious disease.

The field of infectious disease, in this discourse, has become the field of AIDS, transforming a consultant-style practice based on treating acute, curable conditions into a primary care practice based on treating a chronic, progressive condition.

Infectious disease has never really had a chronic life-threatening illness to take care of. And we never really had an outpatient practice for the most part. So this [AIDS] completely changed the two most basic aspects of infectious diseases.

Thus, in the context of AIDS, infectious disease is caught up in a struggle to maintain its boundaries as a separate field:

I think that the field of infectious disease has become the field of AIDS, pretty much. . . . Our infectious disease society in the Bay Area, we had a moratorium on AIDS cases being presented at the bimonthly rounds. You know, you weren't allowed to present AIDS cases [laugh]. And you are pretty hard-pressed to find something interesting that's not HIV related.

A conversation between a Northlake resident and Dr. Holtzman underscores this definitional conflict. The resident was interested in finding an infectious disease fellowship program that focused on HIV. Dr. Holtzman replied, "Traditional infectious disease services that are interested in bacterial infections, the *Staph. aureus* [a bacteria], don't seem really interested in HIV. Some people have suggested that it should be a separate specialty."

With the advent of AIDS, ID specialists find themselves in increasing demand. Their specialized knowledge is now paradoxically relevant at a time when medicine, as one informant put it, "means managing chronic disease." Far from being a "cushy" consultation service, the field of infectious disease is now constructed as continuous managing of complex conditions.

Well, Dr. Petersdorf wrote a paper, I've forgotten how long ago, saying that we are producing too many infectious disease specialists and they would end up culturing each other's throats. That was pre-AIDS. And that was obviously wrong, so that there's now a demand by hospital, by group practices, clinics, for persons who are trained in infectious disease. . . . It's turned it around from a field which was primarily a consultation practice, hospital based, to a field which now has large primary care responsibilities and much greater ambulatory activity. . . . That's all AIDS. It's had a major impact."

For my American informants, what was once a classic specialty practice is emerging as primary care, in part because of the continued social stigma of AIDS and, as discussed previously, the uncertainty of the usual primary care physicians in dealing with the mysteries of AIDS medicine.

It is certainly different with HIV, where ID has become sort of the primary care specialty for this group of patients, in part because other doctors don't feel comfortable or don't want to care for them. I'm speaking in generalities. But we have become a primary care specialty for HIV patients.

At Northlake, many of the patients utilized the clinic physicians for all of their health care needs, not only those related to HIV. The construction of AIDS as a disease that can affect every organ system reinforces this practice as well. Even the Northlake ophthalmologist, geographically separate from the clinic, talked about his increasing primary care role. At a clinic presentation, he told the story of a new patient, diagnosed with an opportunistic eye infection, who did not know he was HIV-positive. The doctor remarked, "It was a double whammy. Not only did I have to tell him that he had CMV, I had to counsel him about HIV." Thus, even non-ID specialists find that they must do a little primary care work. Additionally, as the patient load has increased, more general internists have been added to the clinic staff on a part-time basis.

At Northlake and other US clinics, the "turf" boundaries become even more confused when the patient develops an AIDS-related cancer. The oncologist takes over the cancer treatment, which often involves substantial decision-making powers regarding the patient's overall care. The question of who is the primary care provider becomes increasingly tangled in the context of AIDS. For example, the Northlake HIV team saw a patient with Kaposi's sarcoma of the lungs and a fever, which may be from *Pneumocystis* or the KS. A fierce discussion ensued between the HIV team and the oncologist. The oncologist refused to do chemotherapy unless infection was ruled out or the fever dissipated, while the HIV team felt that the fever was due to the KS and thus could only be relieved by chemotherapy. This turf battle lasted for over a day and was eventually resolved through a change in the patient's condition. Turf issues such as this are renegotiated with every encounter, as the role of the specialties continues to evolve through AIDS.

The kind of turf battle described above is, in contrast, quite rare at the Rousseau clinic. Instead, arguments over the treatment for inpatients were fairly common, due to the clinic doctors having no formal authority over inpatient care. In Paris, AIDS seems to be treated largely by ID specialists or general practitioners,[5] while the role of other specialists, including oncologists, is limited to consults for specific events instead of overall chronic treatment. Rather than the specialties reemerging as primary care, primary care and infectious disease are incorporating the knowledge and practices of other fields.

For example, according to the Rousseau physicians and my own observations, an eye exam using an ophthalmoscope, known as a *funduscopic exam*, is considered the sole province of ophthalmology specialists. In the United States, in contrast, this exam is a routine part of almost every physical. Given the potential for infections involving the eye in AIDS, Dr. Bernard encourages his staff to become proficient in performing funduscopic exams. Similarly, Rousseau physicians manage Kaposi's sarcoma chemotherapy. Thus, via AIDS, Rousseau physicians cross the boundaries of two specialties, incorporating specialist knowledge into a primary care foundation.

In France particularly, AIDS serves as a medium for redefining the role of the general practitioner (GP). Many of the Rousseau physicians are general practitioners who developed an interest in AIDS, usually through seeing a number of AIDS patients in their own offices. In an experimental program, Dr. Bernard has trained them regarding HIV disease and incorporated them into the clinic on a part-time basis. As one such generalist explained, AZT can only be distributed at the hospital, not at the GP's office or a standard pharmacy. He remarked that this is inconvenient for asymptomatic patients, since it forces them to arrange a visit to the hospital clinic simply to refill medication.[6] He stated that the follow-up for these patients could be done by the *médecins de ville*, freeing the hospital-based specialists to care for sicker patients: "At least 25 percent of the patients could be followed in town." Through discourse on AIDS, the role of the general practitioner takes on new significance in the French health care system.

It is true that until the moment that AIDS had appeared, the hospital was very removed from the concerns of the town doctors. . . . Because the town doctors became patient recruiters, we became interesting for the hospitals, and the hospitals made a lot of effort to go out and meet us. And there was the effect of meeting people like Dr. Bernard, who has a wonderfully open mind for meeting others, allowing us to be trained, allowing us another discourse, another way of conceiving medicine.

In France, there are plenty of primary care physicians, but they have been limited in power by the structure of the French health care system. In the United States, there are relatively fewer primary care physicians, and their involvement with AIDS seems hampered by the ambiguity of AIDS itself, defined as a primary care problem requiring specialist knowledge. A New York family practitioner described a typical day:

I have a patient knocking on the door, asking for Motrin [an analgesic], "because it hurts when I pee. I have a fever, cough, and night sweats, but just give me the Motrin." Then a minute later, a woman comes in the office and falls on her face because she's having a seizure and left-sided hemiplegia [paralysis] because of her cerebral toxoplasmosis. This is not what they said I'd be doing when you go into family practice.

The result in both the French and American cases is patient overload. As the number of AIDS patients and the standardization of treatments increase, the role of generalists takes on greater significance.

Because as the numbers continue to increase, the general internists are the ones who are going to end up taking care of the majority of the population. And there is nothing really magical about caring for AIDS patients as long as you understand the disease process. You don't have to be an infectious disease—trained expert to take care of AIDS patients.

In effect, the bulk of inpatient care is already being done by general internists with subspecialty consultation from infectious disease and the AIDS service. I would say that's the right way to go. We can't continue to try and just expand infectious disease to handle the enormous caseload. It's just not practical.

The experience of AIDS thus continues to act as a vehicle, both in discourse and in practice, for redefining the nature of various medical specialties, their interactions, and the role of primary care.

Medicine is more than the sum of its specialties. My informants often talk about how AIDS has fundamentally changed the nature of medical practice. Just as the boundaries of the specialties are reconfigured through discourse, so are the boundaries of medicine itself, the distinction between medical and nonmedical problems. Biomedicine is more and more the chosen explanatory framework, coexisting with or even supplanting moralistic models of many phenomena (Foucault 1972). However, as Hahn (1985, 97) observes, a strong dichotomy between medical and nonmedical pervades physicians' discourse. Medical problems are generally considered to be organic and physiological in nature. They are objective phenomena which can be validated by one or more outside observers. Nonmedical problems, in contrast, are characterized as subjective, having little or no physical manifestation. They are often spoken of as "emotional" or "social" in nature.

My informants, like other physicians, recognize that many medical conditions have significant nonmedical components, and often address their patients' emotional and social status. Still, these clinicians seem most comfortable with what are constructed as strictly medical problems, such as diagnosing an infection and finding the appropriate antibiotic. As discussed previously, activities such as managing a patient's financial access to said antibiotic emerge as dissatisfying, taking time away from the physician's "real work." In my informants' discourse, AIDS expands and highlights this problematic boundary between medical and social problems.

It [AIDS] challenged all of our attitudes yet again about homosexuality and chemical dependency principally. I think it has also changed medicine in terms of requiring medicine to confront and deal with social implications of the disease and not pretend that medicine was a very limited context diagnosis and treatment, because it is clear that many of the things that make the most difference for our patients in clinic or in hospital are nonmedical interventions that involve entitlements or housing or, you know, other related nonmedical issues.

While the above American speaker classes housing and such as nonmedical issues, he nevertheless places them in the purview of the clinic's activities. AIDS blurs the boundaries between the medical and the social, requiring physicians to expertly straddle that boundary. Chemical dependency—drug abuse—is one of the social issues that, through AIDS, is drawn further into the medical domain.

There has really been sort of this orphan situation in terms of medicine in general and substance abuse treatment. And there has been a movement over the last few years to try and incorporate it more into the medical training education or at least medical practice. . . . So I think what AIDS has done in a sense has both shed light on the potentially important role of drug abuse treatment and the AIDS epidemic, but it has also at the same time exposed the weaknesses of that system.

Most of my informants, however, have had little or no training in handling drug abuse, particularly on other than an individual scale. During a staff meeting at Rousseau, a visiting speaker introduced the topic of incorporating recently imprisoned drug users and prostitutes into the clinic. Dr. Bernard remarked that the problem of drug use is ultimately a collective and social one and cannot be solved on an individual basis. AIDS acts as a medium for redefining social problems and brings the social smack into the medical. Doctors now are expected to talk expertly about the issues of prostitution and drug abuse, and while some do, many feel uncomfortable, even resentful, of this new responsibility.

In the clinical experience of AIDS, social problems are often inextricably entwined with medical ones, to the point where the physician may feel powerless to affect the situation at all. One patient encounter at Northlake illustrates this experience. The patient was a financially strapped seventeen-year-old woman, six and a half months pregnant with her second child. She had tested HIV-positive when she was pregnant with her first child, born less than a year ago. The physician spent over fifteen minutes going over the patient's family history.[7] Two out of three sisters were also HIV-positive, and one had three children who tested positive at birth. There was a history of drug abuse in several family members, as well as diabetes. A family pattern of not seeking or following through with medical assistance for any health problem was central to the patient's narrative. As the patient's sister commented, "We don't like to go to doctors very much." After the patient's visit, the physician shook his head and told me that he did not have much hope for this patient continuing treatment. The implication of this statement, combined with the patient's narrative, is clear: No matter what any of us do, the patient, her baby, her HIV-positive sisters, and their HIV-positive children will quickly develop AIDS and die. The whole encounter evoked a sense of being overwhelmed, of being an insignificant factor in the patient's well-being.

We've pretty much decided that poverty is a problem that we can't solve or don't care to make an attempt to solve. So, in a way we've redlined AIDS, too, and that the problem has gotten too big; it affects people with all kinds of other problems. We can't put a roof over everybody's head, let alone treat this horrible disease.

For some of my informants, experiences such as these spark attempts to accept the larger boundary, incorporating the social into the medical, and vice versa.

In France, it [AIDS] is really something very important because it made people get moving, those who are interested; it motivated them, it forced them to get training, to involve themselves in other than medical problems, to take in charge [*prise en charge*] the social problems, the problems of society. . . . One has gone past, a little, the medical arena.

As we have seen before, the AIDS epidemic can be considered a rite of passage for the medical community, a liminal time in which boundaries are more fluid, fostering a reshaping of the meanings of medicine. As one French physician concluded:

AIDS is an example of the necessity to see a sickness with all the aspects in the life of someone. I mean, that we can nevermore see a sickness with only the side of medicine. A sickness in the life of someone now has psychological aspects, familial aspects, social aspects, work aspects, and medical aspects, and all that are one in many things for the sick people.

AIDS has not only changed what constitutes medical work but how that work is carried out, primarily due to the institution of universal precautions—treating the bodily fluids of all patients as if they contained HIV.

I think it [AIDS] has made us aware of transmissibility to a greater extent than anything else. We instituted things like universal precautions on every patient that is admitted to the hospital. We now bag blood and all specimens. That was never done before. The procedure in the operating room has changed—double gloving, goggles, no passing of sharp instruments from person to person. All of that has changed with the AIDS epidemic.

It's [medicine] changed dramatically. I mean, the consciousness of universal precautions and the consciousness of the fear of blood transfusions . . . wearing of gloves by everyone practically. Initially when all of this started, having to wear gloves and masks and gowns to examine patients.

A conversation between three Northlake physicians illustrates how protective practices are incorporated in the daily life of the clinic. Dr. Landry was carrying the needle-stick pager, which notifies him when an exposure incident has occurred, as required by hospital policy. He remarked on how low the threshold is for people to call in:

> *Dr. Landry*: A nurse called me the other day, saying, "I had a needle-stick eight months ago, and I never really got tested or anything."
> *Dr. Holtzman*: Tell her to take a bath in AZT.
> *Dr. Landry*: Really, the threshold is getting lower and lower. A bunch of security guards had to restrain a patient in adolescent psych [psychiatric unit] the other day. One guy got scratched on the hand, and he called me, wanting AZT.
> *Dr. Holtzman*: Did you see that article in *JAMA* [*Journal of the American Medical Association*] about the person who got splashed in the eye and seroconverted?

A doctor from the adjacent Veterans hospital jumped in the discussion. He had recently cut his palm, and his hand was wrapped in two bandages. He remarked:

"Yeah, now I can see all my people walking around wearing goggles. You know, though, I wrapped my hand up like this because I'm constantly seeing HIV patients. Before, I wouldn't have done it this way." While universal precautions are not practiced in the same way by everyone in the medical community, nearly everyone has implemented some type of protective practice, be it using gloves on physical exam or immediate disposal of used syringes in marked boxes. Thus, AIDS has changed how medicine is done on a daily basis.

The practice and its accompanying discourse construct medicine as a dangerous enterprise, marked with the potential for contagion and even death. Talk about occupational exposure to HIV was a large portion of the health care forum on transmission in Paris and an even more common topic of discussion among my American informants.

It's [AIDS] certainly kept a lot of people out of internal medicine and out of the various specialties in internal medicine because they are fearful of contagion. It's showed us that as physicians we cannot be as isolated and dogmatic and stick to old principles and say, "Well, we do this because this is the way we have always done it."

My informants often use this discourse to situate medicine historically, constructing a longitudinal view of the nature of the profession.

First, it [AIDS] has reminded us that we are at some personal risk in the course of doing our work. That's been a really important reminder. It wasn't a huge period of time that we forgot that, but we forgot it very thoroughly in the period from, say, 1945 to 1981. And now it's back.

In this discourse, medicine has always been dangerous, and the antibiotic era of the recent past emerges as a mere aberration. The theme is consistent: AIDS reminds us of the true nature of medicine.

I think it [AIDS] has brought back some old things associated with medicine. There was a very brief period between the late '50s and the AIDS epidemic where there were very few dangerous infectious diseases left in the developed nations. . . . I mean, there wasn't a lot of threat to health care workers, patients weren't dying from these things, everything was treatable. So, we got lulled into this sort of complacent type of attitude.

It is in this historically framed discourse about the nature of medicine that my informants draw on the analogy of plague.

It's [AIDS] let everybody know that we haven't conquered all the infectious diseases in the world. It caused doctors to realize that there may be some very dangerous diseases out there that they're going to have to take care of. Go back to the bubonic plague. It's brought forward some new diseases that no one ever thought of.

You look historically, doctors were always on the front. They were always getting TB or bubonic plague. The doctors ran out of the major hospitals of London and left the doors open and head for the hills of Wales and hid out for a year. . . . I mean, doctors have always been at risk in the past; it's only been recently that they really haven't had any risk. So now there is risk again. Now there is a deadly infectious disease again. We are kind of back to how it used to be.

The discourse of danger constructs physicians as individuals as well as the medical community as a whole. Physicians are and have always been afraid. They, too, run for the hills in times of plague, and the ones that stay behind are not always the best suited for the job:[8] "It's [AIDS] also given the perspective that physicians are human beings, and that some don't want to treat AIDS patients. Some do, and some know how to do it and do it, and some don't know how to do it, and do it."

Discourse on AIDS acts as a medium for reexamining the nature of being a physician. AIDS invokes a question of the medical community that is perhaps fundamental to all human experience: "Why are you here?"

Absolutely, it [AIDS] brings fear back to medicine. Fear has always been in medicine, we always take chances, and some choose lines of work that take more chances than others. It really kind of shakes some basic questions of why you are in medicine.

Taken together, the discourse constructs AIDS as a trial by fire for the medical community. Some will turn away from the challenge:

I think it [AIDS] is affecting a lot of occupational choices. . . . That's been pretty well shown that people will often base their residency choice based on the perceived incidence of HIV in that particular hospital or within that particular field.

I think that [AIDS] has changed medicine substantially because people are now making alternative career choices rather than going into medicine. So people have to think about what they are doing in a much different light.

Ultimately, those who remain will emerge from the trial stronger for the experience.

One of the things that's clearly happened in AIDS is that health care providers are confronted with a disease to which they might be at risk. And having lived through that period where we were intensely afraid to catch AIDS ourselves from our patients and nevertheless having decided to continue seeing patients during that period, those of us who went through that said, "Well, yeah. Maybe we really are willing to give ourselves for our patients, even at the expense of being willing to assume personal risk of mortality in the process." And I think that's something that had completely been lost from medicine. . . . I think we've realized that we still are like doctors of old in the sense of being willing to do that.

In talking about AIDS, my informants establish a link with their professional history, enabling them to renew their identity as physicians in the face of a dangerous enterprise.

In sum, discourse on AIDS refashions the nature and practice of medicine, its specialties, and its dangers. The plague becomes an opportunity for rebirth, a fire enabling the phoenix of medicine to rise once more.

AIDS has given medicine a new reason to be enthusiastic about itself. I think we have achieved incredible successes with AIDS. We have shown the value of clinical research. We have shown the value of an interactive system of medical care, of focusing on community issues, of interactions between patients and the health care providers. And I certainly hope all those things continue to be with us long after AIDS is gone.

NOTES

1. This figure varies considerably, depending on the study. The cost has been lessened over the course of the epidemic with the development of prophylaxis for opportunistic infections and the increased use of home care. The efficient integration and use of all health care services, with increased reliance on outpatient treatment, have come to be known as the "San Francisco model" and have been adapted for use throughout the United States. See Volberding's (1988) "Caring for the Patient with AIDS: An Integrated Approach."

2. If an insurance company refuses to pay for additional days of hospitalization, or certain equipment or procedures, the hospital is forced to "eat" the bill. Thus, poorly insured or uninsured patients cost hospitals money. Many American hospitals have departments dedicated to utilization review, with the goal of cutting these costs.

3. *Codes* refers to diagnostic codes, known as DRGs (diagnostic-related groups), which guide billing and reimbursement by insurance, particularly Medicaid and Medicare. Each patient stay is assigned a code or set of codes theoretically appropriate to their actual disease. The hospital and physicians are then reimbursed on the basis of the average length of hospitalization (and complexity of care) for that category rather than the actual hospitalization. In 1991, codes for AIDS and AIDS-related sicknesses were both inaccurate and inadequate in terms describing the patient's condition. For some AIDS-related diagnoses, appropriate codes did not exist. Although coding has improved since then, it still lags behind the rapidly changing medical models of AIDS.

4. When I mentioned the level of American bureaucracy to the Rousseau physicians, they remained skeptical. Then Dr. Martine was sent some forms by the California public aid office for an American patient she had last seen four months ago. After going through the six forms, she exclaimed to me, "American bureaucracy is just as bad as in France!"

5. HIV infection is not uncommonly diagnosed and even treated by dermatologists in France, who historically have covered care of sexually transmitted diseases.

6. As of 1991, French general practitioners were allowed to renew, but not initiate, AZT prescriptions.

7. To put this in perspective, new patient visits generally last an hour in total, including patient history, past medical history, family history, physical exam, diagnosis, and discussion. To spend a quarter of this time on family history alone is significant.

8. Historically, civic authorities relied on a variety of incentives, including increased payment and citizenship, to attract physicians during epidemics (Fox 1988b).

10

Good Science, Bad Science

What was great for me is that when I think to these years, back to 1982, 1983, '84, '85, I learned a great deal. I learned about viruses, I learned about politics, I learned about science in general, I learned about human beings. It was great because AIDS was so *mediatique*.

French researcher

Just as clinicians refashion the practice of medicine through discourse on AIDS, so my research informants use AIDS as a medium for talking about the scientific enterprise. As the above quote suggests, discourse on AIDS serves to reinterpret the nature of science, communication with the lay public, and the relations between science, politics, and clinical medicine. A central theme in this discourse is the distinction between "good science" and "bad science," increasingly problematic in the context of AIDS.

In talking about their work on AIDS and HIV, many of my research informants expand their discourse to cover the nature of scientific research itself.

The bottom line is there's no dogma in this disease [AIDS]. . . . I have to tell people, in science and nature, one of the most exciting things is to take something that's so tried and true and ask other questions. Is it really? Are there exceptions? That's how you decipher new concepts that may have you make even more common denominators.

Science is defined by the American researcher above as challenging the obvious, unscrambling the code to reveal fundamental relationships. The challenge comes not only from nature but from colleagues.

You know, science is not about making a pronouncement and having everybody say, "Oh, that's nice," and go along. It's about being challenged. . . . Scientists are taught that you take data apart, you rip it to shreds, you analyze it, you look for holes in it. And if the presenter hasn't seen these obvious, or perhaps not so obvious, deficiencies, you call it to their attention. . . . That's what science is all about.

In this sense, science is often contrasted with religion or magic.

Science ultimately is charged with being the antithesis of witchcraft. Witchcraft plays on the dark side of the human persona. That's what it's about, and that's what voodoo and all that stuff does, plays on the irrational side of the human. Science tries to play on the rational.

Science, specifically good science, thus is about challenging and accepting challenge in order to promote objectivity. According to my informants, bad science rejects challenge, abandons objectivity, and thus, dangerously, leaves the realm of the rational. The researcher below uses the work of Peter Duesberg as an example of bad science.

The thing that annoys me about Peter is that he is not by my view practicing the tools of science. He's not looking at all the data objectively and drawing conclusions. He's looking for those things that support his point of view, and selectively presenting those.

However, as another American researcher noted, even good science requires an element of the magical: "I think that the lesson I learned from that [set of experiments], in retrospect, is that science really depends on a lot of luck, as well as good science. We did good science, and we had bad luck.

Good science, in the discourse of my informants, is not a sudden discovery made in a blaze of inspiration. Rather, it is methodical and repetitive.

It's the old Beethoven remark, actually: It's 90 percent perspiration and 10 percent inspiration. I'd say we're 98 percent perspiration. There are very few new ideas. . . . What we did was to clone the sequence of the genome, and it's not a new idea at all. But it had to be done. It's like stamp collecting.

Any experiment you're designing in your lab, if it's a good experiment, then a dozen other groups are also doing exactly the same thing.

Bad science, predictably, is characterized by quick, dramatic conclusions that have not undergone repetitive challenge.

One of the things that concerned me was that you did not make a statement of importance, such as "We found the virus that causes AIDS," unless you covered your territory. It was too demeaning as a scientist. . . . I learned as well, you don't make conclusions on theory; you do the experiment.

AIDS research, as characterized by both French and American informants, has been particularly plagued by bad science.

I believe that still the AIDS research is a little more respected than it used to be, in '86, '87. . . . The first years it was really terrible; it was the worst groups in virology that started on the AIDS virus. And the real good groups in virology wouldn't touch it, for it was second-grade research, easily published.

The other thing which has changed is that not only do we have these great scientists that are working, but also a lot of other scientists are working on AIDS. . . . All the scientists have to get grants to work, doing experiments and writing up papers, and I think in the AIDS fields so many papers are just bullshit.

As seen in the first narrative above, there were few scientists working on AIDS early in the epidemic, enabling mediocre papers to be published due to a lack of outside challenge. Later in the epidemic, as presented in the second example, there are more scientists of all calibers involved, leading to increased competition and promoting quick announcements of insufficiently challenged experiments.

That's another thing that has changed. Too many people working on AIDS, trying to get money, trying to have a paper published, even before the experiment is completely done. . . . I don't think it's working very well these days. Too many papers, not very careful experiments.

Thus, researchers' discourse on AIDS and science appears to construct a no-win situation, such that no matter how many scientists of whatever caliber are involved in AIDS, there will be an unusual amount of bad science.

Why is AIDS intrinsically linked to bad science in these narratives? Three major themes of AIDS research, all interrelated, emerge out of the discourse: money, public visibility, and politics. The excerpt immediately above mentions competition for research money as an integral element in the production of bad science. In 1987, many of my French informants spoke about the lack of money, particularly in the early days of the epidemic. In 1991, my American informants expressed similar recollections, noting that funding increased substantially after 1985, when Rock Hudson died.

Now the discourse is opposite. Too much money has flooded the system, encouraging bad science in AIDS as well as reducing money for good science in other fields.

The government has been very successful at spending money, and they are able to come back and tell Congress year after year that, yes, they've increased the budget as Congress has requested and spent the money. But they really spend it very often on projects that are just spinning the wheels.

We had a lot of money poured into AIDS, and it's actually hurt the scientific community. Just remember, before this disease became in the forefront of the limelight, a lot of other people were working on a lot of other clearly important things. . . . A friend of mine who actually does that [genetic research] is a very capable scientist, has had a lot of publications in very big journals, only to lose funding because all of the money is going into HIV.

For my French informants particularly, the large increase in money for AIDS seems to taint the scientific enterprise itself:

It is very hard to communicate. Everybody keeps everything a secret and is very protective of their work. It's getting worse. I guess when too much money is involved, you get that kind of competition. That's not real science.

There is a lot more money. Too much I think. . . . And research on AIDS is not so well liked by the other people. If you ask for a position at INSERM or CNRS, they often say, "Ah, but with AIDS you don't need it; you have a lot of money." Someone who is working on AIDS is seen as a bit of a *profiteur*. It has a bad reputation, and you have to fight against this bad reputation.

Money, particularly talk about money, is a disreputable subject among the French (Carroll 1988). This French scientific discourse is similar to that regarding money in the clinical setting. As the practice of medicine is constructed as being above commercial considerations,[1] so, too, is the practice of science. For the French informants, too much money not only promotes bad science; it is bad science.

Americans, in contrast, are more ambivalent regarding money and will often cite the benefits of increased funding:

There's a lot of money in it [AIDS]. I understand that it's a significant health problem—and I'm not questioning that—but just the fact that there were no established research groups, nothing out here in the scientific community that had traditionally focused on this problem. And then all of a sudden, people are—it's sort of a vacuum that's filled with money. People are being sucked into it generally for the positive reasons of having a chance to have an impact, to express good ideas.

By having this kind of Manhattan Project for AIDS, it is doing for my discipline—infectious diseases and immunology and epidemiology—what the Manhattan Project did for physicists in the 1940s. It is giving the whole field a huge intellectual and financial boost. So it's a very good place to be in my field right now because it is where the money is and it is where a lot of the intellectual resources are.

AIDS makes the role of money in science problematic. The urgent nature of the epidemic allows for an increased acceptance of money, at least in the United States, as a means of directing research without tainting its objectivity.

They say the best thing to do in science is to put out the money, let smart people do their work within the basic science approach. And there's no doubt in my mind that there's merit to that. Some of the greatest scientific discoveries have been made in basic research. But in the AIDS field, we do have to do somewhat more directed research, because of its declared priority in the public health.

Besides carrying the taint of money, AIDS research contradicts the tenet that good science is slow and unspectacular. AIDS research makes headlines, from the torrid reports of the Gallo-Montagnier dispute to the weekly announcements of new treatments. Thus, AIDS carries with it great potential for bad science on both sides of the Atlantic.

The problem with the media has been an interest in the eye-catching headline and so, for instance, the media has been caught up in the whole Gallo-Montagnier story. And certainly the history of science has been replete with that sort of interest. But that fact is a sideshow to what's going on in HIV. It has no relevance to where we need to go or need to be doing. It may have relevance to who gets royalties and to the lawyers, but it has no relevance to science or in taking care of people.

I just wish they [physicians] were more suspicious of what is still said, because there are still groups who are publishing, in scientific journals or in the press, results with no basis. And I think this still gets a lot of attention from media, and it's regrettable. I'm not sure the story of *Mycoplasma* [causing AIDS] could have existed for another field.

The last example, from a French researcher, points to Montagnier's recent research on *Mycoplasma* as an example of bad science, a result of its high visibility. A spectacular announcement, for most of my informants, indicates bad science, suggesting that the researcher did not adequately challenge the data. Dr. Bernard at Rousseau spoke similarly about Montagnier's *Mycoplasma* research: "The error is arriving at premature conclusions. . . . One must have a certain prudence, and keep to scientific rigor." Gallo's highly publicized announcement of his discovery of HIV and the French physicians' announcement of cyclosporin as a treatment for AIDS were also among the stories used by my informants to construct the nature of bad science and its relationship to publicity.[2]

Such announcements are linked structurally to money in both countries. In France, young researchers need to publish spectacular results quickly in order to have access to positions, while researchers in the United States need dramatic findings in order to get funding for their projects. A young French researcher commented: "A very hot subject [AIDS], very competitive. There is a little advantage to working on AIDS. You get money; publications are easier, too." The money and spectacle inherent in AIDS research provides opportunities to overcome these structural obstacles, which then lead to bad science or, as Jay Winsten (1985, 15) terms it, "science by press conference." Cook and Colby (1992, 84) note that the media's priorities, as well as the researcher's fiscal needs, can thus serve to frame research questions.

The most telling theme in discourse on AIDS and science concerns the role of politics. Scientific ideology holds that science is an apolitical discovery of truth, of "the way things really are." That science *is* a political process, involving relationships of power and authority, is rendered visible by the spectacle of AIDS, much to the unease of French and American informants alike. A few of the references were to political pressures from outside the scientific community, as in this American example:

Really extremist politicians, for some reason in this disease, because of the embarrassment of other more mainline politicians, tend to get involved in AIDS. These extremists often wield a ridiculous amount of power, because there's a vacuum left from other people who just don't stand up and say, "Come on, you guys. We need to know about this."

Most of the discourse, however, focuses on power relations within the scientific community.

I think what we're doing is carrying it [new experiments] over to the extent that it is HIV and it's very political, it gets the limelight, and it's all this historical stuff. . . . It's an extremely political thing. And I think that's probably far more important than anything else. It's as political scientific-wise as it is political at the politics level.

The American researcher cited above also provided the following narrative:

It's difficult to obtain reagents, for instance, in a case where you might want to obtain a reagent from a lab that's been working in the field of HIV for a number of years, and it may be a government lab. . . The bottom line is that it's really difficult to obtain the reagents that you may want to use. And it's a scientific thing. It's: "I have it. I want to do the work on it. I don't want to give it to anybody else, because they may do this thing."

Politics in science means control: over material resources, over funding, over information. While American informants did talk about these issues to some extent, they were a central theme among the French. Within the French labs I visited, stories about competition, conflict, and bureaucracy abound, recounting and reconstituting the identity of the lab, the research institute, or the French scientific community as a whole.

I think it is a moral obligation to publish quickly, to give information. We also give all the material to other groups if they want it. Some people hold on to information so only they can make further discoveries. I think this is morally wrong.

In France, money is given essentially because you are very powerful in the system and you don't have to have results. You just have to know the good person to get money.

So they're [INSERM] starting now raising money, and the money is going to be going to fundamental biotechnology applied to viruses. It's going to go to groups already proficient in that thing; they don't fund new groups, for sure. That's also part of the French story—they don't fund you unless you've already been established, and you're only established if you're part of the institution. It's a circle.

Several common themes emerge from these examples. There is a sense of restriction, in regard to who is allowed to do research and what research they are allowed to perform. Research efforts are further confined by a large, dominant bureaucracy. Access to power is thus limited, reinforced by a lack of cohesion and extreme individualism among members of the scientific community and characterized by secrecy and competition. This discourse thus reinforces, and is reinforced by, the structure of French scientific research, with its fierce competition for a small number of tenured positions and the power of those occupying those positions.

The synthesis of restriction and individualism results in the creation of "star scientists," powerful people who have access to money, resources, and most important, information. These stars have the bureaucracy on their side and, indeed, may be portrayed as part of it. Gallo and Montagnier, for example, have emerged as such stars: "Even if they generate an idea that doesn't pan out, just because they're Montagnier and Gallo it's worth paying attention to, because they are extremely bright people. And major players in the AIDS field and will be for a long time.

For both French and American AIDS researchers, represented below, the Gallo-Montagnier dispute remains the primary parable on the dangers of politics in science.

I'm very well aware of Montagnier-Gallo story. For me, it's simple—you've got two people who made fundamental contributions. It's very similar to Salk and Sabin. Both get tremendous credit in my book for fundamental contributions to polio. The fact that Salk and Sabin duked it out in public for thirty years prevented them from getting a Nobel Prize, and Montagnier and Gallo aren't going to get the Nobel Prize either. They're digging their own grave, and they're jumping in it. The hell with them, as far as I'm concerned.

Then, of course, they [Gallo and Montagnier] got in the whole division that the rest of the world did between the Pasteur Institute and NCI [National Cancer Institute] on the study of the virus and they kind of divided everyone. It divided the French. It divided the Americans. It divided the rest of the world. It was a very bad thing, and the French sometimes had it worse within the Institut Pasteur even.

Political infighting on the level seen in the Gallo-Montagnier dispute is constructed by my informants as grotesquely inappropriate and damaging to the scientific community. It is the epitome of bad science. It makes visible that science is not done apart from politics, national identity, personal identity, or economic motivations. In terms of the Gallo-Montagnier dispute,[3] this inhibited the scientific community from countering Gallo's (or for that matter, Montagnier's) narratives, because to do so would have required public participation in what is characterized as a "political" dispute. Thus, it was left to nonscientists such as Randy Shilts and particularly John Crewdson to forge a coherent alternative narrative (J. Feldman 1992c).

In the French scientific community, the divisions over Montagnier's Mycoplasma theory emerge as another narrative linking politics and bad science. At a Rousseau conference, for example, Dr. Bernard commented: "I told Montagnier directly that he is perhaps on an erroneous track. But he is isolated, not out in the field, in the reality. It is something political." To Bernard, a clinician, laboratory science in itself is isolated from reality, but the political influence in science is even further afield. To another French researcher, the conflict over Montagnier's new theory exemplifies power relationships inherent within the structure of the French scientific community.

Maybe you know Montagnier now is convinced that HIV is not the cause of AIDS, and he is trying to include his views to the rest of the team. And for us, there is no scientific evidence; he was unable to provide us with scientific evidence. So we're not interested on working on this, and it has created some conflict. And in France, labs are run by the director, who has every right to the money. . . . The money is granted to the director of the lab, who is able to redistribute it as he wishes.

Money and publicity are interwoven in the discourse on politics, to the point that they often appear as an inextricable troika, a hallmark of bad science.

If someone stepped up and said, "I've discovered that *Mycoplasma* is the cause of tuberculosis," for example, probably everyone would say this guy is crazy. But it's Montagnier, and it's absurd, and so I think that everything said about AIDS research is picked up by the press and amplified.

The moral of all these stories, particularly among the French, is that good science gets done in spite of the stars, in spite of the political infighting.

There is the world of "bosses." We don't need it. And there is the world of scientists underneath. I think it's functioning correctly, just like any other field of research, even if there are conflicts between institutes that prevent us from working with people.

In fact, the mark of good science is its separation from politics: "There isn't anything to study about how people study AIDS. There is, on the other hand, a lot of politics and inefficiency. . . . In France, AIDS is *very* political—it's all political. We must keep politics out of science." It is a separation my informants have yet to find—indeed, may never find in the world of AIDS.

Equally important to my informants, AIDS has brought scientific research, bad and good, out from behind the bench and into the public domain.

The amount of interest of nonscientific people in the science of what we're doing is completely unprecedented. And the involvement that they are insisting on having, that degree of involvement in the process is totally unprecedented in the history of science.

This involvement draws researchers into a communicative role similar to that of clinicians, since they, too, provide the authoritative story on AIDS. Many of my informants were surprisingly reflexive about speaking with the lay public.

Scientists are notoriously stupid when it comes to expressing themselves; [they] don't realize the implications. . . . There is a great reluctance to explain science. We think it's too complicated, takes too much time. . . . I think you've got to go from the premise that science has to be open. You say, "Oh I can't be bothered now," and in the long run, it's not good. You're just contributing to ignorance.

It's part of the world of science. It should be more high-profile than it is. Unless you get your ideas across to people, in your grant writing, in your papers, to the public. I mean, I'm a taxpayer, and if you can't explain to me what you are going to do with my money, I'm not going to give it to you.

Researchers recognize a necessity for sharing discourse with the lay public, yet this very publicity contravenes the tenets of good science.

At one point I thought it was wrong to talk to the press; it was again not what a respectable scientist does. . . . You do your work. You don't go for publicity. I now realize that I'm in a disease that is highly public minded. The money I am using is coming from the public. So I have to be able to talk to the public.

Communication is problematic, yet essential. Scientific narratives must be conveyed not only to the lay public but to the clinical side of the medical community as well.

That's what AIDS is about. We need to communicate very sophisticated messages to our elite audience because we have to drive science with them. We have to keep them all informed about the state of the art and where things are moving. We have to communicate to our second rung, which is our nursing, our physician, our nonscientific professional—not basic science but more pragmatic applied science rung. We've got to communicate to our politicians, to our educated laypeople who don't have any scientific background but have to know enough about the issue to make policy.

Discourse on AIDS thus constructs a scientific enterprise that, by nature and necessity, is public, political, and interdisciplinary.

If AIDS research is haunted by the specter of politics, it is also blessed by an unprecedented level of international and interdisciplinary cooperation. Good science, by the definition of my informants, is international in nature. One Chicago researcher commented:

Research is something that you can do anywhere, except if you look at large patient samples. Most of our baby work [finding HIV in infants] is done on samples we get from Miami. Most of my collaborators—I have collaborators in Belgium—I have hardly anyone in the Midwest. It's such a fluid field that you just pick up the phone. The Fed Ex guy's here at least twice a day; he nearly lives here. Samples move within a day. That's how real science meets these days.

Researchers in French labs also construct a global scientific enterprise.

Science is too international. You can't really pin it down. You know, in the States, it's done by Indians and Chinese and Japs and Germans and Americans and god knows what. And in this lab here [in France], there's a Chilean, a Czech who's been here three months; I'm British, my colleague's Colombian, we've got a Brazilian, we might get another Brazilian, and there's a Spaniard.

AIDS seems to highlight the international ties of the various scientific communities. One need only leaf through recent abstracts of the International AIDS Conferences to recognize the extraordinary level of this exchange, which literally covers the world.

Even more striking is the cross-disciplinary nature of AIDS research, particularly between bench research and clinical medicine. My informants construct this quality as being fundamental, even unique to AIDS, and they value it highly.

I had always thought that one of the reasons that we had such big advances in research in the AIDS field was that because of the confrontation of different aspects, *c'est l'observation, le même phénomène et différente éclairage.* It's the observation of this phenomenon with different types of light.

In the area of AIDS, there has probably been the best two-way communication [between medicine and research] as anything I have ever seen. . . . And certainly at the international meetings, there is a great attempt to cross boundaries.

We [the French study group on AIDS] were very multidisciplinary. We had everything, immunologists, virologists, epidemiologists, clinicians, general practitioners, gay physicians. It was very open.

I think that certainly in the beginning, when we were all working on this major puzzle, there was a huge amount of interaction. We all used to get together all the time, the clinicians and the basic scientists. We used to have meetings at least once a month. . . . Now there are a few programs bringing the basic sciences under the same umbrella as the clinical arenas, but I think it's much less of a marriage than it used to be.

In the histories of AIDS research told by my informants, this interdisciplinary camaraderie has tapered off over time, a victim of the increasing size of the AIDS research community and its responsibilities. Those involved in AIDS the longest, particularly among the French informants, expressed nostalgia for the equality and intimacy of those early days.

There are many people who work in social science and so on, and I don't know everybody anymore. I used to know everybody—it was a small group. In '82, '83,'84, we had a small group and everybody was close together, on friendly terms. After, it was less strong. But now, even people who are my friends, I don't see them anymore; I have no time.

It's more or less natural, because everybody has more and more work, so we have less time to discuss, to meet, and so on. . . . I think that the time we have to spend to just share experiences is becoming fewer and fewer.

This discourse is evocative of Turner's (1969) descriptions of *communitas*, those liminal experiences in which relationships emerge outside of people's usual structural positions, emphasizing unity and equality. Communitas is also filled with a sense of power, almost magical in nature, and one can find its echoes in the stories of my informants.

The people who initially got interested in HIV were, at least in France, quite atypical. When we started this first study group, the group of clinicians, virologists, immunologists back in 1982, we were all quite young doctors, in our thirties. There was no big shot, no professor. Because nobody was interested in AIDS. . . . And I think that was great because since nobody was interested in this disease, we had enough time to work and do what we were interested in doing.

Communitas, according to Turner, "is a phase, a moment, not a permanent condition" (140). In AIDS discourse, as in Turner's, participants eventually return to the "real," structural world, but they mourn the loss of those magic days.

The experience of communitas is not lost forever to my informants but is now integrated into an annual ritual known as the International AIDS Conference. Since 1984, members of the medical community, researchers and clinicians alike, have been meeting annually at various international sites, ostensibly to share information on AIDS. Over time, the conference has drawn increasing numbers of nonmedical people involved with AIDS: social workers, health educators, policy analysts—what might be termed "adjunct" health care professionals—as well as lay activists and the media.

The Montreal Conference in 1989, which I attended, drew over 10,000 people. At Montreal and the San Francisco Conference the following year, activists, nonbiomedical healers, and assorted other groups set up "anticonferences" in opposition, both physically and discursively. The conference itself lasts over four or five days, beginning with an opening session attended by all participants. The opening speakers may not even be members of the medical community—at Montreal, for example, the prime minister of Canada was among these speakers. The conference then breaks up into meetings and poster presentations categorized into several "tracks," including epidemiology, clinical science, basic science, and as of 1989, social science. These meetings, containing usually four to eight presentations at a time, are, in theory, where the science gets done. Researchers present their data and then are challenged by their peers, bringing both one step closer to knowing the facts of AIDS. At the more recent conferences, activists would often attend formal presentations, questioning the fundamental goals of the presented research and sometimes utilizing question-answer time to make political/social statements. Out and out demonstrations during the proceedings are not uncommon.

The discourse of my informants and their practice as participants in the International Conference constructs three distinct yet interwoven conferences, all occurring simultaneously. The first is the authoritative, formal, structured conference, with its strict schedule of reviewed speakers and presenters; the second is the "anticonference" mentioned above, set up in opposition to the "authoritative" conference and presenting alternative narratives. Finally, there are the informal meetings that take place between presentations or at the end of the day, including talks in the hall between colleagues in the same field, meetings of friends, and finally, meetings between cooperative groups that rarely are able to assemble face to face (such as those that are international or national in scope). The third conference is the one that virtually all my informants identify as the most important, where the "real work" gets done.

You have to make a decision when you go that you're going to take advantage of the opportunity to talk to people and pursue collaborations and opportunities. And there will be less opportunity to have as much time as one would like to ingest a lot of information. . . . But, you know, we just have a lot of collaboration, and a lot of meetings are better than the meeting itself. . . . There's sort of a tension there, because you want to go to some of the formal stuff.

They're always good meetings to go to because of the contacts—the stuff that goes on out in the hallways. . . . There's almost nothing that is presented that we didn't know about. But it's the hallway stuff, and the meetings and the opportunity to brainstorm, that's the real value for us of a conference like that.

I think that it's a nice place to get together with friends from all over the world that are dealing with the same problem and perhaps have interactions and conversations outside of the meeting halls that may be fruitful for networking or learning what's happening somewhere else, but I don't think that the science is that particularly earth-shattering.

Thus, members of the medical community do not see the formal presentations as being or doing "real science" but rather those dialogues that are informal and of the moment. There can be no anticonference to this because of its spontaneous, informal nature. The value of the International AIDS Conference lies not in information per se but in communitas.

Why isn't the conference a forum for good science? Not surprisingly, my informants, French and American, cite many of the same reasons that the field of AIDS itself does not make for good science: too many people, too much publicity, and far too much politics.

If you had an audience that was twenty to fifty people that was just there, you could discuss one on one. At the International you can't discuss. . . . It's like a couple thousand people in the audience, and somebody raises their hand and says, "Oh." I gave sort of a white bread–type talk. You can't really give a talk that's going to raise too much data, because otherwise you don't get the chance. They can't interact.

Sometimes you want to listen to one paper in a session, and you go to another session a few doors farther and listen to some other papers, and if there are too many people, you cannot [get in] because the rooms are crowded. You lose your time, so you stay at the session and listen to things that don't interest you. So this is really a problem. I think the conferences are too big and should be split into social science and biology, clinic and—it should not be split completely, but with an overlap.

As seen in the above examples, the sheer size of the conference creates logistical problems that inhibit the doing of good science, namely, the intimacy needed for challenge and defense. More problematic is the interdisciplinary nature of the conference, particularly after Montreal and its addition of the social science category. While many of my informants acknowledge a need for broad interdisciplinary communication, it may, in their view, interfere with the doing of good science. On the other hand, several informants present the interdisciplinary nature of the International Conferences as a highlight of the meetings, essential to AIDS science, if not all science.

The meetings are highly professional, very well organized for the most part. They have maintained some of the good parts of AIDS meetings, which are the multidisciplinary flavor. People from the infected community and from the community-based organizations can make the dialogue vary research. And the strong blending of clinical, epidemiologic, and laboratory-based science.

I think it's also been very critical that we have said, "This disease requires a meeting that is both international, because the disease is international, and a meeting where people from widely different academic disciplines get together." Even if the getting together is kind of token at some level, they're meeting in the same place, and I think interchanges occur. But it also hopefully sends out a message to people working in the area and people watching the epidemic that it is important for behavioral scientists to be aware of the basic science and also for the basic scientists to be aware of epidemiology trends and changes in clinical care. I don't think it has been addressed, and I think it is really critical for this kind of an epidemic.

The ambivalence toward the interdisciplinary nature of the meetings extends to its international character as well.

There has been an extraordinary effort to put forward the Third World presence in these conferences, often, I think, not to the great benefit of science itself. I think there's this effort to do this for social reasons that have little to do with science.

Paula Treichler (1992b), in her analysis of discourse at the Montreal Conference, discusses Robert Gallo's comments (below) on that conference's emphasis on social concerns:

I must have heard fifty or one hundred scientists yesterday say there wasn't enough time for science. . . . We didn't expect this amount of diversity. People from the Third World nations need a chance to get together, but is here the best place? You can't even find the people you want to talk to here. (78)

Treichler observes that the term *social* for Gallo refers to a range of issues: the amount of time allotted to social science research, the sociocultural diversity of conference participants, and the visible participation of AIDS activists. There exists in my informants' discourse, as Treichler noted in her own analysis, "conflation of conventional academic social science with political activism" (79).

Even more than the crossing of disciplinary boundaries, political activism emerges as an ambivalent force in this discourse.

It irritates me, maybe just because I'm in the trenches working. It's good in the sense that without it, probably we wouldn't focus so much of our time and energy on having to do with HIV. But the pitfalls from that are it's effectively rerouted some other diseases that don't get worked on as hard, which are probably equally, if not more, important—heart disease, cancer kill a lot more people than HIV here in America. So you start rerouting the money. That's where the politics comes in.

Researchers, as in the above example, sometimes interpret the actions of lay activists as being an attack on their dedication and integrity, both as scientists and as human beings. Activism is constructed as opposing and challenging the scientific enterprise at the same time, hence, the ambivalence. Activism also emerges as injecting politics into research, thus promoting bad science. The International Conferences, like AIDS itself, make the encounter between science and politics not only highly public but sometimes physically disruptive. As one clinical researcher noted:

San Francisco had so much circus and all those protestors. . . . They have every right to protest. The protest at this meeting is, I think, crazy. All it does is turn off people to the whole AIDS program. They should be protesting the politicians. They should have all those people out in force hitting them, hitting the insurance companies and the government people that are not responding to this crisis. That's where the emphasis in this country should be, not the workers. I mean, there is some legitimate question that they have, and I think they should go to the meeting. I think we should have them there, but that thing with all the whistles and getting up—It was hard to concentrate at that meeting.

The primary metaphor for these meetings is that of "a circus," evoking a sense of spectacle without substance, or as one French researcher put it, "too much show business." In this way, the conference counters the tenets of good science, yet is intrinsically part of the experience of AIDS.

I encourage the junior staff to go to them, partially for the information exchange but also partly because I want them to experience the circus atmosphere that surrounds the science and medicine of HIV. To get at least even a small sense of the political activism, the emotionalism that surrounds the entire AIDS issue. And that any work they do has to be filtered through that political and emotional context before it will actually be translated into anything, and that it is important for bench docs to know that. It shouldn't really influence what they do, but I do think that it is useful for them.[4]

Lay activism emerges from the discourse, like many issues in AIDS, as a paradox. It is political and brings publicity, the enemies of good science. Yet activism also brings challenge, the potential for questioning the obvious that lies at the heart of the scientific enterprise.

People who are affected by the disease want to be involved in what happens. They want to be there to make sure the sense of urgency that they feel is right there, in front of everybody . . . and that has created a whole set of challenges for science that science has never had to deal with before. . . . I think an equally exciting part of it is having somebody sit there who is not a scientist and say, "Well, why do you do it that way?" And sometimes the only answer you can give back is, "Because that's the way it's done." They say, "Why don't you do it this way instead of that way?" And sometimes you don't have an answer. So that sort of challenging of assumption that's gone on, I think that's worked both ways. It's been very fascinating and very good for science.

The International AIDS Conferences are not, by the definitions of my informants, good science. However, they serve an equal if not greater purpose in the medical community, that of getting researchers, clinicians, activists, and policy makers together. Sitting in the opening session at Montreal, I looked around myself and gasped. The room was filled, end to end, with over 10,000 people, each having one goal in common: resisting the onslaught of AIDS. The experience of that moment, awesome and powerful, emerges out of my informants' words as well.

Since the time of the Olympic Games, people have sort of sensed that if you bring people together and make them compete with each other, good things come of that. . . . It gives people an opportunity to see old friends and to network and to build those kinds of bridges as well. And it gives the Third World an opportunity to let us share some of their agony and to see this disease through a different light, out different eyes.[5]

The best part of the meeting is stepping away from your work, looking at what everyone else is doing, and seeing all the work that is being done. It's kind of an army of world people who are out there doing remarkably good stuff, all over the world—Africa, urban Paris—there's good stuff going on. And little pieces fit together. That's really the good part of them. The bad part is the shared frustration that everyone has from every country, talking about their government. And the other thing, especially for us old-timers, is seeing everybody. Saying hello. Still alive. If you can make it, I can make it. It kind of reinvigorates you.

The International AIDS Conference can be viewed as an annual rite of passage in the world of AIDS. As in van Gennep's (1960) classic description, there is separation of the subjects from workings of everyday society to enter the ambiguous, nominally egalitarian state of "participant." It is in this liminal phase that AIDS and those involved with it are made anew, reshaping meanings for their experiences. The International AIDS Conference stands for AIDS in all its power and paradox. During those few days, in a sense, it *is* the AIDS community: patients, clinicians, researchers, journalists. We are all there because of AIDS.

NOTES

1. This attitude, to be discussed later in detail, is evidenced by France's nationalized health care system and the respect accorded physicians working in public hospitals versus private, "for-profit" institutions.

2. The Gallo-Montagnier dispute exemplifies not only the process of how scientific facts are made but the interrelationships of political power, cultural identity, and the structural forces inherent to the scientific enterprise. See J. Feldman (1992c) for a detailed analysis.

3. And, more recently, the Duesberg "anti-HIV" narratives.

4. Here, a researcher constructs the scientific enterprise as ideally uninfluenced by politics, yet in this discourse, the scientist is encouraged to be informed about it. The researcher's duty in this narrative is to venture forth from the ivory tower, though not necessarily to invite the masses back in.

5. Another informant, a French clinician, also used the Olympics as a metaphor for the International AIDS Conference: "The question of course, Is the AIDS Conference useful? Are the Olympic Games useful? I don't know."

11

Identity and the AIDS Doctor

Pasteur said, "*La science n'a pas de patrie.*" "Science has no homeland."
You all represent the entire world (more than ten countries) and so, your
presence here today is proof of this statement. But Pasteur paradoxically
added soon after: "*La science droit être la plus haut personification de la
patrie.*" "Science should be the greatest symbol of one's homeland." And
thus, it is the essence of scientific competition that you also represent here.
Jeanne-Marie Lecomte, President-Director of Pasteur Vaccins
(Girard and Vallette 1987, vii)

Embedded within all of my informants' discourse are commentaries on the cultural
identity of the speaker. Geertz (1973) says of the Balinese cockfight: "In the
cockfight, then, the Balinese forms and discovers his temperament and his society's
temper at the same time. Or, more exactly, he forms and discovers a particular facet
of them" (451). In becoming involved with AIDS, and more important, in talking
about becoming involved with AIDS, these men and women form the temper of
being medical scientists in French and American contexts and of being French and
American in a medical context.

NATIONAL IDENTITY: FIRST STORIES, HARDSHIP STORIES

Outside of talk on the health care system, my American informants are as likely
to talk about their city or region as the whole United States. My French informants,
in comparison, never spoke about Paris specifically and rarely referred to the
provinces. This may well be due to the centrality of Paris in the French world view
(Ardagh 1987). Paris stands for France in a way that has no American parallel. In
contrast, regional affiliation appears as a significant element in American discourse.[1]

Discourse on regional affiliation may serve another purpose, constructing a key element of American identity. As seen in one of its founding mottoes, *E pluribus unum*, the American whole is established through the coming together of disparate parts. By asserting their regional identity, my informants are also refashioning their national identity as well.[2] Perhaps because of the US' internal diversity and relatively short history as a nation, the American identity appears somewhat diffuse in my informants' discourse. However, as the United States is more than the sum of its regions, so a fundamentally American identity emerges from these narratives.

Occasionally, when asked, American informants would offer up comments on French medicine or research. An American identity often lies implicit in this discourse, a sounding board against which the French are defined.

My immediate reaction is to say that they are probably a little more infatuated with theory and less concerned with applications. That's my immediate reaction. I will admit that the reason I was hesitating for so long was trying to decide if that was fair or not.

By implication, Americans emerge as pragmatic, more interested in doing than thinking. This dichotomy—French thought versus American action—has been noted by Payer (1988) as well, and is a common theme in American comments on French research.

I don't think that we [Americans] have quite the freedom to explore new stuff. . . . And secondly, it forces us to focus on what's really important. This is not specific to France exactly; this applies to other countries, all other countries. But I think where you get this opportunity to, if you will, chase willow wisps, most of the time you're going to be chasing exactly that, a willow wisp, which disappears on you and there's nothing really there.

Americans find real solutions, while the French chase intellectual ghosts, unfettered by rigorous, standardized controls.

I think in general my impression is that research in France isn't quite as rigid or regulated or controlled as in this country. That the standards of conducting clinical trials and analyzing and approving drugs are maybe a little looser than here. I think there's often times a lot of anecdote that gets accepted more readily in France.

In talking about French medicine, Americans reinterpret their own experiences. Americans in this discourse function under fierce legal restraints, a marked contrast to the relaxed French environment.

I think the French, by virtue of their law, probably are much more able to take chances that few people in the United States would dare to do. And Europeans in general have more lax laws about drug therapy, about introducing new ideas of drugs, about even vaccine trials, things like that, that most scientists in the United States would be afraid to do it because of the regulatory restrictions. We may think that it's a good idea, but we wouldn't dare to do it because there are so many formal steps, and boy, Congress will hang you if you step out of line. Your agency will let them do it, too.

For the Americans, French "laxness," a sense of relaxed tolerance, extends beyond the realm of research, emerging as a defining characteristic of the French way of life. As one American researcher observed:

I think they [French researchers] are much more relaxed. They come in late and they leave early and they take their lunch. It's revealed when they come and work with me here. I don't have very many French scientists who put in the hours that I think Americans do.

This discourse evokes not only skepticism but envy: "They may have their priorities correct. If I lived in Paris, I might also want to get out to the cafe and have my wine." Americans, in reference to the French, construct themselves as hardworking, both internally and externally constrained from the lenient approach of their French counterparts. Two common symbols used in this discourse are food and sex. For example, one New York physician compared French and US hospital food:

Here, each tray of food is presented to the patient, often outside the door. In many hospitals, if they're in isolation, a knock on the door and they pick up this disposable cardboard tray and enjoy their meal. In France, there was a guy with a chef hat at the hospital. He had a real plate, real silverware, and would show the entrees and scoop out individual servings.

Tolerance of sexual diversity is seen as a French hallmark and its lack as an American shortcoming: "I think they do better with sex than we do. Even though it's a Catholic country, you'd think that it would be harder to do. I think they do better with homosexuality than we deal with it." Food and sex act as symbols for identifying what is French, as well as metaphors by which the American identity can be distinguished from the Other.

Despite the above examples of contrast, French and Americans often appear as opposite ends of the same rope:

I think the French have a similar and sometimes worse problem than we have in their public health system. They do not have a CDC-type organization, only the state, which would be provincial local authorities, and so it's even more haphazard in terms of getting public health policy than ours. . . . You'd think this country should do beautifully with its fed-state-local health department. But with the Reagan administration totally undermining the CDC and not allowing it to do what it should, it really wasn't that much different than the French. So it was sort of forced into the same decentralized approach that the local communities do it. . . . And so in a way, the French and Americans have suffered from that. We had the structure and couldn't use it, and the French didn't have the structure, and it's all chaos.

As a number of informants emphasized, France is "just like here."

I mean, it's [the French medical community] very nonmonolithic, as it is in the United States. This is not a smear on the French; it's just like every place else. There is no such thing as a unity of the French community of scientists about this issue. I probably would have to say I don't have enough experience to give you the range of opinions in France, but the ones that I've contacted, and you'd find lots of different variation. But it's probably in the same range as the colleagues that I talk to in the United States. I don't see a lot of difference, frankly.

This example constructs not only the uniformity of science but the internationality of a fundamental American characteristic: diversity within unity. America is everywhere, and everywhere is America.

Few, if any, of my American informants offered unsolicited observations on the French, and even when I asked them about the French medical community, most said they did not know or had no opinion. The Americans thus do not seem to define themselves primarily in terms of an Other, at least not a French Other, but in terms of their own actions and accomplishments. As one American researcher remarked, "The US has had the most cases and has done the most research, the most everything. The most problems."

The American identity is grounded in superlatives; the most, the best, the first. This is evidenced in the remarkable proliferation of what I call "first stories," discourse about seeing or doing things before anyone else. These stories are common to virtually all the American speakers across all regions, while being comparatively rare among French informants.

The first prospective cohort that was ever set up was the cohort we set up in Denmark, and it was also the first cohort to publish that prospectively you had to have the virus before you got AIDS. . . . We had the first publication to ever prove that you had to have the virus before you got AIDS.

I'm going to be immodest here. The first institution in the world to believe that early diagnosis of HIV was a good way to approach the AIDS epidemic was ours. . . . At those times, those [early diagnosis policies] were visionary compared to the rest of society, and by *society*, I mean the world.

Then we applied for and received one of the first twelve of the AIDS clinical trial units here. At that time they were called ATEU's—AIDS Treatment Evaluation Units—and we were one of the first six to give a drug discovery grant for the development of anti-AIDS compounds. . . . Also some of the first work with interferon was done here.

Even my Midwest informants utilize "firsts" to establish their place in the American AIDS community, as in the examples below.

We were the first to report *Mycobacteria kansasii* in disseminated form of HIV disease.

That's why we were successful in competing for one of the first federal AIDS Treatment and Evaluation Units. I think because we probably had as good as, if not better, multidisciplinary clinic or service than anybody in the country.

One popular first story is that of seeing the first AIDS patients, either in the world, country, region, or institution, while only later recognizing the significance of the event.

I was chief resident at San Francisco General Hospital from mid-1980 to mid-1981, at which time we saw several gay men with what appeared to be acute clinical problems, and their presentations were distinct enough that it was clear with even just one or two patients that they had a new disease. . . . So I would say probably six months before the Gottleib *New England Journal* paper describing the Los Angeles *Pneumocystis* cases, we realized that we were seeing some new disease that was occurring in gay men that was also being appreciated in New York.

In my second rotation as an attending physician, my residents presented a case of young homosexually active black man who was short of breath after jogging a mile and was unable to complete his usual exertion. This was in February of 1982. And he proved to be our first patient at this hospital with *Pneumocystis* pneumonia and AIDS.

By far the most common first stories are those about starting prophylaxis, usually aerosolized pentamidine, for *Pneumocystis* pneumonia.[3] From a clinical perspective, there is little question this practice has improved mortality and morbidity, and informants from nearly every institution I visited claim credit for it. At one New York hospital, I was introduced to a researcher and told that "he invented aerosol prophylaxis for PCP." Variations on this claim are ubiquitous in the discourse, as in the following New York, Chicago, and San Francisco narratives:

We've done some of the opportunistic infection trials also. We were the first to use the aerosol pentamidine and had studied a large group of patients who were in that.

We worked with the initial fluconazole studies for the long-term treatment of cryptoccocal meningitis . . . trimethotrexate for *Pneumocystis* pneumonia, aerosol pentamidine. We were among the first to bring that capability to Chicago.

We did very well with *Pneumocystis*. Our group was the first group that showed inhalation pentamidine worked.

Next to AZT, the institution of prophylaxis emerges as a watershed in the medical community's experience with AIDS. Aerosolized pentamidine, in particular, seems to signify innovation under pressure and, when placed in a discourse of firsts, establishes a distinctly American approach to the world.

The American informants thus utilize three discursive techniques to construct their identity as Americans. First, by constructing a significant regional identity, they establish the distinctive value of diversity within unity. Second, though less common, American identity emerges by comparison to an Other—in this case, the French. The Other, in turn, is sometimes represented as not being different at all, thus developing a theme of "Americanism" as universal, at least in the medical community. Most important, these informants rely on the description or listing of accomplishments, made significant by their superlative character as seen in the proliferation of first stories. Identity is thus constructed by reference to individual action rather than through opposition, the hallmark of French discourse.

Conflict plays a strong part in the discourse of my French informants, as seen previously in narratives about scientific research. Individualism is paramount.

It is very difficult to get a group of French around a table and get them to work together, as a team. . . . When we were at the other hospital, we had lots of problems with the rest of the department. This is very common in France. This is too bad because AIDS needs teamwork.

Generally, stories of competition and dissension are generically located, simply "taking place" out there in the world of French medicine. It is an assertion of a French identity, a French way of doing medicine, revolving around themes of individual struggle against bureaucratic restriction and the power of personal contacts. An excellent example is found in one physician's narrative about attempting to establish a high school–level education program on AIDS.

No one asked me anything. I had no money, nothing, and I started a big project. It was very difficult. I had to see many people to get authorization, several hundred. The Ministry of Education didn't give me a penny.

I call these narratives "hardship stories," in which the predominant theme is one of overcoming impossible obstacles to achieve a measure of success. Whereas American first stories concentrate on what you did and when you did it, French hardship stories focus on how you got there, the end result made meaningful by the preceding struggle. These narratives are pervasive in the discourse of my French informants and, like the first stories of the Americans, act as a fundamental expression of French identity.

The focus on the individual and the theme of a restrictive, powerful, central "establishment" are also common to French discourse in general (Ardagh 1987). There is no comparable discourse among the Americans, who tend to focus on regional tensions or the lack of a strong center. As Beriss (1991, 3–4) notes, "In the dominant model for French identity, the central element that defines a member of French society is his or her relationship to the state. This relationship provides the basic symbolic framework for defining what is, and is not, French." However, these motifs unfold with new vitality in the stories on the beginning of AIDS research in France. It is the story of underdogs, unknown and underfinanced, fighting against a powerful and stagnant establishment who sought, and still seeks, to control them.

By March '82, we formed a group of approximately ten people to study AIDS in France, to see whether it was the same thing described in the States where there were approximately 100 cases at the time. We called it "The French Study Group on AIDS." It was very informal, we were unknown people and young. I was the oldest, the only professor, and we had very frequent meetings where we discussed the new cases, exchanged information. . . . I tell you where I think it is interesting, because everything in France started from the bottom. It did not start from the government or from the high officials, who were not aware of the problem. . . . What is interesting is that no big shot was with us.

The youth, informality, and almost grass-roots character of the original study group are emphasized throughout this researcher's narrative. By their wits, open minds, and personal contacts, the study group is able to maneuver around the monolithic French bureaucracy and the entrenched scientific establishment.

The first one we contacted was a guy who specialized in cytomegalovirus. He came to one or two of our meetings and left, saying that this is not a cytomegalovirus, because we thought at the beginning—we thought it could be a cytomegalovirus. . . . We had another guy, who is a specialist in EBV [Epstein-Barr virus]. And he said, "This is not EBV," and he left. But one of our friends contacted a guy who is very powerful in France, who was an immunologist working on animal tumors, so his lab was working with animal retroviruses. And this guy was not interested; he did not want to work with unknown people.

Conflict between the imaginative upstarts and the established authorities is an intrinsic element in the French AIDS research narrative. The study group eventually wins the conflict by turning away from the big shots and enlisting the help of Montagnier, who was himself relatively unknown at the time. Another informant associated with the initial study group develops a similar theme, one of "us" against the rest of the scientific world.

I started to work on AIDS in 1983, the beginning of 1983. . . . And at the end of 1982, the idea that a retrovirus can be involved in the disease was not accepted but was in the mind of a lot of scientists in the world. . . . We thought we should begin to work on an antiviral drug, which is impossible to work on cells which are immortalized by a retrovirus like HTLV-I. But it was really difficult for us to make the medical and scientific community admit that it was a different virus and that we can maybe have a treatment.

The point of the narratives is not only one of unknown upstarts struggling to prove a new breakthrough but that these are *French* upstarts. The ultimate individualists, their countrymen are among their most vocal opponents.

The big French immunologists discovered AIDS in August '83, at an International Immunology meeting which was taking place in Japan. They began to be interested, and they were not convinced it was important. They were interested and they were very shocked to see that David Klatzman [a French associate] presented some of the data we got with Montagnier at the time. At the meeting, they said, "It is scandalous. Someone is presenting a new virus, telling people how to work, that they don't know how to work." It was a real scandal. . . . People couldn't understand perhaps that the virus was a French virus, found in French patients, because it had been studied at that time in French patients. . . . And that is, I think, one thing we live through in France, is that all the powerful people were excluded from AIDS research. So first they rejected our results, and after, they became jealous of the results, and now they are trying to get the direction of the research, not only the direction but to control the AIDS research. And they are almost successful.

The study group's detractors are French, specifically the big shots of French immunology. Although the virus has now been acknowledged and its discoverers have attained world recognition, the struggle continues.

By the way, do you know that some people are so mad at us in France that we applied almost one year for a grant from a society which supports research on cancer, and they didn't give us the money. So I wrote to ask them why, because the project had been judged very good by the scientists. And I had the answer from a great French oncologist who said, "This association has to deal with cancer and not with retroviruses." I keep the letter because I think it something of a caricature. Because retroviruses are the cause of cancer.

In the above narrative, two elements stand out. First, the conceptual link again forged between AIDS and cancer. Second, the search for financial and scholarly support requires patience—waiting a year to hear from the society—and negotiating the necessary bureaucratic channels. The ending, by now, is somewhat predictable. The money is denied, and the scholarly support undermined by "a *great French oncologist*" (emphasis mine). Some six years later, the underdogs remain the underdogs, outside the establishment, scrapping and winning against those with money and power.

The clinical half of the story is not quite so fraught with conflict, but the same elements are present. Dr. Bernard offered the following narrative about how he became involved with AIDS.

And so the story began. And it was very strange because I have a friend, a good colleague, we had a good relation, and in August we discussed about this case, and he did not want to trust this history. He said, "Your patient has a lymphoma; you have to try to find it. I'm sure that he has it." But, I told him, "You know, in the States, there are strange stories about homosexuals who have PCP without any cause.

Dr. Bernard eventually convinces his colleague that AIDS is at work in Paris. He begins to gather epidemiological data on the disease in France and continues to treat increasing numbers of AIDS patients at his consultation. Conflict with the hospital establishment follows.

After that, it was in '82, and at my consultation, half the patients were homosexuals, and the boss there told me that if I want to continue to take care of homosexuals, I'd have to go to another hospital. It was not the position of himself, or not much, but it was all my colleagues who looked very bad at things. First, because it was much noise. They told me that I did too much noise [publicity]. Also that it's not the problem of this hospital to take care of homosexuals. They told me like that.

The homosexual component of this narrative seems subordinate to the theme of conflict between the audacious young physician and the restrictive medical hierarchy. This is better demonstrated by the story of Bernard's experiences at his next hospital.

When I came in, I talked to the boss, the chief of the department, and the only thing that I ask is just to work on my subject, and my subject was the control system survey, and also a new disease, AIDS, that perhaps he had heard of. So I began. And two years after, when 90 percent of the beds were full of AIDS, conflict again. And when I received about 100 calls a day, and the secretary—he had five secretaries, but more than half was because of Dr. Bernard. And when he received a call, "Okay, you are Professeur Michel. May I speak to Professeur Bernard? To your chief." When he began to see Dr. Bernard on the TV and—[trails off]. . . . You know, he never asked me to leave, but he turned off the water, the electricity, the gas. So I left.

But one of the great ironies that seems so characteristic of the French way of doing things, Dr. Bernard ended up back at his original hospital before opening the clinic at Rousseau.

From story to story, from researcher to clinician, the message is consistently one of unknowns, against all odds, outsmarting the established authorities. Americans are classed with the authorities. Like their French counterparts, they emerge from these narratives as members of a dominating organization with easy access to financial and informational resources. French identity is again constructed, this time not in the more individualistic conflict of French versus French but of French versus American. The Gallo-Montagnier controversy is but a part of this larger discourse and perhaps exemplifies it.

It was two groups; they were French groups—it was a small team [laughter]. The American group was a very big team known for a long time. In this way, it is difficult for people to make their own opinions.

In the following narrative, Gallo and Montagnier become symbolic of American and French identities, and their conflict reenacts the adversarial nature of the larger relationship.

That's what Montagnier did with Gallo, and two years later, he was in a position to acknowledge it [where he had gotten his information from]; therefore, he acknowledged it. But he had to lie for two years and mount such a campaign, an aggressive campaign to balance the desire of the Americans to crush him. I must say also on the other side, Gallo was not very elegant; he tried to knock him off. Gallo also acknowledged two years later that he had made a big mistake by mocking the French. He did, despising them, telling them, "Get out of the way. This is mine." He touched off something.

Another French informant recalled:

The guy who is a big shot in French biology didn't believe the virus, the Pasteur virus. All the other people working either in immunology or virology, they say it must be a lab contaminant. And their argument was that it could not be the AIDS virus because if it were, the Americans would have discovered it first.

In the last excerpt, the Americans are identified with the French big shot, scoffing at the little French team. In fact, Americans become the ultimate "big shot," for even the French scientific establishment believes they will discover the virus first. In these narratives, however, the French researchers, as a group, tend to become more and more distinct from Americans, seeking to provide, as one researcher put it, a different "angle of vision on what would later be called AIDS."

The identity of the researchers emerges from their stories, constructed against a background of the American Other. Their words are at the same time an assertion and a construction. It is thus not a simple case of segmental opposition à la Evans-Pritchard (1940)—"We are French because we fight with Americans"—but a commentary on what is involved in being French, in doing French medicine, in discovering a French (in terms of invention and not epidemiology) virus. The identity of the researchers and the identity of the virus, French or American, are closely linked. To have lost the battle over HIV would have meant a loss of cultural identity as well. The relative triumph, on the other, was quite literally a rebirth.

The contrast of French versus American does not end with the settlement on the identity of the virus.

It is a competition. Before I came to the lab, I didn't know the spirit of the researchers. I didn't know about the competition between the French and the US. It is a very intense battle. The head of the lab tells us, "Work! Write papers because the Americans will write it before us!"

Even those researchers and clinicians who have only been involved with AIDS for a year or two have plenty of stories and observations about American science and its practitioners. In 1987, one such researcher had this to say about the Third International AIDS Conference in Washington, DC:

At this time, it seems there is a new struggle in progress, for HIV-2, like for HIV-1 in 1983. The HIV-2 was isolated in 1986 at Pasteur and sequenced and was published in *Nature* by the Pasteur team. Gallo and collaborators want to make HIV-2 their own virus. I didn't really understand strategy; for that, it is cloudy. We have to be careful, to look for an appearance of a new virus named perhaps HTLV-4, 5, 24, with the same sequence as HIV-2.[4]

Thus, the opposition between French upstarts and the American establishment continues, a never ending production of what it means to be French.

French clinicians, like their research colleagues, make extensive use of the American Other in their discourse, not only as an opposing force but as a humorous foil. For example, at a Rousseau journal meeting, Dr. Farsi discussed a US study on *Camplyobacter* infection, a gastrointestinal infection, in HIV positive men. Controls, who didn't have the infection, were "challenged" with the bacteria and their antibody response checked. Dr. Bernard then quipped, "They were challenged? How? By the mouth?" The implication is that they were tested with the bacteria through eating feces. Bernard then told a story of another US study of a resistant *Salmonella* strain in "volunteers"—the emphasis is Bernard's—from prison. He mentioned that type of study is now illegal in the United States, but added, laughing, "Even in Iraq, they don't do this." Americans emerge through these stories as being so caught up in the scientific enterprise that they will do anything, from the scatological to the unethical.

In this discourse, Americans attempt all manner of strange and silly practices, not only in the name of science. At a Rousseau staff meeting, the social worker made an announcement about meeting with the families of patients, listing several families that are already involved.

> *Bernard*: You mean "family" in the large sense?
> *Social worker*: Whoever the patient refers to: mothers and fathers, mothers alone, brothers, friends, lovers.
> *Bernard* [*laughing*]: What about their dogs?
> *Social worker*: Not dogs, since I've found that they don't speak very well.
> *Bernard* [*looking at me*]: There are psychiatrists for dogs in the US, no?

This example reconstructs the meaning of family, using the American Other to mark the extreme boundary. Americans will accept anyone as family, even sending the dog to therapy. By implication, the French are more selective in who is counted among family. The French family, like the French home, must be protected from those outside its circle (Carroll 1988), and this may be a model for French identity as well. Americans are careless with their intimacy; the French, scrupulous. My American presence, of course, provided the perfect opportunity—and target—for these sociologic musings.

Unlike my American informants, French commentary on the United States was extremely common and often unsolicited. The French first stories on PCP prophylaxis are constructed like hardship stories, using the American Other as the powerful opposition.

So the main treatment has not changed, but prevention of *Pneumocystis* and so on is something new, and in fact we were one of the first to have the idea. . . . We started that in '87 or '88, when we first had the idea there maybe should be the possibility towards treatment and prevention for PCP. And I remember at that time nobody was even for secondary prevention. Even in the States, many people were against secondary prevention for PCP. And now, everybody says that.

I think the primary prevention [of PCP], and secondary prevention, because this was not accepted before, it's a big step forward. This was because of the personal philosophy of Dr. Bernard, who since '85 in fact started secondary prevention of *Pneumocystis*, and primary prevention later on. Whereas I remember he did an interview on infectious, opportunistic infections during the Paris [International AIDS] conference, he was criticized actually. This was back in 1985, because people in the room said that the data was not conclusive. For instance, primary prevention of *Pneumocystis* during chemotherapy, for Kaposi's sarcoma, was something I have always known. I have never known the contrary. Whereas the first article by Fischl [an American clinical researcher] came out, I think in '87. Now everybody has adopted prevention, and this is a good thing.

At Rousseau, discussions of new treatments often included references to the American medical community: "All the patients in the US are asking for DDI"; "Dapsone is all the fashion in the US."

References to other nationalities exist in the French discourse as well. When one informant traveled to the Washington conference on AIDS, he met with an American physician working on an education program similar to his own. The French physician said of the meeting, "He treated me like an African." The narrative is constructive on two levels. It constructs Americans as condescending, perceiving the French and other Europeans as backward "Third Worlders." On a deeper level, French attitudes toward Africans emerge out of this story: The American treated the Frenchman as the Frenchman might treat an African. The narrative also reveals the impact that France's colonial past and present African immigration have on French life.

By far, however, most commentary revolved around the distinctions between French and American culture. Certainly my presence as an American sparked a measure of this discourse, but the sheer volume of these commentaries suggests that additional factors are at work. By comparison, I spoke often of my French experiences to the Northlake staff, but unsolicited references to the French or even European medical communities were rare. In the field of AIDS, the majority of published research is American in origin, providing yet another impetus for use of the American Other.

I also felt that the Congress [San Francisco conference] was also not an international congress, because there was too much bias towards Americans. If you take the list of speakers for the main conference, in fact they are almost all Americans. So this was not very good.

English speakers, particularly Americans, are constructed as dominating the academic press, leaving the French to develop innovations without recognition.

One problem with, I think with the French was they do have a lot of clinical experience, but little is published. As comparison to maybe to American centers, and I think it's a pity because they have things to say, but they don't say them, or they're not organized right or they don't have access because it is not easy to publish in English. Look, for instance at low-dose AZT. It was published in '88 in *Lancet*, and the big series from Fischl and other people have been coming out just now. Whereas, 300mg of AZT is something we have been doing since '88, and we never published because the basic everyday clinical experience—or common sense, if you like—articles can't just come out in a month or two.

In the midst of the vast American publication machine, French common sense finds little accommodation, much less renown.

The French informants thus construct their national identity through two powerful means: hardship stories, often revolving around the state-controlled scientific establishment, and comparison with the American Other. What may appear on the surface as American-style first stories more closely resemble hardship narratives, even involving powerful Americans in opposition. This discourse of conflict/comparison is a hallmark in constructions of French identity, as David Beriss (1991) notes in his work on French and Antillean identity. "What is striking about the French case, however, is the insistence on being comparative. French national identity is represented as a specific cultural way of being among others" (3). While the Americans construct their identity through emphasizing internal diversity, the French emphasize external difference. As Beriss concludes:

> The reduction of internal diversity to a form of cultural wealth shared by all French people helps to legitimize the notion that France is a nation of individual citizens who share a common culture. These notions are, however, further legitimized by defining the Other in terms that contrast specifically with the individualistic culture of French civilization. (11)

For French clinicians and researchers involved with AIDS, that Other is American.

> We all knew that [the disease was transmissible from women to men] ever since the African story was known and we never could understand—it was a joke for us to see the Americans wondering how men get it from women. . . . It was so funny. We had those puns about the "immaculate contamination."

> I think the situation is a little different in the States because I think that you have lobbies, you have political pressure, you have a lot of people who are fighting. In France, we have only some doctors who are taking on this big problem; we have nothing to fight against it, but we are very few and everybody says, "Yes, they are very interested because they want some money, so for that they will say that." . . . By definition it's [research in France and the United States] different because we have no means, so we have to think more. *C'est très impossible*, but in France, every time we are working with "*Système D*."

Ardagh (1987) describes the famous *système D*: "Their [French] lives are spent devising ingenious rules and then finding equally cunning ways of evading them. Thus they are able to cut corners and circumvent some of the bureaucratic absurdities, and this is know as *le système D*, a long-standing and cardinal feature of French life" (621). Or as a British friend of Dr. Bernard put it, "It means you are trying to work with rubberbands and paperclips." Americans, wealthy, renowned, and homophobic, do not have *le système D*. It and the AIDS virus are French inventions, and AIDS itself provides the medium for discovering anew the French identity.

PROFESSIONAL IDENTITY: THE MAKING OF AN AIDS DOCTOR

> A plague doctor was regarded as a contact and all contacts had to live in isolation.
>
>   Carlo Cipolla (1977, 71)

As much as hardship stories tell of being French, they also tell of being a scientific professional working on AIDS. In many of the above narratives, the themes of individualism, youth, and struggle can be interpreted not only as constructing French or American character but as developing an identity for this distinct group of people independent of national affiliation. While stories involving struggle between the speaker and a powerful opposition are more common among French informants, narratives involving some form of conflict are extensive among all informants. A number of these revolve around finding a niche for themselves within their local medical contexts. Dr. Bernard's narrative, for example, can be interpreted in this regard. One San Francisco physician recounted a similar tale of being shuttled between hospitals after becoming involved with AIDS.

So a decision was made that all patients newly diagnosed with Kaposi's sarcoma, wherever they were diagnosed within the University system, should be sent over to the public hospital. I was a little disturbed about that because, you know, the facility is not the same. I mean the University structure is very nice, very cushy, and very elegant—most of our patients had insurance. This hospital has always been the charity hospital, and it takes all comers, including people off the street. . . . So I sort of fought that and became a little loud and a little vocal. . . . By this time, people are started to be concerned about, "What is this disease?" And should these patients be sitting in the waiting room with all the cancer and leukemia patients at the heme/onc [hematology/oncology] clinic at the University? Probably better to move him and all of his lymphadenopathy patients and everybody else over to the city's hospital to be coordinated under that umbrella. I really fought that, but again, slightly because I thought that gay men in the city should have a choice from where they got their health care. . . . It was something that I thought that there was homophobia in the University Administration in sort of getting me off campus and over to here and getting my patients off campus and over to here. Ironically, I was here only six months, and I loved it, and I got a call from one of the people saying, "You know, we think the University really needs to have an AIDS clinic at the University Hospital. How would you like to come back and be in charge?" And I said, "I'm no yo-yo." They had just sent me over here, and now they wanted me back. I said, "Never mind, I like it here."

The physician, like his patients, is shuttled around the local health care system until a niche is established. Rather than becoming absorbed into one department or another, a separate space develops for AIDS doctors. Refusing to become a "yo-yo," the speaker establishes his identity as part of the community at the city's public hospital.

One of the Northlake directors, Dr. O'Neill, tells a comparable story. In this example, instead of being physically separated from the original institutional framework, the speaker takes on new roles and responsibilities distinct from other physicians.

We had a little clinic. It was called the NIH clinic, because we didn't want to use "AIDS" or we didn't know what had caused AIDS at the time. So we called it the NIH clinic, and I would relieve everybody's fears. At that time, everybody was really weird about getting HIV, even though we didn't know what it was. . . . We were sharing with geriatrics and oncology simultaneously, and there was no further time. At this time, we were actually keeping their records separate in our research offices and lugging them over there every time we had clinic. We were taking over these file cabinets every day. It just wasn't working out. And then we were going over one o'clock, our allotted time span, and the other doctors were nice but not that nice. . . . I was taking care of all of these patients myself at that time here primarily in our department anyway. And it became painfully obvious after a couple of years that I was taking care of all of these patients, but the infectious disease service was really unwilling. They didn't really have the manpower to take care of them. I practiced in a call group [a group of physicians sharing on-call duties], and the internists didn't like me anymore because of all of my patients in the hospital. I would have three to six patients in the hospital, and between the three of them that I was sharing call with, they would have three to five patients in the hospital. Of course, mine were the sickest, and they were all infectious related. They just couldn't handle it and basically threw me out of the call group.

The story ends with the AIDS clinic gaining separate hospital space, as well as funding to hire additional physicians and support staff. The separation of AIDS from other hospital services—arising out of fear of contagion, homophobia, or sheer overwork—begins as a conflict and ends as a success. This separation is not isolation but the emergence of a distinct medical practice involving a recognizable assembly of physicians.

The issue of AIDS as a separate medical specialty, mentioned previously, is relevant here as well. While my informants infrequently referred to themselves as "AIDS doctors," their discourse constructs a clear divergence between themselves and other physicians. One of the elements of this discourse concerns fear of AIDS, which can be presented as fear of contagion, fear of homosexuality, and fear of complexity. Surgeons as a group are constructed as being afraid of working with AIDS patients due to fear of contagion.

There are a lot of doctors who are just as ignorant as the general population in that regard, who I don't think are ever going to be convinced or who are always going to be frightened, especially surgeons. I have had some of my surgical colleagues here not so subtly tell me that they do not want to see any of my AIDS patients in consultation. And I have not so subtly informed them that they will not see any of my patients for consultation.

There's sometimes surgical consultants—you'll meet a lot of resistance in terms of getting them to see the patient. And it's hard to pin them down as to a reason, so one has to think, "Gee, it's because of HIV." They are conscious of these individuals; they have made decisions to try to avoid HIV-infected people. It's very rare that a surgeon will say, "I will not see your HIV patient." They are usually not that direct about it. . . . One example, I had a patient with squamous cancer of the lung, was a surgical candidate, who was otherwise doing well. Basically, thoracic surgery refused to operate on him. They couched it in terms of "Well, he's a smoker and his pulmonary function isn't very good and he's kind of wasted, and we don't think he would do very well. We were going to recommend radiation therapy." Which all sounded reasonable, but I have seen them operate on much sicker patients than this with all the same things going on. So it was bogus. And the one guy surprised me because he showed his colors.

This old senior surgeon says, "And I don't think it is fair that we expose everyone in the operating room to this guy's virus and who knows what. And that risk is unacceptable."

Conversations among Northlake physicians are another source of this construction. After a clinic presentation, several doctors began talking about particular surgical intervention for a patient. Dr. O'Neill commented, while the rest nodded their heads, on how reluctant the surgeons were to do anything with AIDS patients. One doctor asked, "Because they are HIV-positive?" Dr. O'Neill replied: "Yes. They'd do it if their backs were against the wall, but not before." Still, several informants expressed sympathy with surgeons' fears.

I think it becomes to some individuals a definite fear, especially if they are in a surgical subspecialty. And I can empathize with those people who are up to their elbows in blood and doing blind suturing and getting stuck with bone spicules. I think those are heroic people and actually are putting their lives on the line to have that kind of activity, and I think they are sort of brave people.

Most of my informants stated they had little or no fear of contagion from their patients. One French physician gave a particularly dramatic story to illustrate this:

I remember I had some patients, straight people, a couple, and the woman couldn't believe that you could drink [from the same glass], because it's easy to say, "You can drink, you can touch the knife of your husband, you risk nothing." It's easy to say, but it's not so obvious to patients. So I did it many times—I give a glass of water to a patient with Kaposi's sarcoma, obvious AIDS, and I drink after, so to show it's not something just I say, but I do it.

However, my informants—French and American, clinicians and researchers—also acknowledge going through a period of fear when they began working with AIDS/HIV.

At some point, it became very difficult, because it was like an obsession. When it became clear that there was something infectious, that we're working with virus, at some point I had some fears. There was one time I actually stuck myself with a needle when I was manipulating HIV. Well, I think I could not sleep for at least a year. I mean, I was sure I had contaminated myself with the virus.

Then the house staff started coming to me and saying, "This really scares me." And it was only when other people said, "This really scares me" that I was able to say, "Oh, it's going to be normal to be scared of this."

Like most of the people that I work with, I have had sort of my own AIDS paranoias and concerns, and I have gone sort of through my own process of initially—which was one of the hardest decisions I felt I would have to make after a needle stick . . . five or six years ago—deciding whether I wanted to be in HIV, started mapping out my whole life, my family, and everything else. And so I had to go through that a couple of times. . . . I don't think I would ever characterize it as something that has interfered with my ability to be with patients or be willing to work in that environment.

As seen in this last example, what distinguishes a medical professional in AIDS from others in the community is getting beyond that fear, or at least working with it.

I had a cardiac surgeon stop me in the hall the other day, and we were talking about a case of infected endocarditis and the valve had to come out, and the patient was HIV infected. She's going, "You know, I have two children." I just looked at her and said, "I have two children." Now we both have—between us we have four children. I mean, if they need their valve taken out, what's going to happen? If you don't take the valve out, the patient is going to die. What is your risk? Your risk is very low. You have to take it out, or you need another job.

I witnessed the process of working through fear at Northlake with one of the new infectious disease fellows. When he began, he wore gloves throughout the entire physical examination. As time went on, he utilized the gloves less and less until he reached a level commensurate with the other clinic physicians. As another Northlake physician remarked:

When the AIDS clinic first started, we drew our own blood. We didn't have a phlebotomist. I guess the fact was always in the back of your mind that you could make a mistake and stick yourself and become an exposure, and I think that was a little worrisome, but I think sometimes familiarity breeds a little bit of laxity. I guess if you are a firefighter and you keep on going to fires, you don't have the same kind of emotional impact if you never did it.

AIDS doctors, like firefighters, keep on going back into the fire, perhaps for the same reason—that's where the action is: "Someone once said that I and other physicians who work in AIDS would want to work in a MASH unit."

Another fear prominent in the discourse is homophobia, fear or dislike of homosexuality, seen previously in Dr. Bernard's and the San Francisco narratives. Though a less common element of this discourse, it remains significant, as evidenced in these two French examples.

It's small, but perhaps 20 percent of my correspondents, I have left them for this reason [refusing to see seropositive patients]. Or for the reason that they have racist attitudes, vis-à-vis homosexuals. That is to say, people who, in the wake of this disease, have declared their racism in regards to homosexuals. There are some people who, a priori, did not think they had a position of this type but who made it clearly known. So I left them as correspondents.

But, some doctors are afraid of AIDS because they are maybe concerned with AIDS, too: they [the patients] are gay and so on, and they don't want to take care of gay patients. It's happened sometimes. . . . I remember once a guy gave me a telephone call because he had a patient, obviously gay because he looked like a queen and so on, and so he said, "I took his blood pressure with two apparatus." He was afraid of getting AIDS or giving it to his patients with just a stethoscope.

Again, what separates AIDS physicians is lack of homophobia or getting beyond it.

I mentioned earlier that the early epidemiologic work made people actually ask gay men what they did. And I think that was, for a lot of people, very horrifying. The disease really flushed out homosexuality even before the level of what the specific sexual practices were. And we [San Francisco] have our share of gay physicians, but overall physicians are overwhelmingly straight and quite conservative. And people were forced, including myself, to recognize that our patients have sexual lives and that often their sexual lives are not what we would assume based on the patient's appearance. So people would say to me, "Gee, I never realized so many people were gay." And it really forced physicians to confront the whole area of their patients' sexuality, which is not the physicians'. Despite the fact that we are trained to be clinical, it's still a very difficult area for us.

For some of my American informants, this separation from other physicians emerges not from simple acceptance of homosexuality but from their identity as gay men. Interestingly, none of the French identified themselves as gay, though some mentioned having gay friends. Overall, however, the discourse constructs AIDS doctors as a distinct group due to the nature of their medical practice and not primarily the sexual orientation of themselves or their patients.

The most interesting element of the discourse on fear concerns fear of complexity. Physicians not in the AIDS field emerge as afraid that the disease is too complicated, fast-paced or unfamiliar for them to treat with confidence. Dr. O'Neill uses this discourse in regard to his original call group, who had asked him to leave:

Well, also they felt that it was not only more work—that I think they would take. They wouldn't have thrown me out just because it was more work. But it was all very complicated—very sick, dying patients with AIDS before there was any treatment available. And it wasn't easy. It was really pretty hard. So they just really didn't feel like they could handle it. And we didn't know what we were doing ourselves, at the time basically. . . . Everything was ultraexperimental at the time. A lot of drug reactions and complications and deaths, and it was just overwhelming. They couldn't handle even that small number.

In this narrative, Dr. O'Neill becomes separated from the other physicians by his ability to treat these patients in spite of not knowing "what we were doing ourselves." General practitioners and physicians in smaller towns are singled out in many of these narratives as being particularly afraid of the complexities of AIDS. At Northlake, for example, Dr. Fields recalled speaking recently to doctors in a medium-size town in Indiana about AIDS treatment, noting that they have about 500 cases in the area, but none of the doctors want to treat them "if they can help it. And that's where they make the damn DDI!"

Dr. Westin: What could you tell them that would possibly change their minds?
Dr. Fields: Well, I gave the HIV 101 [basic lecture on AIDS] talk and stressed that there's no magic to managing these patients. Except for the terminal phase, it's like dealing

with hypertension or diabetes. I think some of these doctors just didn't feel comfortable—they needed a framework.

He added that before the talk only one doctor said he would take referrals, and afterward, seven more agreed to see AIDS patients. A French intern told me a similar story, stating that many generalists send the patients off to a specialist as soon as things get the least bit complicated, for fear of doing the wrong thing.

The fear of complexity is not limited to general practitioners or small-town doctors. As seen in the following narrative, even physicians from a hospital with a large AIDS patient population are susceptible.

Now this was probably in about 1987 when on the fifth floor we had been taking care of HIV-infected patients for six years. . . . And they first began to see HIV-infected women upstairs on the sixth floor, coming in to have babies. And the Ob-Gyn people went absolutely crazy. When you go upstairs and say, "We have a lot of experience with this disease in this hospital," people would say, "We knew you guys had it, but we didn't think we were going to have to deal with it."

Again, physicians in AIDS are not constructed as magically immune to this fear but emerge as distinct by their ability to overcome it. A young French resident explained: "[I don't have] any fear in any physical case, nor of contact. The only fear, in fact, is of not being up to the task technically because the treatments, etcetera, are something very new and a little difficult for me."

In daily experience of AIDS, these fears are not isolated from one another but are intertwined in distinguishing physicians in AIDS from other medical personnel. The fear of complexity and the fear of contagion are two sides of the same coin:

The service that I was in before, a general medicine service, the chief came in with gloves and a mask in the room of a patient with AIDS. And me, I came without anything, and he told me, "You are crazy." Me, I came in without anything, I examined him without gloves, without anything. But him, in addition, he is a dermatologist, and he absolutely does not know the disease; he doesn't want to be interested. I find this dangerous even—it's crazy.

As Dr. O'Neill summarized, "They don't know enough, nor do they want to know enough." Physicians in AIDS, in contrast, must continually strive to "know enough" and can be characterized by this desire.

AIDS physicians distinguish themselves from other physicians through the nature of their medical practice as well as through their response to fear. One element of this practice is the rate of change regarding new information or new techniques for treating AIDS. In the discourse of American informants especially, time passes differently for those in the AIDS field. A Northlake patient remarked that she read a book on AIDS from 1986, "and it was very depressing." Dr. Westin responded, "So much has changed in just the last two or three years. 1986 is like two centuries ago with this disease." A conversation between Dr. Holtzman and a resident also develops this theme:

> *Resident*: I was looking back in some of the charts and I was amazed, comparing what
> we used to do to what we do now. I remember we used to spend all this time trying
> to keep people on 1,200 [*mg*] of AZT.
> *Dr. Holtzman*: Yeah, that's ancient history now.

AIDS physicians are distinguished by their ability to keep up with the differential
time stream. For example, Dr. O'Neill described a non-AIDS colleague to another
clinic doctor: "He'd be good on general ID, but not on the HIV service. It's too fast;
you need to be there twenty-four hours." During inpatient rounds, a patient pointed
out an article in the newspaper on Bactrim being approved by the FDA to treat PCP.
Dr. Peters commented, "It's interesting because we've been using Bactrim for a long
time. . . . This is the only field where if you're not in it, you're out-of-date."

Experts are made in a matter of a few years. A resident asked Dr. O'Neill about
the use of a drug in treating *Pneumocystis*. Afterward, the resident commented, "Well,
that's ten years of experience talking." Dr. O'Neill replied, "Ten years makes you an
old-timer with this disease." The resident shot back, "No, six months."

My informants identify themselves by their ability to thrive in the ever-
changing world of AIDS.

I like taking care of sick people. I couldn't imagine seeing people with sore throats and, you
know, UTI's [urinary tract infections] all day long; I just couldn't imagine doing that. . . . It's
changing constantly, so there's a lot to keep up with. Intellectually, it's challenging. The patients
are complicated, which is challenging. But apart from the sort of cerebral pleasures of it—that's
kind of sick isn't it?—I like the patients—you know, I really do like the patients.

In a reflexive moment, Dr. O'Neill remarked:

Most medicine, like cardiology, for example, is so fixed. I mean, there are new drugs coming
out, but slowly, a sort of 4 percent change. In fact, I went into ID because there is always
something new coming out. In the 70s and 80s, there were new drugs, but they weren't really
very different from what we had. AIDS, though, is a whole wild thing.

For these physicians, AIDS is "a whole wild thing" rather than an unfamiliar source
of fear. Not only do my informants distinguish themselves in this fashion, so do their
non-AIDS colleagues. After a patient visit at Northlake, one general internist
discussed the case with the HIV team for a while. The internist remarked: "You
know, I consider the role of the general internist like myself in AIDS, and I'm damn
glad that there are guys like you around. I can't keep up."

AIDS medicine is distinguished by its character as well as its pace, and in
treating AIDS, physicians cease being internists or ID specialists and become AIDS
doctors. On rounds, the Northlake HIV team noted that a patient has tested positively
for bacterial pneumonia rather than PCP. Dr. O'Neill then joked about forgetting how
to recognize "typical" infectious disease. Dr. Holtzman added that if the team were
to go back to the ID service, they would "see a fever spike and order MAI
[*Mycobacterium avium-intracellulare*, also known as MAC] cultures and a serum

Crypto[coccus] antigen," the exotic AIDS fever work-up instead of the mundane tests appropriate to general infectious disease. HIV medicine is thus clearly distinguished from "typical" medicine, with its own list of differential diagnoses, categories, and thought patterns. In the process of treating AIDS, the doctors of the HIV team are no longer good ID specialists or internists or oncologists. They have become AIDS specialists.

I think a lot of it has more to do with the clinician's interest in the disease rather than his or her background. I know oncologists who are AIDS specialists; I know dermatologists; I know pediatricians; in Europe, I know a couple of psychiatrists. So, I really think it has more to do with the interest of the practitioner than with the training the practitioner has.

One type of discourse shared by almost all my informants is a narrative about their introduction to AIDS. These stories evoke a sense of initiation, as if into some secret society:

I've been in the retrovirus field since 1970—that's before reverse transcriptase. . . . So when I saw the HIV virus, I just became intrigued about how to make a vaccine for it. And I knew it would be difficult. So, I just got this inspiration. I don't know, I call it inspiration.

You just realize the magnitude of the scope of the epidemic—it made me a believer. It evolved my research closer and closer to AIDS. I ended up taking this job, which was the most unlikely thing for me because I wasn't a known AIDS researcher.

Well, I came here in 1981, in November, to work in the Department of Cancer Prevention with a friend of mine who was director of the department. And in that month, someone who worked for us came and asked me if I could help him, because he was having difficulties swallowing and was losing weight and had fever and didn't feel well. And it turned out after a couple of weeks of investigation and wondering what was wrong with him that he actually had the esophageal candidiasis and in fact had AIDS. Although I had seen some cases in Miami earlier that year where I was working before, it never really occurred to me that AIDS sort of actually happened to people you knew.

I heard in the summer of 1981 about the outbreak of Kaposi's in homosexual men. After a short period of scoffing at the idea, which I thought was a ridiculous concept, I soon became convinced in fact that it was real and jumped right in, basically in August of 1981. So I was right at the beginning. . . . But the really convincing people were the clinicians out in the field, particularly Michael Gottlieb, some of these people who said, "Guys, this is real." You listen to these people, you see their pictures, and you believe, or at least I believed.

These stories of initiation into the world of AIDS are imbued with mystic qualities, invoking themes of inspiration, recognition, belief.

The introduction to AIDS emerges as a moment of truth, when the speakers recognized AIDS as a significant force in the world. For many of my informants, American and French, that moment came with their first encounter with an AIDS patient and forms a significant part of these initiation stories.

So I did medicine in June and July of 1981, and as a second-year medical student, first time on the ward, my very first patient as a new student was this gay male from Florida who had come up to North Carolina with this article that he had got out of some gay magazine, talking about this new gay disease. It was about Kaposi's. That's what he had—he had these purple lesions all over him. Anyway, he just walks into the emergency room with this article and says, "I think I have this." . . . And obviously that was at the very beginning of the whole process, and it has just been sort of fascinating. I mean, in first-year medical school when you are reading all of this stuff, you sort of view medicine like you are learning an art that is already here and developed, and all of a sudden, I realized that this was a new disease.

I saw this report, with five PCP in homosexuals, and I read it and it was like nothing public at this time. And the same day, in the afternoon, I had a consultation, and one of the patients I saw was a steward, and he told me that he was a homosexual, and he came with cough, with fever, with diarrhea, with exactly the same symptoms that I had read in the morning for this famous PCP. . . . At this time, I think it was in August '81, I remember one of my patients I saw in '79, and who died in '80 or at the beginning of '81, who had exactly the same symptoms: with anemia deficiency that we never found why, who had PCP, neurological symptoms, who was a Portuguese and who died of unknown cause, who was with the Portuguese army in Angola in '74, '75. And I make the connection between the two cases because it was also PCP of unknown cause.

As a reporter in the *New York Times* noted, "Doctors remember vividly when and where they saw their first AIDS patient. It is an event burned in their minds like the assassination of President Kennedy" (Kolata 1991, A11). The event itself, if not the thoughts at the time, is etched in the memory, and thus the discourse, of my informants.

Sometimes the speaker is drawn into the AIDS world by the illness of a friend, relative, or colleague.

I worked with a doctor, when you're a student working with doctors. And that doctor died of AIDS after I started. . . . I was supposed to replace him one week, and the last day he had an epilepsy [seizure] and his friend called me to keep on working for him because his friend [the doctor] was sick. And he died six months later; I worked in AIDS six months later.

I was doing internal medicine basically in San Francisco, which has a lot of AIDS patients. So I was interested in that, and also I think to a large degree, I think my interest was spurred on by the fact that my brothers are both HIV-positive.

Other informants talk of being drawn into AIDS by chance, by being in the right—or wrong—place at the right time.

[I got involved in AIDS] by accident, like everybody else. We got started in December 1981, because the first patient, who would be ignored in France, was followed by Dr. Bernard, who is one of my friends.

[I got started in AIDS by] bad luck. I and several other people were working in the STD [sexually transmitted disease] division in 1981 when the first case reports of AIDS came in.

I was in the right place at the right time, or I was in the wrong place at the wrong time. I guess that just depends on your perspective.

In many cases, as the narrative unfolds, the chance emerges as something more akin to fate than luck. For many informants, AIDS is the disease that they have been training for all their lives, literally what they have been destined to do as medical professionals.

But the HIV thing sort of—I was trained for it. It's an epidemic. It's a disease of the latter half of this century that's far in importance of developing nations—even underdeveloped nations now—and I feel that it's a challenge to one's career. If you are trained in this field, to just sort of ignore it or whatever I think is just such an incredible waste.

Again, as a gay man, I often sometimes feel that I'm on a mission and that I've always been in the right place at the right time, starting with learning about how to do clinical trials in an intelligent way and why they need to be done that way. . . . So, I've just always felt like this is what I am supposed to be doing. Not to be too mystical in California about it, but it seems like this is it. This is what I was meant to do.

Everything interests me about it, but the thing that is important, that keeps me riveted, is that I almost feel like I have a calling. That never comes out sounding right. But my background was working in infectious diseases, and I spent many years working on other epidemic virus diseases. . . . So you put those together, my background and the position—it's almost as if I have a—calling is the only word, and that implies a religious overtone, but it is not intended to be religious, just the idea that what I have been doing all my life if I can't take on the most important epidemic virus disease to come along in a while.

Through their discourse, physicians and researchers in AIDS construct themselves as being a part of something larger, an epic phenomenon that few people experience within their lifetime.

I was drawn to it initially because it struck me that this is going to have an enormous public health impact. There's no question about that in my mind. That's what pulled me into this. I thought, "Wow, we really have a problem, and this is going to be the most important thing in my scientific lifetime."

My initial interest was based upon the fact that I had a long-standing investigative interest of the impact of infection upon the immune system. As the decade went by, it became apparent that this was, for someone in infectious disease, an extremely important problem. And that for someone of my age, there was probably never going to be another infectious disease of equal importance that I will ever deal with—certainly none prior to this.

The challenge is both social and intellectual:

When you say "drawn to it," there's various levels. There's the level of saying, "There's part of me that is this good soul, and I'm going to go out there and save the world." And that says, "Oh, it's a big problem. You have to do something about this." There's another part of me, which is up in my head, which says something to the effect that, "God this is an issue to know." I'm sorry people are dying, but it's a fascinating problem, and it's just an extraordinarily interesting virus in its own right, and we don't know anything about it. It's terra incognita, and just as an intellectual problem, it's extraordinary.

It suddenly occurred to me that with AIDS we didn't have that luxury, because while herpes is terrible, and it will ruin your sex life, it won't kill you, and AIDS will. And it wasn't enough to sit up here and tell these kids when they came up with their Kaposi's sarcoma that, "Oh, yea, you've got this fatal disease, and there's nothing we can do. Have a nice day." And once that dawns on you, you become socially very active. So it did dawn, and I did.

It is a shattering epidemic. By far the worst epidemic of the twentieth century, and it is likely to change the history books. So as a public health problem, it is devastatingly overwhelming. I think that for those two reasons, both the magnitude of the epidemic and the sense that I don't have to get up in the morning and wonder if what I'm doing for a living is worthwhile, you have an inherent sense of self-worth coming from a job like this. . . . And then the selfish reasons, the intellectual gratifications, the ability to have an idea and make it happen.

This discourse of calling, of being part of a broadly significant phenomenon, separates my informants from their non-AIDS colleagues as much as any other narrative. As one clinician put it, "My professional life has been, and will be, dominated by this disease." Often their personal life becomes enmeshed in AIDS as well:

You have to realize we were all spending our life thinking of working on AIDS, because from 1982 until at least 1985, 1986, every dinner I went to—where I was not myself saying anything on AIDS—even when I was going out, having dinner with friends, we knew what I was doing, so people were immediately asking me questions. . . . Finally, they realized I was working on AIDS, and immediately the whole discussion for the rest of dinner or the rest of the evening was on AIDS.

By chance or by choice, they have entered the HIV community, and it has changed them irrevocably.

Just as doctor-patient relationships in the AIDS clinics tend to be warm and informal, so are relations between medical colleagues. As one French physician explained:

Maybe the human relation is different here. It is much more friendly, much less strict, less academic than in another hospital. If you visit another hospital, some of the departments are very rigid, very strict, like in the old days for infectious disease.

The residents at Rousseau spoke similarly about the AIDS clinic compared to the other medical services they had experienced.

I think the fact that the structure is very small, everyone can communicate very easily, from Bernard to the nurses. And it's so easy, people get closer and it works much easier than services when you have the professor who is coming one visit a week and if you have to ask something to the professor, you have to wait if he's here or at the visit. . . . And the lowest person has to ask the intern, and the intern has to ask the professor, the assistant, and then the professor says yes, and you do the exam.

This intimacy may be grounded in the history of AIDS medicine. In Paris, the original study group was informal and multidisciplinary in nature, often meeting over dinner at a member's house. At many American sites, similar groups arose, informal at first, then later evolving into formal organizations. As described previously, the experience of these informal groups emerges as a significant element in my informants' discourse, both clinicians and researchers.

When I was speaking a few minutes ago of the first meeting we made in '84, I can assure you that I will still remember it all my life, these first dinners where we started to speak of AIDS, on the epidemiological plane, of what we had seen, of what struck us. We started at nine o'clock in the morning and finished at three, four o'clock [in the morning]! We were very excited, very enthusiastic. . . . In '84, there was a wild enthusiasm; it was truly wild. And that is the truly remarkable. It was a period that I found extraordinary.

These narratives form a creation story about the birth of the medical HIV community and the strength of the ties among its members.

In this discourse, AIDS clinicians and researchers, from whatever their initial backgrounds, have more in common with each other than with colleagues outside of AIDS. As Dr. O'Neill relates:

I was telling the former chief of staff, who is a friend of mine—we're neighbors. I occasionally ride to work with him. He said, "Well, how are things going? I heard you got the new grant, blah, blah, blah." And I said, "Yea, I'm going up to the NIH to present some data we have put together. And I was sort of happy. I finally got promoted—not promoted, but appointed to a committee—Pneumocystis Pathogen Study Group Committee within the Opportunistic Infection Committee of the whole ACTG." [Laugh] So this guy starts laughing his head off. He goes, "Now I have heard everything. Now you are specializing in one organism in one kind of patient. That's like your whole specialty now." It was really kind of funny that it is so focused. I never really looked at it that way.

As Dr. O'Neill talks about his professional life, he constructs his identity as a member of the HIV community, signified here by the AIDS Clinical Trials Groups, while at the same time becoming increasingly distant from other medical circles.

Because actually now, one of the things really very attractive to me is that people at my level at the various centers around the country are all people basically about my same age, within five or ten years. They've all got the same sort of training/education background, and they've all written their little share of papers, everyone has got their little niche, and we see each other constantly. . . . So it's a different circle. It's not anything that is rarified or anything. We're all human and it's all the same. But it's really kind of a different blend of people. It's not actually people you would pick out as your friends. But as far as colleagues go, it's [the ACTG meetings] the only place where you are going to find your real peers in this funny niche that we found ourselves in.

Physicians in AIDS thus look within the HIV community, "this funny niche that we found ourselves in," for their professional identity. On a daily basis, that identity is found within the clinic itself.

At Northlake and Rousseau, all physicians, including residents, were on a first-name basis. Residents and fellows at both clinics confirmed that this practice is unusual in other medical departments. Additionally, most of the nurses addressed the physicians by first or last name (not as "Doctor"). This may be an effect of developing a close team that works together in dealing with a complex and emotionally charged disease.

I experienced this sense of closeness more fully at two clinic-wide celebrations, one at Northlake and one at Rousseau. At the end of the infectious disease fellows' rotation through the Northlake clinic, everyone—nurses, receptionists, and physicians—went out to a restaurant to celebrate. With scarcely controlled solemnity, the staff presented each of the fellows with corsages made of flowers, a condom, latex gloves, a mask and a viral culture tube as an award for their service. The fellows, in turn, presented everyone else with small gag gifts, appropriate to their personality or job, as well as a "Golden Condom Award": a certificate with a gold condom attached to it. I even received one.[5] The clinic members had all put a significant measure of time and effort into this celebration, making sure that none were excluded from recognition. This level of warmth and familiarity, unimpeded by formal rank within the medical community, appears distinctive of AIDS medicine.

A similar celebration took place at Rousseau. Ostensibly a New Year's party, it was also a farewell celebration for two visiting clinicians and myself. The entire afternoon had been set aside for this party, patient visits having been rescheduled around it. Lunch was prepared by the nurses and secretaries and served in the day hospital, with plenty of wine and various desserts brought in by clinic members.[6] At the end, I received proper French good-byes—a kiss on each cheek—from everyone, the nurses, secretaries, and Dr. Bernard himself. While the styles of the two celebrations differ, they each reconstruct an unusually intimate set of social ties, evoking a sense of familiarity and warmth recognized by participants as distinct from other professional interactions.

While few informants directly refer to themselves as "AIDS specialists" or "AIDSologists," this identity emerges through the stories they choose to tell about themselves and their work. They have become AIDS doctors, and this designation is carried with them wherever they go.

I do a lot of lecturing for other infectious disease topics and AIDS always comes up, because when they introduce me, it's always as medical director of the AIDS Clinic, and they wonder why they're hearing a story about ciprofloxacin [an antibiotic]. And they always ask about their AIDS patients.

Outside of a few postdoctoral researchers, all of my informants have made AIDS treatment and/or research a strong, even exclusive aspect of their professional lives. Their dedication and fascination with AIDS touch those who meet them, as was the case between Dr. Bernard and the Rousseau general practitioners, and Dr. O'Neill and the internists at Northlake. Involvement with AIDS is thus contagious and often incurable. At the farewell celebration at Rousseau, Dr. Farsi and I talked awhile about my future plans. He said we would, of course, be seeing each other in the future, "because now you, too, have been bitten by the AIDS." And so I have.

CONCLUSION

> That is my dream, that the AIDS epidemic does alert the society we live in to some of its defects. And that it wakes people up to appreciate that we have to do something about it. If there's a crumbling bridge, you've got to fix the bridge. And I think that people have got to think about the human bridge at least as articulately as they think about the bridge that may go over the East River.
>
> San Francisco clinician

As seen throughout this section, my informants use AIDS to talk about a broad variety of experiences: the body, patients, health care, science, medical relationships, and their own identity as French and American medical professionals. All of these experiences, and the discourse they engender, are integral to the lives of these men and women. Taken together, they redefine the medical community in the context of AIDS.

AIDS is thus more than a disease, the constructed object of medical science. It is rather a medium for reconstructing the fundamental character of the medical world, material, historical, and social. Through AIDS, death can be a "good outcome," medicine is and has always been a dangerous enterprise, and good science can be done amidst publicity and politics. As discussed earlier, AIDS can be interpreted as a yet-incomplete rite of passage, filled with the paradox and *communitas* characteristic of liminal experiences. Physicians and researchers of disparate backgrounds enter through the door of AIDS and are transformed into AIDS doctors/researchers, members of the HIV community. Their regional and national affiliations are simultaneously a part of this process and renewed by it.

The medical community is not transformed in isolation to the rest of society. The relationships, that is, the discourse and practices between the medical community, patients, and the lay public, are also reconstructed via AIDS. Patients emerge more fully as partners, ascribed a level of knowledge and power approaching expertise. The lay involvement in decision making in research and therapeutics is unprecedented. At the same time, social problems are being redefined as medical ones, such that medical professionals are becoming, perhaps reluctantly, participants in discourse on housing, access to social services, substance abuse, and education. The boundaries between medical and nonmedical practices are increasingly blurred. As one epidemiologist concluded: "To me, AIDS is a mirror of many things. It's really a foundation, the strength of the building that we are building in terms of a society."AIDS is thus perhaps a rite of passage not only for the medical community but for entire societies as well.

NOTES

1. Each region emerges from the discourse with varying degrees of power in the AIDS field, as well as definitive sociocultural characteristics highlighted by the epidemic. For a thorough analysis, see J. Feldman (1993).

2. I use the term *national* rather than *ethnic* to avoid confusion with the latter's more common meaning of ancestral ties, such as Italian-American or Hispanic. Rather, I am interested in the construction of an American or French identity, as distinct from other such affiliations. The concept of ethnic or cultural groups is a tricky one, and discerning boundaries between such groups is problematic at the least (Barth 1984). Thus, my separation between ethnic and national identity is, as always, an artificial device intended to open up new meanings, not to assert a truth about life as lived.

3. Interestingly enough, the rare "first stories" I encountered in France were almost always about PCP prophylaxis, though, as described below, they are somewhat different from the American versions in their construction.

4. In fact, colleagues of Gallo did isolate another virus in 1987, which they christened HTLV-IV. By the end of the year, however, the isolate was determined to be a lab contaminant.

5. My certificate also came with a little Sherlock Holmes detective book, in recognition of my research at the clinic.

6. The two celebrations provide interesting cultural comparisons outside of AIDS as well. The American party was held at a restaurant, which perhaps carries a higher status in the United States than celebrations in the home. The French party was held within the clinic itself—the value placed on privacy—and the food was prepared by the clinic staff, suggesting the personal commitment common to French interactions between friends. The personalized gag gifts presented by the Americans could be interpreted as an American version of a similar bond.

Part IV

MEDICAL DIFFERENCES, DIFFERENT MEDICINES

12

French and American Differences

If the general will is to be able to express itself, it is essential that there should be no partial society within the State and that each citizen should think only his own thoughts.
                    Jean-Jacques Rousseau (quoted in Wilsford 1991, 30)

If American physicians were to enter a Paris clinic, they would initially feel comfortable. All the tools of the trade are present—thermometers, blood pressure cuffs, the X-ray view box. Their French colleagues would be speaking in recognizable terms, of pneumonia and blood counts and brisk reflexes. Little by little, however, a certain unease would develop. Americans would notice that temperatures are taken rectally or under the arm but never orally. Drugs are almost never called by the generic name, but by an entirely distinct set of trade names, including a vast number of antibiotics American doctors have never encountered. Powders and suppositories are popular drug forms, and it is the patient, not the doctor, who carries the prescription pad. A routine checkup does not usually include a urinalysis, and the French physician rarely inquires about smoking or alcohol.

One may well brush off these differences as "local color," interesting but unimportant in the face of the overarching common ideas of biomedicine. As seen in the previous sections, however, biomedicine is hardly uniform, and some key differences exist between French and American medicine surrounding AIDS. It is, after all, through these differences in what people say and do that culture is continually reshaped. The expression of culture in French biomedicine can be found in how health care is structured, in the relationship between doctors and patients, and even in conceptualizations of health and disease, as in the case of AIDS. During my field experiences, I discovered a wide variety of differences in the structure, values, and practices of French medical care and in the stories that help to fashion them. Many of these differences are not specific to AIDS, but rather, AIDS serves to exemplify them and to act as a medium for expressing what makes French medicine, indeed French identity, distinct.

One of the first differences that confronted me in Paris was that of nationalized health care, described previously, where patients are reimbursed by the Securité Sociale for 75 to 100 percent of the costs of care, including medication. On my second day at the clinic, a nurse-administrator asked me, "Is it true that you have people in America going without care because they don't have money?" This question was repeated many times by many people during my stay, accompanied by looks of either indignation or complete bafflement. The fact that everyone is *prise en charge*, literally "taken in charge," by the French health care system acts as an expression of social values, a belief in basic health care as a right and that the state, rather than corporate groups or individuals as in the United States, is the appropriate guarantor of this right. In fact, the term *prise en charge* has no single counterpart in English. It most closely incorporates two American concepts, that of a physician "following" a patient over the course of a disease or as part of a lifetime relationship, plus that of being "covered" by some form of health insurance. To be *prise en charge* in France encompasses not only the individual doctor-patient relationship but that between the state, as guarantor of access to care, and all patients as a group. It is at once a professional, economic, and social obligation, distinctively French in character.

This fundamental structural difference immediately affects the encounter between doctor and patient. In sharp contrast to everyday practice in the United States, patients in France, except for foreign visitors, are never asked how they are paying for their care, while patients themselves almost never request a different medication because of concern over cost. When I asked a resident at the Paris clinic about differences between the United States and France, she replied:

Well, I would say the first point is maybe a social point, because patients here, as soon as they get AZT, they are 100 percent taken in charge by the Social Security. I don't really know how it goes on in America, but maybe that's a very important part because that changes, I think, completely the relationship between the doctors and the patients.

The role of money, for the French resident, changes this fundamental relationship in a critical way. Raymonde Carroll (1988) suggests that French attitudes toward talk of money are quite similar in character to American responses to talk of sexuality. Americans express repugnance toward public talk of sexual experiences, while talk of financial conquests is quite acceptable. In France, the reverse holds. People may openly vaunt their sexual exploits, while bragging about one's wealth is considered to be in "bad taste" (Carroll 1988, 128–131). In developing a nationalized system of health care, the French are able to remove talk about money, an ambivalent and distasteful topic, from the medical encounter. What on the surface appears a simple difference in health care policy is, on a deeper level, an essential difference in culture.

If one now places AIDS within the milieu of the two health care systems, the differential impact on physician discourse is notable. As mentioned in the discussion of discourse constructing AIDS, my American informants used the phrase "CDC-defined AIDS" on a regular basis. Whether a patient had "AIDS" was, for them, an important question. In France, on the other hand, the term "CDC-[or WHO] defined AIDS" was not only unimportant but nonexistent outside of a WHO survey form and a few international clinical trials. Not surprisingly, in order for HIV-positive patients in the United States to qualify for certain important health benefits including disability, they must carry an AIDS diagnosis as determined by CDC criteria. Under the French system, this distinction is irrelevant in regard to access to health benefits. However, the correlation is not simply one of cause and effect, since my American informants would ask this question about patients outside the issue of access to benefits, such as in the case of patients already on disability or having no need to pursue it. Nonetheless, the differing structure of the two health care systems certainly plays its role.

Another aspect of the interaction of health care structure and discourse lies in AIDS-related discourse about the system itself. As discussed earlier, AIDS is presented by both French and American informants as a "highlighter" of systemwide problems, showing up defects or even as the straw breaking the system's back. The latter is especially common in American discourse, with many of these informants calling for nationalized health care. The French informants, on the other hand, are less likely to criticize the system of care per se, and some in fact spoke of increased admiration for their Securité Sociale.

What my French informants did talk about was centralized control over health care and research resources. Through their stories, they construct a narrative of a stifling centralized bureaucracy that controls from the top, resulting in stagnation and immobility. In contrast, American informants construct a fragmented, chaotic system operating from the bottom, resulting in confusion and lack of direction. Thus, both sets of informants produce themes in which they themselves lack power and control, but through virtually opposite mechanisms. These stories appear directly tied to the structure of health care in their respective countries and, when put together with narratives on how informants develop new approaches, such as community research initiatives, act as models of and models for these same health care structures.

Another structural difference, that of the roles of generalist and specialist, is also highlighted by AIDS. As noted before, most patients with HIV infection in France are referred to hospital-based specialists rather than general practitioners, and those that do are not allowed to prescribe AZT. The rules governing distribution of AZT are set by multihospital committees, made up of clinicians and pharmacists. At one such meeting I attended, a physician brought up the idea of expanding AZT-prescribing privileges to generalists. The pharmacists expressed skepticism that generalists would know how to manage the drug appropriately, as well as concern that patients would go from doctor to doctor, pharmacy to pharmacy, stockpiling prescriptions for AZT. The committee finally agreed that certain generalists who "were known" to the hospital would be allowed to prescribe the drug, but patients could only obtain the medication at that hospital's pharmacy.

In this instance, AIDS serves as a vehicle for talking about the role of the generalist physician in France. It also underlines the power of pharmacists in dictating access to medications, as well as the importance of personal ties, of "being known" in the French medical community. The AIDS epidemic does not merely reflect the role of the generalist but reconstructs it. There simply are not enough specialists in France to handle the volume of cases, which in turn creates potential for expansion of the generalist role, first in AIDS care and then perhaps in other areas as well.[1] As one general practitioner put it:

The town doctors had always been kept apart. The general practitioner had always been someone who has not been well viewed in France. He is someone who is there to prescribe for sore throats, do certificates, but he has not, I find, had a sufficient impact. It is true that AIDS has come to transform somewhat this way of seeing the town doctor.

In French medical practice, strong boundaries seem to exist not only between generalists and specialists but between specialties themselves. As noted previously, physicians in the Paris clinic, for example, rarely performed funduscopic exams on patients, considered the province of ophthalmologists.[2] When I explained that this was not the case in the United States, I was informally designated the funduscopic exam specialist for the clinic and was encouraged to help the residents practice this skill.

As in so many areas of medicine, this strong differentiation, too, is changing in response to AIDS. As we have seen, the administration of chemotherapy and increasing practice of eye exams by Rousseau physicians are two such examples. The trend in France seems to be one of generalists or infectious disease specialists incorporating more and more knowledge and abilities from outside their previous role. They have become *sidalogues*, AIDS specialists.

In the United States, in contrast, there are no general practitioners in the French sense of the term, and a higher proportion of specialists than in the French system. Treatment of AIDS in the United States has historically been handled by a number of different specialties, most commonly infectious disease, but oncologists and dermatologists also entered the field early on. In the course of the epidemic, these specialists have assumed much of the primary care associated with their patients rather than maintaining their purely consultant role.

For example, a New York informant, working in a tertiary center devoted mainly to cancer treatment and research, stated: "When I came here in 1983, we saw only ten patients a day, total. We actually had to share patients. Now each of us sees seven to ten patients each afternoon." He added that this increase is due solely to the increase in AIDS patients. He concluded, "We're no longer consultants; we've become primary care for these HIV patients." Given the highly specialized nature of his institution as a whole, this is a telling commentary on the transformative nature of AIDS in American medicine. As we have seen, this new role with its new responsibilities and boundaries is the subject of my American informants' discourse.

They have become AIDS doctors, a type of primary care doctor who utilizes other specialists such as oncologists to handle specific tasks.

Thus, as was the case with health care system narratives, French and American clinicians involved with AIDS have come to similar conclusions by way of quite different paths. They have ceased being what they were and have become, more or less, AIDS doctors. In France, they are specialists, former infectious disease doctors, internists, or generalists who by way of new experience and training have adopted a variety of knowledge and techniques formerly appropriate only to other specialties. In the United States, they are primary care doctors, responsible for the total care of their patient, utilizing outside specialists when needed. Obviously, the distinctions between the two are not nearly so clear-cut, either in discourse or practice. They are fluid and changeable, as with all social phenomena. Yet differences are discernible and useful for understanding both French and American experiences.

As seen in the discussion of money and health care, the doctor-patient relationship in France is another element immediately recognizable as different from that in the United States. My American informants who have had contact with French medicine invariably describe it as "paternalistic," with the doctor assuming most of the control over decision making. Indeed, on the surface, this description appears to be accurate. The important question, however, is, What sociocultural values are involved in the French doctor-patient relationship? As one might guess, it goes beyond a simple question of doctors maintaining control over patients.

The treatment of persons with AIDS provides an excellent setting to analyze this relationship. As demonstrated by several encounters at Northlake, the American physician almost invariably tells the patient of the diagnosis of AIDS, while the French clinician often will choose not to do so. This was especially true nearer the beginning of the epidemic, when few therapies existed. As one French clinician said in 1987:

Sometimes we may say to a patient, "You are an AIDS patient." Sometimes we cannot because we feel they know what it means, but they don't want to hear the word. They want to hear, for example, "Kaposi's sarcoma"; they want to hear "toxoplasmosis," "*Pneumocystis*," but they don't want to know the AIDS. The word "AIDS."

The value expressed in this discourse is not one of maintaining control or of saying, "I know best," but rather one of caring for the patient, of trying to ascertain what the patient may wish to know or not to know. While the issue of power is certainly involved in control of information, it is not the sole factor at work. Rather, I would suggest that, unlike Americans, both the French physician and patient are tending to value the social tie over the gaining of information as the predominant feature of the doctor-patient relationship.

Although Carroll (1988) does not explore the doctor-patient relationship specifically, she notes that French people seek information on any topic differently than Americans, privileging information gained from trusted people in a face-to-face encounter. "The preceding suggests that when I (a French person) ask for information, I am, in a sense, delegating power. I temporarily put myself in someone else's hands, I undertake to follow his or her directions. This is why I will not ask just anyone" (116). In fact, French patients will often change doctors until they can establish this sense of trust with a provider (Escande 1975).

In this regard, the doctor-patient relationship in France takes on some aspects of friendship as described by Carroll (1988). A friend is expected, in an emergency such as illness, to take burdens off the ill person to the point of temporarily taking charge of the person's life. The French physician, by not fully informing the patient of the diagnosis, is perhaps doing as might a trusted friend (75). In contrast, the values expressed in the American doctor-patient relationship, as seen in the context of AIDS, are those of information sharing and patient empowerment.

The French doctor-patient relationship also shares some characteristics with the relationship between parent and child, as constructed through the medical decision-making process. In the United States, as seen previously, the stereotypical person with AIDS is constructed by physicians as well informed about the disease, taking an extremely active role in treatment, to the point of suggesting or refusing specific therapies in accordance with his or her own knowledge and desires. The French patient, on the other hand, rarely questions the prescribed treatments and virtually never suggests alternatives. French doctors, unlike their American counterparts, rarely lay out several options for the patient's decision but rather recommend a path of therapy and explain the reasons for that recommendation.

In one such observed encounter, a French clinician had discovered the rapid spread of a patient's Kaposi's sarcoma. The doctor told the patient: "Because they are nodular lesions, you can't treat them locally [with radiation]; you must use general [systemic] treatment." The doctor then outlined the chemotherapy agents he favors. The patient's questions were procedural—how often must he come in, will he be able to work during this time—rather than questioning the proposed therapy itself. This example serves as interesting contrast to an encounter between one of the French clinicians and an American patient. When the doctor informed the patient that he needed to be hospitalized to treat an infection, the American quickly suggested that he could receive the intravenous antibiotics at home. This sparked an uncomfortable negotiation between the two, a result of differences not only between doctor and patient explanations but between French and American expectations of doctors and patients.

As seen in the way the French medical system is structured, health care is more clearly a social act incorporating social, rather than individual, values. Carroll (1988) explains that having and raising a child is a social act for the French as well, that the child is a link between the parent and the society (47). The parent constantly must demonstrate that he or she is performing the social obligation of raising a new, responsible member of that society. It is through the bond of love between parent and child that the child is likely to comply. If we apply this to the French doctor-patient relationship, the patient is the link between the doctor and society, and it is a social obligation to help produce a well, or at least compliant, patient. The patient, like the child, complies not out of love in this case but out of trust. Patients, like the French adolescent described by Carroll, may know too that they will be able to ultimately follow their own inclinations in peace if they allow the doctor to play out such a quasi-parental role (52).

Another, complementary interpretation is also available. According to Wilsford (1991), the French privilege the discourse of experts, especially in the areas of government and administration. This is due not simply to a belief in a rational paradigm where only experts can participate in specialized narratives but also to a belief that expert bureaucrats speak *for France*, not as individuals or as a partisan interest group. Extending this to French medicine, a doctor's discourse is privileged because he speaks not only as an individual expert but as *French medicine* in its entirety, representing the whole of society rather than the partisan group "doctors," as is commonly designated in the United States.

This set of meanings could also be tied into French ambivalence about money, mentioned above. According to some of my informants, French public hospital doctors carry more respect than private hospital doctors. This is in part because they are not "in it for the money" but are motivated and trained to speak for French medicine rather than private interests.[3]

As in the parent/child analogy used earlier, the emphasis here is on the manifestly social character of French medicine, in comparison with the individual or associative group character of American medicine.[4] In the United States, doctors are an interest group. The government may be seen as another interest group, insurance companies as yet another, and recently, patients and activists as yet another. All of these are social in the sense that they incorporate relationships between people, yet only when taken all together do you approach a sense of American society as a whole. In France, as evidenced in Rousseau's eloquent pronouncement, there is the individual and there is France—French society as a collective identity/entity—and not much in between.

As discussed earlier, AIDS is changing the doctor-patient relationship in France. AIDS patients are perceived as more active and questioning about their treatment than other patients, and that AIDS, in turn, has changed my informants' approach to advising patients about their disease. The central issue remains maintaining a relationship of trust. A similar sense of change is found in the American discourse, voiced as varying degrees of acceptance of patient activism and empowerment in relation to the medical community as a whole, as well as in the relationship between individual doctor and patient. The theme of both French and American narratives on the doctor-patient relationship in the age of AIDS is one of partnership: in France, through physician honesty; in America, through patient autonomy.

Differences between French and American biomedicine are found not only in how medical care is structured, or how doctors relate to patients, but in how the body and its ills are constituted. These differences are subtle but telling, and the context of AIDS provides us again with a remarkable example.

Earlier, I noted that the French clinicians I encountered administered some types of chemotherapy themselves, unlike any of my American informants. This difference appears to be rooted in the history of AIDS in both countries. At the beginning of the epidemic, the vast majority of French clinicians who became involved with AIDS were general internists or infectious disease specialists. Research on AIDS followed this pattern, coming out of hospital-based laboratories or basic biological research centers such as the Pasteur Institute. Clinical research arose as an outgrowth of treating AIDS patients. In the United States, however, a significant number of research and clinical informants began their careers in oncology. A large number of well-known cancer centers have included AIDS research and treatment into their mission, such as Memorial Sloan-Kettering in New York City and the Dana Farber Cancer Institute in Boston. Certain clinics, particularly in these specialized institutions, began solely as vehicles for conducting clinical research rather than providing treatment for large numbers of patients.

These origins have a profound impact on how AIDS is viewed and treated in each country. One American clinician described a "turf battle" over AIDS between infectious disease specialists and oncologists. In his view, the infectious disease specialists technically won but have themselves ended up employing an oncological model of the disease. As Rothman and Edgar (1992) demonstrate, extensive debate over the role of placebo, randomized control trials was framed in terms of whether AIDS was like an infectious disease or a cancer. The initial ID-supported placebo trials, such as with AZT, have since given way to comparative treatment trials.

In both the Northlake and Rousseau clinics, courses of treatment would be influenced by the patient's symptoms, if any, and the number of CD4 lymphocytes. However, in the Northlake clinic, clinicians would distinguish whether or not the patient has had an "AIDS-defining illness." In contrast, when epidemiologists asked the Rousseau clinic for a count of patients with CDC-defined AIDS, the staff had to spend several minutes reviewing a patient's chart before deciding whether he indeed had AIDS. AIDS in France is consistently addressed as a continuous spectrum of disease rather than in the discrete stages more common to American models.

As seen in previous chapters, American clinicians tend to approach AIDS much like cancer: diagnose early and treat aggressively. Once the external threat has entered the body (or the body has taken on alien qualities, as in the case of a cancer), health is lost and can only be regained by attacking the threat directly through medication or surgery. As Payer (1988) suggests, the body, for Americans, is akin to a machine: It does not fix itself but requires external intervention.

While cancer remains a powerful point of reference for clinicians treating AIDS in France, their models of AIDS retain elements of an infectious disease paradigm even today. As we have seen, themes of toxicity and development of resistance to drugs, both important concepts in treating infectious diseases, are common in how French clinicians speak of AIDS, especially in reference to the use of AZT. The French practice of prescribing AZT at a lower CD4 count reinforces this construction.

Why the French emphasis on the problem of resistance? As cancer is a primary model for AIDS in America, so tuberculosis may be a strong model for AIDS in France. Historically, the two countries have had extremely divergent experiences with and approaches to this chronic infectious disease. The American approach is to screen the population for exposure to TB using skin tests, then provide prophylaxis with the drug isoniazid (INH) to those known to have been exposed. In contrast, the French have long had a high prevalence of tuberculosis and now vaccinate most of their population, negating the value of skin tests. Additionally, resistance to INH and other therapies is not uncommon.[5] As Dr. Bernard informed his staff during a meeting:

The approach to tuberculosis in the US and Europe is totally different. For one thing, they don't have vaccination. In the US, their approach to prevention is to treat exposed people with isoniazid by itself, which seems to me not very good. French mycobacteriologists would be horrified. It is a function of the epidemiology of tuberculosis in the US, not like Europe, Africa, where resistance is rampant.

Thus, French experience with tuberculosis seems to inform their approach to AIDS, itself a chronic, difficult-to-treat infection. Concerned over the development of resistant strains of HIV in the population, the French intervene later in the individual. Yet another factor besides epidemiological experience may be driving this difference in treatment for both diseases—the distinctly French concept of *terrain*. As Lynn Payer (1988) notes, "It makes the French leaders in fields that concentrate on shoring up the *terrain*, such as immunotherapy for cancer. And it results in a decidedly more casual attitude toward the elimination of dirt and germs than that seen in many other countries" (62). Surprisingly enough, I rarely heard the term used in the clinic, though it may well be so fundamentally understood that it would not often be encountered in daily discourse.

Herzlich (1973) observes that, for the French, illness is exogenous in origin, while health is composed of the person's innate resistance to such threats. She also presents the concept of toxicity as being central to the French understanding of how illness develops:

Toxicity is the mechanism which particularly expresses the conflict involved in the encounter between the unhealthy way of life and the threatened individual. Firstly it may be viewed as a process extending over time. By virtue of its quality of slow accumulation its full effects only appear in the long term; decline in health is an intermediate stage in the process of the "release" of the illness. (43)

This analysis is consistent with my French informants' concern over the long-term toxicity of AZT, and their construction of the process from asymptomatic HIV infection to AIDS as a continuum. Working from the concept of *terrain*, it would be reasonable to emphasize vaccines for both tuberculosis and, experimentally, for AIDS, exposing the body to the disease agent and enabling the *terrain* to defend against subsequent infection. Also, it would make sense in this model to let a relatively healthy *terrain* do its work as long as possible before damaging both it and the disease agent with relatively toxic drugs—as seen in the French approach to the use of AZT. Finally, immune modulators, such as Imuthiol and interferon, would be considered a significant form of therapy, as reflected in their use early in the AIDS epidemic and continuing to a lesser extent today. Thus, French biomedical models and treatment practices regarding AIDS arise out of culturally distinct conceptualizations of how the body works in response to disease.

The French emphasis on vaccines and immunomodulators seems to have decreased over time, because the French medical community is, after all, not fully isolated from other such biomedical communities. Some isolation exists as a number of French physicians, especially general practitioners, do not or cannot read the "Anglo-Saxon" medical literature, and few can afford visits to the United States, even for conferences. In turn, articles published in the French medical journals rarely ever see the light of day in their English-language counterparts. Yet there is consistent exchange of ideas, people, and technologies between the two biomedicines, particularly between university or research oriented institutions such as Northlake and Rousseau, though certainly more prevalent in the area of bench research than in clinical medicine.[6] Despite their differences, there is no doubt that French and American biomedicine share many commonalities, both being based on a cellular-biochemical definition of disease. While their approaches to AIDS vary, they remain, for the most part, mutually comprehensible, utilizing similar therapies such as AZT and extrapolating from overlapping diseases of reference, such as cancer and tuberculosis.

In this regard, a certain standardization of models and approaches to AIDS seems to be taking place. In light of the Concord study, American clinical researchers are reexamining when to begin AZT therapy, while French physicians are abandoning certain immunological therapies, given their equivocal results in clinical trials. An almost paradigmatic shift appears to be in motion, with both biomedicines moving from a wide variety of constructions early on toward a more unified paradigm of AIDS, emerging out of a strong analogy with life-shortening chronic diseases such as diabetes or heart disease. Biomedical order—standard, meaningful patterns—thus arise on both sides of the Atlantic out of ambiguity, uncertainty, creativity. As we have seen, however, standardization is never complete in biomedicine, and French and American conceptualizations of how the body works will continue to inform how AIDS is treated in each country.

Up until now, we have looked at the subjects of French and American medical discourse, that is, what is directly constructed, be it the roles of specialists or the nature of AIDS itself. However, not only are the subjects of discourse different in France and the United States, but the nature of the discourse itself also differs. The type of narrative is particularly distinctive. In the previous chapter, we have seen that the Americans often relied on "first" stories—seeing the first patients, being the first clinic to use a particular treatment—while French informants frequently utilized "hardship" stories, narratives of overcoming tremendous obstacles and intense opposition in the course of their work with AIDS/HIV. Each of these types of narratives was especially common in relation to constructing issues of identity, be they personal, professional, or notable among the French, national. As always, one can find American hardship stories and French first narratives, but overall the difference is strikingly consistent. The question, of course, is, "Why?" or in theoretical terms, "What valid, meaningful interpretations are available for us as anthropologists?"

Remembering that any biomedicine is intrinsic to its sociocultural context, one can look for answers beyond biomedical paradigms and the myriad influences of the AIDS epidemic to their ethnographic surroundings. Atwood Gaines (1986) views France as part of the "Mediterranean Culture Area" proposed by Gilmore (1982) and characterized by such commonalities as patronage, parochialism, "structural dualism," authoritarian religion, dotal marriage, and the honor-shame complex. Gaines himself adds a "rhetoric of complaint," a type of discourse that communicates the suffering and misfortune and therefore the worthiness of the speaker. It also serves to protect oneself from the jealousy of others.[7] "One does not talk of glowing possibilities, plans and goals, and how well things are going; one complains" (Gaines 1986, 305). Narratives and commentaries about personal sickness are part of this discourse and contribute to a culturally specific French view of the self (Gaines 1982). The narratives of French physicians and researchers involved with AIDS, centering on this theme of hardship, might well be an example of this "rhetoric of complaint."

While I encountered no evidence of authoritarian religion—in fact, religious references or related practices were strikingly absent in the Rousseau clinic—one could interpret some of the AIDS discourse as "parochial" in the sense of continually emphasizing the French national identity, usually in opposition to American nationality, in a variety of narratives. In the stories of the early days of the AIDS epidemic, the French, as a group, are the underdog heroes of hardship stories, accomplishing great medical advances with little money or recognition. The Gallo-Montagnier dispute is, of course, the ultimate narrative in this regard. If we expand Gilmore's (1982) view of parochialism, we can see this discourse as constructive of France as one village, defined against and in opposition to other "villages" of the world.

There is evidence for Gilmore's "structural dualism" as well. Gilmore speaks as a structuralist when he refers to this "underlying theme of a dynamic tension between contrasting elements," found in "both conscious and unconscious processes" (180). Translating this structurally framed concept into a interpretive theme of ambivalence, Rousseau's statement and the hardship narratives open themselves up to new meanings. There emerges from both, on the one hand, the construction of a unified France, the subject of parochialism discussed above. On the other hand, there exists the individual, the French man or woman thinking his or her own thoughts, often in vociferous opposition to other such individuals. As we have seen in the hardship narratives, some of the greatest opposition the protagonists face is from their compatriots.

One of my American research informants visits France regularly and related a story of how one French virologist would get up on the table at the Pasteur Institute cafeteria, shouting invectives about Montagnier: "He said, 'I'll talk about Montagnier any way I please!' And the amazing thing is that no one even looked up." The American researcher is not only constructing his French counterparts but also commenting on how the French construct themselves as passionate, even fanatic individualists. French stories of secrecy and refusal to share data also support this construction. Thus, in terms of medical discourse surrounding the AIDS epidemic, we can see this dynamic tension about which Gilmore talks, pulling between the all-encompassing French society, on one hand, and the French individual, on the other.

Finally, the cultural importance of patronage emerges out of the data as well, though perhaps not in the strict patron-client sense in which Gilmore utilizes the term. Rather, I was continually struck by the overt importance of personal contacts in the French medical community. For example, whenever I first encountered a new informant, particularly those heading a lab or clinic, they almost always asked about who else I had spoken with, and what they had to say. After I would tell them a few names, my new informant would generally offer commentary, sometimes quite cutting, about my earlier contacts, and my credentials having been accepted, the interview would proceed.

The role of personal contacts also crops up frequently in the narratives about the original working group on AIDS, highlighted by a former student asking Montagnier to work on AIDS. Personal contacts emerge as a means of accessing material resources and expertise outside of the usual bureaucratic channels. Personal charisma seems to play an important role in the clinic as well. Several doctors and nurses at Rousseau told me they agreed to join or continue with the clinic mainly because of Dr. Bernard, not out of his status as a well-known AIDS doctor or as *chef de service* but because of their personal rapport and respect for him.

This is not to say that personal contacts do not play a role in the American medical community as well, but there is less discourse about them, outside of a general sense of camaraderie and increased sharing of information. With the American value placed on individual ability, I suspect the power of personal contacts in the United States is more covert. Gaining access to resources through individual or institutional status is thus emphasized in the discourse, while personal ties are recognized but not advertised as important. As Dr. O'Neill, head of the Northlake clinic, comments:

You can get inferior stuff published if you are the right person in the right place. . . . But overall, I don't think it's a problem. We have had some very good work that has been rejected from the first-rung journals. But, on the other hand, we have made some inroads. And now being on these national committees, maybe one of us someday will get a name enough so that when the editors at least see it that it will fly a little easier.

The fit between Gilmore's model and the French data presented here is an imperfect one, and indeed one might make a case for a "Northern European Culture Area" at work as well. The point is not to decide whether Gilmore's model is the true one for France but to utilize its constructions to open up a range of interpretations of French medical discourse. Looking at the data through Gilmore's framework brings home the point that biomedicine is not a thing apart from culture but is enmeshed within it while emerging out of it. French biomedical discourse on AIDS is inherently different from American discourse because it is French. What it means to be French, to do things in a French way, is constructed in how health care is delivered, how doctors and patients relate, the roles and relations within the medical community, how the body and its ills are constituted, and how clinicians and researchers talk about their experiences with AIDS. In contrast to the American focus on information sharing and individual empowerment, the French value is placed on the social, even as it exists in tension with the individual.

As we have seen, AIDS in France is a different disease than AIDS in the United States, constructed and acted upon as a continuous spectrum of disease, requiring, like tuberculosis, attention to the problem of resistance in both the population and the individual. AIDS in France is, above all, an infectious disease affecting the *terrain*. In addition to differences in a mutually recognized disease such as AIDS, Gaines (1987) and Payer (1988) both note that there are illnesses accepted as somatic disturbances by French biomedicine that have no counterpart in American lay or professional medicine. Gaines concludes that the two biomedicines are not units of a universal, empirical system but are distinct, locally influenced symbolic systems, continuously being reinterpreted. French and American biomedicines are not monoparadigmatic but "multiparadigmatic cultural realities, realities created and grounded in local cultural knowledge and history and expressed as biology" (22). In the end, American and French physicians may speak to one another, but true translation requires not just a dictionary but an anthropological perspective.

NOTES

1.   A relatively new agency, Centres d'Information et de Soins de l'Immunodéfience Humaine (CISIH) has been established to educate medical personnel about AIDS and its treatment.

2. This may be a result of a long history of "turf" battles over the field of eye care (Wilsford 1991).

3. French physicians are barred from having a financial interest in laboratory or radiological facilities and cannot charge for biochemical tests done in the office (Fielding and Lancry 1993). This is again consistent with the separation of financial interests from the medical encounter.

4. As Ardagh (1987) observes, the French tend not to join clubs or associations, outside of political or union groups. The size of AIDES, the French AIDS support association, is thus an unusual accomplishment.

5. There are 12,000 cases of tuberculosis annually in France, and resistance to INH approaches 5 percent (Association des Professeurs de Pathologie Infectieuse 1990).

6. While the Rousseau clinic had a few visiting European physicians, the French laboratories I visited consistently had researchers from around the world. My research informants spoke of regular contact with American counterparts, either through working in joint projects or at least in the exchanging of information and reagents.

7. In some Mediterranean cultures, particularly Arabic ones, such jealousy is expressed as "the evil eye."

13

The Meanings of AIDS—Conclusions

All diseases have particular meanings—meanings that are both historically
and culturally specific. These meanings reflect our ability to make sense of
the disease scientifically, culturally, and politically; they reflect our notions
of the physical and social qualities of the specific disease and its victims.
Allan Brandt (1988, 415)

All of us—physicians, social scientists, laypersons—are trying to make meaning of
AIDS. As we have seen, the uncertainty and ambiguity surrounding AIDS are fertile
ground for the proliferation of multiple voices, even within the medical community
itself. By examining AIDS as a continuous construction of these voices rather than
as a static object, we are better able to understand the process by which biomedical
knowledge emerges and how AIDS is like and unlike other diseases in this regard.

As we have seen, narrative plays an important role in the construction of AIDS.
Medical discourse on AIDS appears in accord with Latour and Woolgar's (1979)
description of how the process of constructing scientific facts is eventually divorced
from the fact itself. In this regard, AIDS is like any other scientific object. As
evidenced throughout this study, however, medical constructions of AIDS are fluid,
dynamic, and highly context sensitive. For example, to interpret French physicians'
talk of resistance in AIDS, one must recognize the French experience with
tuberculosis.

Context, however, is only the beginning. My informants use a variety of
discursive techniques for understanding AIDS as a disease, sketching the outlines of
AIDS utilizing smaller, more knowable elements of the medical experience. Analogy
is one of the most common techniques, used to construct a set of medically and
historically situated meanings for AIDS, informed by experiences with hepatitis B,
syphilis, diabetes, tuberculosis, and cancer. As we have seen, given the historical lack
of standardized treatment for AIDS, a multiplicity of natural histories has emerged
over the last decade, often built around particular disease analogies. Some have fallen

out of use, while others persist in lay discourse or that of medical personnel outside the field of AIDS. The analogies of tuberculosis and cancer particularly have had a profound impact on how the natural history and associated treatments for AIDS have emerged in both countries. Thus, how diseases are constructed through discourse and practice has a direct and significant effect on people's lives. Working models of AIDS have changed significantly since the beginning of the epidemic, again demonstrating the importance of incorporating change into anthropological understandings of the constructive process.

The nature of AIDS that emerges out of medical discourse is inherently ambiguous, even paradoxical. Neither a cancer nor an infectious disease but containing elements of both, AIDS is conceptually more powerful. At the same time that medical discourse and practice are striving to build a uniform, standardized AIDS, my informants rely on innovation and improvisation in their daily practice. As we have seen, the very practice of AIDS medicine is an inversion of usual medical practice, and AIDS is thus medically dangerous, not merely through the possibility of contagion and death but to the entire order of the medical world. It may be fear of this ambiguity, along with fear of contagion and homosexuality, that keeps many physicians from becoming involved with AIDS. It also serves to separate "AIDS doctors" from other physicians, such that they constitute an identifiable group of physicians practicing a distinctive type of medicine.

Necessarily, patients' and physicians' constructions of AIDS appear different, and negotiation between the two is a significant part of daily life at the clinic. Patient discourse on AIDS appears marked by its close encounters with medical discourse, utilizing much of past and present medical terminology, as in the case of ARC. These terms have emerged from the discourse with significantly different meanings, meanings that order the experience of patients and sometimes disorder the experience of clinicians. The paradoxical nature of AIDS opens the way for the proliferation of alternative narratives, particularly about AIDS transmission. Thus, though medical and lay models may share a similar terminology, the constructions are ultimately different, requiring continual negotiation between physicians, researchers, and laypersons. The gap is never completely bridged but becomes incorporated into the ongoing process of making sense of AIDS. Nonetheless, AIDS doctors and AIDS patients are an integral part of each other's lives, each part of the HIV community.

Discourse within the medical community is not univocal but, rather, is composed of interacting discourses that sometimes compete, as seen, for example, those regarding the use of AZT, or HIV as the cause of AIDS. This proliferation of discourses is fed by the inherent ambiguity of AIDS. This ambiguity opens up the narrative field to the lay public, including patients and activists. As seen, for example, at the International AIDS Conference at Montreal, lay participants may develop their own narratives and give them equal authority, enabling them to participate in the fact-making process. AIDS challenges the scientific community to recognize political and economic factors as being intrinsic to the process of scientific production. This move from, in W. Fisher's (1987) terms, a "rational" paradigm, in which only experts may tell the story, to a narrative paradigm, in which nonexpert discourse plays an important role, may well be a unique aspect of the AIDS experience. However, this phenomenon may be carrying over into other arenas, such as breast cancer. The ambiguity of AIDS also allows innovation and improvisation to flourish within the medical community, opening up new ways of speaking about disease, medicine, and the human body, as well as acknowledgment of the limitations of medical knowledge.

Medical discourse never only constructs AIDS but simultaneously produces a host of meanings for other experiences. Patients and their bodies are an integral part of medical discourse on AIDS. The interested, educated high-status gay patient is often contrasted with the undeniably low-status IV drug user, both in France and the United States. Gay men emerge as the norm, in terms of both their bodies and their behavior as patients, with other patient groups being constructed in reference to them. The concept of an HIV community also emerges from discourse on patients, ultimately emphasizing the distinctiveness of AIDS patients from other patients, and their unifying social relationships as experienced in the daily life of the clinic.

Additionally, AIDS serves as a context for refashioning the intricate relationship between physicians and patients. My American informants developed central themes of information sharing and empowerment, while the French emphasized the value of trust. Patient activism emerges from this discourse as both a force for constructive change and a disruptive conflict. The relationship between AIDS patients and physicians is characterized in discourse and practice by a greater level of warmth, informality, and partnership than with other diseases. The "experimental" nature of AIDS and its treatments may be an important factor in this regard.

As we have seen, how informants speak of and operate within their health care system is integral to the medical experience of AIDS. The health care system that emerges from French discourse is equitable, monolithic, static, and politically motivated, compared with the American constructions of an inequitable, fragmented, economically motivated system. American physicians in particular use AIDS to talk about the deficiencies of their system. As evidenced by the improvisation regarding clinical trials and the rise of community-based organizations, AIDS becomes a medium for subverting and even changing this system. Still, the discourse of the American informants evokes a sense of powerlessness, of having to struggle against a powerful and fragmented commercial bureaucracy in order to care for their patients.

Discourse on AIDS also serves to reinterpret the nature of science, and the relations between science, politics, and clinical medicine. A central theme in this discourse is the distinction between "good" and "bad" science. AIDS often emerges as being intrinsically linked to bad science through money, public visibility, and politics. Nevertheless, the distinction between the traits of good and bad science appears to be increasingly problematic in the context of the epidemic.

Medical discourse on AIDS ultimately constructs a scientific enterprise that, by nature and necessity, is public, political, and interdisciplinary. This sets AIDS research apart from other scientific endeavors but, as seen with clinical practice, may come to influence the way science is done. "Fast-track" drug trials, community-based research, and the active participation of persons with AIDS in determining the design and focus of studies are important examples of how AIDS transforms scientific practice.

My informants use AIDS to explore significant changes in their everyday experience of medical practice, such as the interaction between various medical specialties and the role of primary care. The boundaries between "medical" and "social" problems are refashioned through discourse, while medicine itself is resituated in a historical context. Invoking a sense of personal danger and professional commitment, medical discourse on AIDS acts as a medium for reexamining the nature of being a physician. This same discourse also constructs the identity of a medical professional in AIDS. Physicians and researchers of disparate backgrounds enter through the door of AIDS and are transformed into AIDS doctors/researchers, members of the HIV community. The International AIDS Conferences have come to be a rite of passage, renewing their dedication against AIDS. For the new "plague doctors," AIDS medicine is not merely what they do, it is who they are. Their national affiliations, expressed in American first stories and French hardship stories, are simultaneously a part of this transformative process and renewed by it.

Throughout this study, we have seen that French constructions of AIDS often, but not always, differ from American ones, though the process of construction is basically the same. AIDS in France is a different disease than AIDS in the United States, constructed and acted upon as a continuous spectrum of disease, requiring, like tuberculosis, attention to the problem of resistance. AIDS in France is, above all, an infectious disease affecting the *terrain*. As important, what it means to be French, to do things in a French way, is constructed in how health care is delivered, how doctors and patients relate, and the roles and relations within the medical community, as well as in how clinicians and researchers talk about their experiences with AIDS. In each circumstance, the value is placed on the social, even as it exists in tension with the individual. Many differences are not specific to AIDS but are exemplified by it, being grounded in differences specific both to the French medical community and to larger culture-wide beliefs and institutional structures. French biomedicine is *not* American biomedicine, but rather, both are distinct, locally influenced symbolic systems, continuously being reinterpreted. Western biomedicine, in turn, is not a single, uniform medical system but a multiplicity of related systems, each arising out of its own cultural and historical contexts.

Several important clinical implications emerge from this last conclusion. First, clinical practice is also cultural practice, whether in Japan, France, or the United States. Physicians across hospitals or across regions may differ in their practice precisely because they practice in different sociohistorical contexts. Second, AIDS is a global epidemic and as such requires international efforts from a variety of health care systems, including biomedicine. The nature of the disease itself may be defined differently among physicians from different countries, entailing extra effort on the part of physicians to reach common understanding. Treatment approaches both successful and acceptable in one biomedical system may not be either in another system, as seen with the tuberculosis vaccine. Finally, the American doctor-patient relationship, based on the cultural values of empowerment and information sharing, may not operate in other biomedical systems, resulting in differences in the protocols for clinical trials, as well as ethical issues such as informed consent and the right to know or not to know certain medical information. The means of empowerment of the patient in each country may well be fashioned out of distinctive cultural values, separate paths to similar goals (J. Feldman 1992a). Each of these areas of concern would benefit from further study.

The strictly theoretical implications of this study are less easily summarized. It does not "prove" that all diseases emerge through a process of social construction. Rather, this analysis of AIDS suggests that a constructionist framework is a valid, coherent, and fruitful way of examining medical knowledge and how it emerges. The fluidity of medical constructions of AIDS over the course of the epidemic underscores the importance of seeing change as integral to this process. Equally significant, we cannot magically extract the object of study from the contextual webs in which it is embedded. As complicated as in situ analysis is, demanding the anthropologist be versed in history, politics or medicine, this approach opens up the possibility for an unmatched breadth and depth of interpretations.

Divorcing French medical discourse from the structural surrounds of the French health care system would have robbed my own constructions of their richness. And, without an intimate knowledge of medicine, detailed interpretations regarding staging, disease analogies, and the cultural implications of variations in treatment would have been unavailable to me. Access to doctor-patient encounters, staff meetings, and other medical experiences would likely have been limited if I had not been recognized as part of the medical community. More important, the experience of actively participating in patient care, of making diagnostic and treatment decisions, and of sharing these experiences with patients and physicians would have been unavailable to the non-MD anthropologist. With my medical training, I stood not only near my informants but with them. This study demonstrates the potential of the physician-anthropologist in ethnographic research. The continued development of this type of approach to ethnography in general and medical anthropology in particular would contribute greatly to the growth of anthropology as a broadly applicable discipline.

Lastly, this research demonstrates that construction is not a single, linear process but a number of interwoven processes occurring simultaneously. Through discourse and practice, AIDS is at once constructed and constructive, used by medical professionals as a vehicle for refashioning their world, indeed their own identities. AIDS is not unique in this regard; the same may be said of any number of shared experiences. Rather, AIDS illustrates the complexity of human experience, and the need for equally sophisticated anthropological understanding.

What of AIDS itself? AIDS appears in many ways to act as a rite of passage for both the French and American medical communities, characterized by ambiguity, inversion, and a sense of *communitas*. This experience may not be limited to the medical community, but medicine lies at the heart of it: "Today our vision of illness and the institution which takes it in charge, medicine, is in a certain way at the epicenter of cultural and social conflicts" (Herzlich 1984, 207). By developing a greater understanding of biomedical discourse, we can appreciate the role it plays in how people cope with AIDS, as an epidemic of physical illness and as an epidemic of meaning. For example, we have seen that medical knowledge and practices regarding AIDS are hardly uniform, and rely extensively on improvisation. Attempts to fully standardize AIDS treatment may hamper physicians and patients in devising biologically and psychosocially appropriate therapy, even as it may overcome some physicians' fear of treating AIDS. Patient and lay discourse on AIDS is informed by medical discourse, past and present. Constructions of AIDS that have become "artifacts" in the medical community remain in use and are refashioned by the lay public in light of their differing experiences, fed by the ambiguity of AIDS as a disease. This study, like that of Elsford (1987), suggests that "misinformation" about AIDS is unlikely to be eliminated, only minimized, by education campaigns. Alternative narratives, in and outside of the medical community, will continue to play an important role in the epidemic.

Susan Sontag (1978) states that we must make medicine and medical talk free from metaphor. Rather, I would suggest that for human beings metaphor is as necessary as air, as water. We cannot live without it because it is essential as a means of making sense of experience. The idea is rather that we become aware of discourse and its constructive power. For physicians, the central rule of medicine is: First, do no harm. We must strive to apply this rule to our discourse, as physicians and as anthropologists alike. Just as with medical treatments, our metaphors must first do no harm.

Appendix: Statistical Description of Informants

Clinician is defined as person whose primary activities revolve around patient care and conducting clinical trials.

Researcher is defined as person whose primary activities involve laboratory or epidemiological research, with little direct patient care.

Note: There were no medical residents or research graduate students among the American informants, resulting in a slightly higher age distribution.

United States (1991)

Total N = 41   Males = 37 Female = 4

Numerical breakdown by city

Chicago = 12
Houston = 5
New York = 5
San Francisco = 7
Washington, DC = 8
Atlanta = 4

Breakdown by age

21–25 = 0
26–30 = 2
31–35 = 7
36–40 = 9
41–45 = 8
46–50 = 7
51–55 = 6
56–60 = 2
61+ = 0

Mean age = 42.4

Breakdown by profession

Clinicians = 22
Researchers = 19

Breakdown by city
C = clinician R = Researcher

Chicago	C = 10	R = 2
Houston	C = 2	R = 3
New York	C = 3	R = 2
San Francisco	C = 6	R = 1
Washington, DC	C= 1	R = 7
Atlanta	C = 0	R = 4

Breakdown of clinicians by specialty

In process of infectious disease specialty training = 4
M.D. family practice/general internal medicine = 5
Infectious disease = 8
Oncology = 3
Dermatology = 1
Immunology = 1

*Breakdown of researchers by degree
and specialty*

MD only = 7
MD/MPH = 3
MD/PhD or Dsc = 2
MD/MS = 1
PhD only = 5
M.S. = 1

Researcher MD (includes dual-degrees) specialties:
Infectious disease = 7
Oncology = 2
Internal medicine = 2
Epidemiology = 2

MS or PhD specialties:
Biochemistry or chemistry = 3
Pharmacology = 1
Sociology = 1
Microbiology = 1

Many of the researchers, including the MD's, have secondary specialties as well, such as epidemiology, immunology, and virology.

Non-Americans = 2 British, 1 Canadian
Informants with professional experience in France = 3
Experience in Europe outside France = 10
Experience elsewhere outside the United States = 9

Paris, France (1987)

Total N = 33   Males = 23 Females =10

Breakdown by age, approximate

20–29 = 15
30–39 = 13
40–49 = 2
50+ = 3

Non-French:
Near East = 5
Other = 6 (3 British, 1 American, 1 Brazilian, 1 Chilean)

Note: Five of these informants received their professional training in France, while three others were educated in the U.S. or Canada.

Breakdown by profession

Research graduate students = 11
Clinicians = 8
Researcher = 14

Note: Data on the specific specialty backgrounds were not gathered during the 1987 study.

Paris, France (1990)

Total N = 26 (13 did not participate in the 1987 study)
Males = 16
Females = 10 (only 3 of which are NOT interns)

Breakdown by age

21–25 = 2
26–30 = 7   Mean age = 35.3
31–35 = 3   Mean age excluding medical interns =
36–40 = 8   39.0
41–45 = 4
46–50 = 2
51+ = 0

Breakdown by profession

Clinicians = 19
Researchers = 7

Clinician breakdown by level and specialty

Interns = 8 (2 in specialty training)
MD generalists = 7
MD specialists = 4 (2 infectious disease, 1 tropical medicine, and 1 dermatology)

Researcher breakdown by degree and speciality

MD only = 3 (epidemiology, 2 immunology specialties)
MD/PhD = 2 (immunology, virology)
PhD only = 2 (biochemistry, virology)

Non-French = 5 (2 trained all professional life in France)
Professional experience in US = 6 (1 clinician only).

Glossary

acyclovir. Drug used to treat infection with herpes simplex virus (HSV).

aerosolized pentamidine. Treatment aimed at preventing occurrence, or recurrence, of *Pneumocystis* pneumonia. Patient inhales the drug on a regular basis.

AIDS. For *acquired immunodeficiency syndrome*. Historically, a syndrome characterized by an increasing depression of the immune system (particularly cell-mediated immunity), with the subsequent development of opportunistic infections and cancers, believed to be caused by the human immunodeficiency virus (HIV). In present medical terminology, AIDS refers only to the most serious phase of this disease process, although is often used informally to refer to the disease as a whole. *See also* **HIV disease**.

AIDS Clinical Trials Groups (ACTG). Federally funded, American association of medical research centers involved in conducting a variety of clinical trials.

anemia. Deficiency in the oxygen-carrying capacity of the blood. Most commonly due to increased destruction of the red blood cells, iron deficiency, or abnormal hemoglobin. Measured by hemoglobin content in blood, among others.

ANRS. Agence Nationale de Recherche sur le SIDA, or the National Agency of AIDS Research. French governmental agency.

antibody. Molecule produced by one's body as part of the humoral immune response. The antibody attaches to "foreign" molecules, helping the body to clear them. Bacteria, or parts of bacteria, for example, can provoke an antibody response. In certain diseases, antibodies may recognize a person's own cells as "foreign," an "autoimmune" reaction.

antigen. That which is bound by the antibody. *See also* **antibody**.

ARC. For AIDS-related complex/condition. Historically, a constellation of less severe symptoms of immunodefiency resulting from HIV infection. Although no longer a part of the basic medical model of AIDS, ARC is used by laypersons, and informally in the medical community to refer to milder phases of HIV infection.

Assitance Publique. Organization consisting of fifty public hospitals in and around Paris. Involved in care, teaching and research, it is one of the largest hospital groups in Europe.

atypical *Mycobacteria* **or atypical tuberculosis (TB)**. Generally systemic disease, which may or may not affect the lungs, caused by a bacteria related to, but not identical with *Mycobacteria tuberculosis*. Usually caused by *M. kansasii* or *M. avium-intracellulare* (also known as MAI or MAC). Until recently, difficult to identify and treat.

AZT. Formerly called *azidothymidine* and now known as *zidovudine* and marketed under the trade name Retrovir. Drug used against HIV directly; targets reverse transcriptase. The first FDA-approved anti-AIDS medication, it was initially developed as a cancer drug.

Bactrim. Trade name of antibiotic used to treat and prevent *Pneumocystis* pneumonia, among other diseases.

Candidiasis. Infection with the fungus *Candida*, usually *C. albicans*. Commonly affects the mouth and esophagus in AIDS patients. *See also* **thrush**.

CD4 lymphocytes. Formerly called *T4* or *T-helper lymphocytes*. A type of T lymphocyte (see **lymphocyte**) involved in "turning on" an immune response. This cell is among the first (if not the first) infected by HIV, which then destroys it. HIV infection is thus characterized by persistent drop in the number of CD4 lymphocytes.

cell-mediated immunity. A type of immune response involving the activation of certain cells of the immune system and without the involvement of antibodies.

Centers for Disease Control (CDC). The national-level American epidemiology center. Collects data on reportable diseases, unusual outbreaks of disease, other related data. Publishes the *Morbidity and Mortality Weekly Report*.

CISIH. Centres d'Information et de Soins de l'Immunodéficience Humaine. Literally, Centers of Information and Care of Human Immunodeficiency. Eight centers set up by the French government in response to the AIDS epidemic to assist medical personnel in learning about and treating AIDS patients.

CITRAS. Centre Interétablissement de Traitement et de Recherche Anti-SIDA. Literally, Interorganization Center of Anti-AIDS Treatment and Research. Another French governmental agency recently developed in response to the epidemic.

CNRS. Centre National de la Recherche Scientifique, or the National Center for Scientific Research. The French equivalent of the United States' National Science Foundation, it is administered through the national government. Unlike the NSF, researchers in public agencies, including universities, must gain membership in CNRS first. CNRS not only grants funding but, through various units, conducts research as well.

cryptococcosis. infection with *Cryptococcus*, a fungus. Most commonly causes meningitis in AIDS patients.

CT scan. For *computerized tomography scan*. Medical imaging technology, often used to scan the brain, abdomen, and chest.

Cytomegalovirus (CMV). Common virus that rarely causes serious disease, with the exception in fetuses, newborns, and the immunocompromised. Often carried by healthy people, it can cause neurological disease and infection of the retina and colon in AIDS patients

DDC. Formerly known as *deoxycytidine*, now called *zalcitabine*. An anti-HIV drug that, like AZT, targets reverse transcriptase, but has different side effects. It was approved for nonexperimental use in 1992.

DDI. *Dideoxyinosine* or *didanosine*. An anti-HIV drug that, like AZT, targets reverse transcriptase, but has different side effects. It was approved for nonexperimental use in 1991.

ELISA. For *enzyme-linked immunosorbent assay*. Lab test designed to detect the presence of antibodies to a particular molecule (bacteria, virus, etc.) in a person's blood. In the case of AIDS, antibodies to HIV. It does not detect the virus directly.

Feline Leukemia Virus (FLV). Virus that causes leukemia in cats, compared by some researchers to HIV.

fluconazole. Antifungal drug developed in Europe.

foscarnet. Drug used to treat CMV-caused diseases, but as of 1994, approved only for treatment of retinitis.

ganciclovir. Drug used to treat CMV-caused diseases, especially retinitis.

hemoglobin. Iron-based molecule in red blood cells that carries oxygen.

hepatitis B virus (HBV). Virus that causes one form of hepatitis, inflammation of the liver. Can lead to cirrhosis and liver cancer. Prevalent among gay men, IV drug users, and in parts of southeast Asia, it is transmitted by sexual and blood contact. Often compared to HIV.

Herpes simplex Virus (HSV). Group of viruses that can cause oral and genital herpes, as well as meningitis and encephalitis among AIDS patients.

HIV disease. Also *HIV infection*. Term used among the medical community (and some lay groups) to refer to the whole spectrum of disease caused by infection with the human immunodeficiency virus (HIV). This includes asymptomatic and mildly symptomatic infections as well as full-blown AIDS.

HTLV-I. A retrovirus, isolated by Robert Gallo and his lab, that infects T lymphocytes, causing a form of leukemia.

HTLV-III. Gallo's name/isolate of HIV.

Human Immunodeficiency Virus (HIV). A retrovirus (types 1 and 2) generally accepted as the ultimate cause of AIDS. Formerly known as: ARV, LAV, HTLV-III.

Human Papilloma Virus (HPV). Virus that causes warts and, likely, cervical cancer in women.

humoral immunity. A type of immune response mediated by antibodies

Imuthiol. Trade name for *DTC* or *ditiocarb*. Experimental drug used to stimulate the immune system. First used in Europe, has declined in popularity.

INSERM. Institut National de la Santé et de la Recherche Medicale, or the National Institute of Health and Medical Research. Similar to National Institutes of Health in the United States, conducting research as well as providing grants. As with CNRS, researchers funded by INSERM are generally tenured members as well.

interferon, alpha-. Molecule produced by the body that stimulates the proliferation of lymphocytes and increases their activity. Used initially to treat AIDS itself, now used primarily to treat Kaposi's sarcoma.

isoniazid. Anti-tuberculosis drug. Used prophylactically in the United States, where it is often referred to as *INH*, short for the trademark for *iso*nicotine *h*ydrazine used in the preparation of isoniazid.

IVDU. For *intravenous drug user*.

Kaposi's sarcoma (KS). Unusual cancer involving the proliferation of cells associated with small blood vessels, resulting in purple lesions on the skin. Can also affect the gastrointestinal tract and lungs.

LAV. For *lymphadenopathy-associated virus*. Luc Montagnier's name/isolate of HIV.

lymphadenopathy. Swelling of lymph nodes. Can be chronic in some people infected with HIV.

lymphocyte. A type of white blood cell (WBC) that functions as part of the body's immune system. There are two main classes of lymphocytes: B and T. The B lymphocytes are involved in humoral (antibody-mediated) immunity, while T lymphocytes, the ones primarily affected in AIDS, are part of cell-mediated immunity.

Medicaid. American program that funds health care for the poor. It is funded partly by the federal government and partly by individual states, who also administer it.

Medicare. American program that funds health care for the elderly and disabled. Funded and administered by the federal government.

Megace. Trade name for a drug used to treat loss of appetite and wasting in cancer and AIDS patients.

mononucleosis. Acute, limited disease caused by Epstein-Barr virus, resulting in proliferation of certain white blood cells, extreme fatigue, fever, swollen lymph nodes. Initial infection with HIV can result in a similar set of symptoms

MRI scan. For *magnetic resonance imaging scan*. Medical imaging technique, used primarily to examine the brain and spinal cord.

Mycobacterium avium-intracellulare (**MAI or MAC**). Organism that can cause "atypical tuberculosis." Common in AIDS patients, usually resulting in unexplained fever and other constitutional symptoms.

Mycoplasma. An unusual bacteria, known mainly as a cause of "walking pneumonia." Has been suggested by Montagnier as a cofactor in the development of AIDS.

National Cancer Institute (NCI). Part of the NIH dedicated to cancer research. Gallo's lab is part of NCI.

National Institutes of Health (NIH). American national-level medical research organization. Federally funded and administered, dispenses grant money across the country.

neutropenia. Abnormal drop in the number of neutrophils (*see also* **neutrophil**) in the blood. Person is then susceptible to certain types of infection. Side effect of several AIDS-related medications (AZT, ganciclovir).

neutrophil. A type of white blood cell, primarily involved with combatting bacterial infections.

Non-Hodgkin's lymphoma. A cancer resulting in proliferation of lymphocytes. Can cause tumors in the brain, as seen in AIDS patients.

PCR. For *polymerase chain reaction*. Sensitive laboratory technique that can detect the presence of particular genetic sequences. Used to detect the presence of HIV in blood, usually for research (rather than screening) purposes.

Pneumocystis carinii **Pneumonia (PCP)**. A protozoan (akin to an amoeba) infection, usually resulting in pneumonia, uncommon in people who are not immunocompromised. Common infection in people with AIDS and was one of the original conditions that led to the recognition of AIDS as a separate disease.

prophylaxis. Prevention of disease, usually by administering a medication. Consists of *secondary prophylaxis*, aimed at preventing recurrence, and *primary prophylaxis*, aimed at preventing (or at least delaying) the initial occurrence. Aerosolized pentamidine treatment is an example of prophylaxis.

RBC. For *red blood cell*. These cells contain **hemoglobin** and carry oxygen throughout the body

retrovirus. A virus characterized by having RNA, rather than DNA, as its genetic material. In order to utilize the cell's machinery to reproduce, the virus must first convert the RNA to DNA (the genetic material in the cell). It utilizes an enzyme, **reverse transcriptase**, to do this. HIV and HTLV-I are both retroviruses.

reverse transcriptase. Characteristic enzyme of retroviruses, used to convert viral RNA to DNA. AZT, DDI, and DDC are drugs that inhibit the activity of reverse transcriptase.

Sécurité Sociale. The French national agency that organizes and funds health care for most of the population. Also administers pensions for the elderly.

sepsis. Serious clinical condition resulting from having bacteria disseminated throughout the bloodstream, rather than isolated in one organ or area of the body.

slim disease. Informal term for the presentation of AIDS as diarrhea, persistent weight loss, and general wasting. Common in, but not limited to, AIDS in many African countries.

stavudine. Also known as *d4T*. An antiretroviral drug approved in 1994 for treatment of advanced HIV infection. Like AZT, it inhibits reverse transcriptase but, unlike AZT, also interferes with viral DNA synthesis by other mechanisms.

T4 lymphocytes. *See* **CD4 lymphocytes**.

thrush. *Candida* infection in the mouth.

toxoplasmosis. A protozoan (akin to an amoeba) infection associated with exposure to cat feces and raw/undercooked meat. In the AIDS patient, can result in brain lesions with neurological symptoms. More common in France than in the United States due to differences in cooking and food storage.

WBC. For *white blood cell*, consisting of several specific types, such as neutrophils and lymphocytes. Together they make up the cells of the immune system. *Also see* **lymphocyte**.

Western blot. Laboratory test that detects antibodies. Used after the ELISA test as a confirmatory test for the presence of HIV antibodies.

World Health Organization (WHO). World organization dedicated to monitoring diseases and promoting health. Sets international criteria for case definition of AIDS as well as assembles international epidemiological data.

Bibliography

Aboulker, Jean-Pierre, and Ann Marie Swart. 1993. "Preliminary Analysis of the Concorde Trial [letter]." *Lancet*. 341:889–890.

Adams, Jad. 1989. *AIDS: The HIV Myth*. New York: St. Martin's Press.

Agar, Michael. 1986. *Speaking of Ethnography*. Newbury Park, CA: Sage Publications.

AIDES-Unaformec. 1987. *SIDA 1987: L'infections par le virus de l'immunodéficience humaine en practique médicale quotidienne*. Paris: Unaformec.

Altman, Dennis. 1986. *AIDS in the Mind of America: The Social, Political, and Psychological Impact of a New Epidemic*. Garden City, NY: Anchor/Doubleday.

Andreoli, Thomas, Charles Carpenter, Fred Plum, and Lloyd Smith, eds. 1986. *Cecil's Essentials of Medicine*. Philadelphia: W. B. Saunders.

Angier, Natalie. 1991. "Who Discovered AIDS?" Book Review. *Chicago Tribune*, 31 March, sec. 14, 3–7.

Ardagh, John. 1987. *France Today*. London: Secker and Warburg.

Association des Professeurs de Pathologie Infectieuse. 1990. *Le POPI: Guide de poche de conduite thérapeutique en pathologie infectieuse*. Paris: Association des Professeurs de Pathologie Infectieuse.

Bachelot, François, and Pierre Lorane. 1988. *Une société au risque du SIDA*. Paris: Albatross.

Bakhtin, Mikhail. 1981. *The Dialogic Imagination*. Austin: University of Texas Press.

Barré-Sinousi, Françoise, J. C. Chermann, F. Rey, M. T. Nugeyre, S. Chamaret, J. Gruest, C. Daugguet, C. Axler-Blin, F. Vézinet-Brun, C. Rouzioux, W. Rozenbaum, and L. Montagnier. 1983. "Isolation of a T-Lymphotrophic Retrovirus from a Patient at Risk for Acquired Immune Deficiency Syndrome (AIDS)." *Science* 220:868–871.

Barré-Sinousi, Françoise, Jean-Claude Chermann, and Willy Rozenbaum. 1987. *Le SIDA en questions*. Paris: Plon

Barré-Sinousi, Françoise, Usha Mathur-Wagh, Françoise Rey, Françoise Brun-Vezinet, Stanley Yancovitz, Christing Rouzioux, Luc Montagnier, Donna Mildvan,and Jean Claude Chermann. 1985. "Isolation of Lymphadenopathy-Associated Virus

(LAV) and Detection of LAV Antibodies from US Patients with AIDS." *Journal of the American Medical Association* 253:1737–1739.

Barth, Frederick. 1984. "Problems in Conceptualizing Cultural Pluralism, with Illustrations from Somar, Oman." In *The Prospects for Plural Societies*. Edited by David Maybury, 77–87. Washington, DC: American Ethnological Society.

Bartlett, J. A. 1992. "Chronic Management and Counseling for Persons with HIV Infection." in *Cecil's Textbook of Medicine*. 19th ed. Edited by J. B. Wyngaarden, L. H. Smith, and J. C. Bennett, 1965–1970. Philadelphia: W. B. Saunders.

Bass, Thomas. 1988. "Interview: AIDS Expert Luc Montagnier." *Omni* 11, no. 3:102–108

Baszanger, Isabelle. 1985. "Professional Socialization and Social Control: From Medical Students to General Practitioners," translated byNoal Mellott, *Social Science and Medicine* 20:133–143.

Bateson, Mary Catherine, and Richard Goldsby. 1988. *Thinking AIDS: The Social Response to the Biological Threat*. Reading, MA: Addison-Wesley.

Bayer, Ronald. 1991. *Private Acts, Social Consequences: AIDS and the Politics of Public Health*. New Brunswick, NJ: Rutgers University Press.

Berger, Peter, and Thomas Luckmann. 1967. *The Social Construction of Reality: A Treatise in the Sociology of Knowledge*. New York: Anchor/Doubleday.

Beriss, David. 1991. "French Identity and the Exotic: Creating the Other in Order to Create the French." Paper presented at the ninetieth annual American Anthropological Association meetings, 20–24 November 1991, Chicago, IL.

Berridge, Virginia, and Philip Strong, eds. 1993. *AIDS and Contemporary History*. Cambridge: Cambridge University Press.

Black, Max. 1962. *Models and Metaphors*. Ithaca, NY: Cornell University Press.

Black, Max. 1979. "More About Metaphor." In *Metaphor and Thought*. Edited by Andrew Ortony, 19–43. Cambridge: Cambridge University Press.

Blumer, H. 1969. *Symbolic Interactionism; Perspective and Method*. Englewood Cliffs, NJ: Prentice-Hall.

Bosk, Charles. 1979. *Forgive and Remember: Managing Medical Failure*. Chicago: University of Chicago Press.

Bosk, Charles, and Joel Fraser. 1991. "AIDS and Its Impact on Medical Work: The Culture and Politics of the Shop Floor." In *A Disease of Society*. Edited by Dorothy Nelkin, David Willis, and Scott Parris, 150–171. Cambridge: Cambridge University Press.

Bourdieu, Pierre. 1977. *Outline of a Theory of Practice*. Cambridge: Cambridge University Press.

Bouvier-Colle, M-H, E. Jougla, and V. Schwoebel. 1993. "Nouvelles définitions du SIDA aux États-Unis et en Europe." *Revue d'Epidémiologie et de Santé Publique* 41:191–193.

Brandt, Allan. 1985. *No Magic Bullet: A Social History of Venereal Disease in the United States Since 1850*. Oxford: Oxford University Press.

Brandt, Allan. 1988. "AIDS and Metaphor: Toward the Social Meaning of Epidemic Disease." *Social Research* 55, no.3:413–432.

Brenky, Dominique, and Olivia Zémor. 1985. *La route du SIDA: Enquête sur une grande peur*. Paris: Londreys.

Brody, Howard. 1988. *Stories of Sickness*. New Haven, CT: Yale University Press.

Bruner, Edward. 1986a. "Ethnography as Narrative." In *The Anthropology of Experience.* Edited by Edward Bruner and Victor Turner, 139–155. Urbana: University of Illinois Press.

Bruner, Edward. 1986b. "Experience and Its Expressions." In *The Anthropology of Experience.* Edited by Edward Bruner and Victor Turner, 1–30. Urbana: University of Illinois Press.

Bruner, Edward, and Phyllis Gorfain. 1984. "Dialogic Narration and the Paradoxes of Masada." In *Text, Play, and Story: The Construction and Reconstruction of Self and Society.* Edited by Edward Bruner, 56–79. Washington, DC: American Ethnological Society.

Buff, Daniel. 1994. "Abbreviations in Medicine: Are We Shortchanging Our Patients and Ourselves?" *AIDS Patient Care* 8, no.3:108–109.

Card, Orson Scott. 1985. *Ender's Game.* New York: TOR.

Carroll, Raymonde. 1988. *Cultural Misunderstandings: The French-American Experience.* Chicago: University of Chicago Press.

Cassell, Eric. 1976. *The Healer's Art: A New Approach to the Doctor-Patient Relationship.* New York: Lippincott.

Centers for Disease Control (CDC). 1981. "*Pneumocystis* Pneumonia—Los Angeles." *Morbidity and Mortality Weekly Report* 30:250–252.

Centers for Disease Control (CDC). 1982a. "*Pneumocystis carinii* Pneumonia Among Persons with Hemophilia A." *Morbidity and Mortality Weekly Report* 31:365–367.

Centers for Disease Control (CDC). 1982b. "Update on Acquired Immune Deficiency Syndrome (AIDS)—United States." *Morbidity and Mortality Weekly Report* 31, no.37:508.

Centers for Disease Control (CDC). 1986a. "Classification System for Human T-lymphotropic Virus Type III/Lymphadenopathy-associated Virus Infections." *Morbidity and Mortality Weekly Report* 35:334–339.

Centers for Disease Control (CDC). 1986b. "Update: Acquired Immunodeficiency Syndrome—Europe." *Morbidity and Mortality Weekly Report* 35, no.3:35–38, 43–46.

Centers for Disease Control (CDC). 1987. "Revision of the CDC Surveillance Case Definition For Acquired Immunuodeficiency Syndrome." *Morbidity and Mortality Weekly Report* 36 suppl. no.1:1S–15S.

Centers for Disease Control (CDC). 1990. *Voluntary HIV Counseling and Testing: Facts, Issues, and Answers.* Atlanta, GA: Centers for Disease Control.

Centers for Disease Control (CDC). 1991. *HIV/AIDS Surveillance: US Cases Reported Through March 1991.* Atlanta, GA: US Department of Health and Human Services.

Centers for Disease Control (CDC). 1992a. "1993 Revised Classification System for HIV Infection and Expanded Surveillance Case Definition for AIDS Among Adolescents and Adults." *Morbidity and Mortality Weekly Report* 41, no.RR-17:1–19.

Centers for Disease Control (CDC). 1992b. "Projections of the Number of Persons Diagnosed with AIDS and the Number of Immunosuppressed HIV-Infected Persons—United States 1992–1994." *Morbidity and Mortality Weekly Report* 41, no.RR-18:1–23.

Christakis, Nicholas. 1989. "Responding to a Pandemic: International Interests in AIDS Control." *Daedalus* 118, no.2:113–134.

Cicourel, Alan. 1974. *Cognitive Sociology: Language and Meaning in Social Interaction.* New York: Free Press.

Cipolla, Carlo. 1977. "A Plague Doctor." In *The Medieval City.* Edited by H. Miskimin, D. Herlihy, and A. L. Udovitch., 65–72 New Haven, CT: Yale University Press.

Clatts, Michael, and Kevin Mutchler. 1989. "AIDS and the Dangerous Other: Metaphors of Sex and Deviance in the Representation of Disease." *Medical Anthropology* 10, nos.2–3:105–114.

Clifford, James. 1986a. "Introduction: Partial Truths." In *Writing Culture: The Poetics and Politics of Ethnography.* Edited by James Clifford and George Marcus, 1–26. Berkeley: University of California Press.

Clifford, James. 1986b. "On Ethnographic Allegory." In *Writing Culture: The Poetics and Politics of Ethnography.* Edited by James Clifford and George Marcus, 98–121. Berkeley: University of California Press.

Clumeck, Nathan, and Stephane De Wit. 1988. "AIDS in Africa." In *The Medical Management of AIDS.* Edited by Merle Sande and Paul Volberding, 331–349. Philadelphia: W. B. Saunders.

Comaroff, Jean. 1982. "Medicine: Symbol and Ideology." In *The Problem of Medical Knowledge: Examining the Social Construction of Medicine.* Edited by Peter Wright and Andrew Treacher, 49–68. Edinburgh: Edinburgh University Press.

Comité Français d'Education Pour la Santé. 1986. *SIDA: Les acteurs de santé en première ligne.* Paris: CFES.

"Controversy over Dr. Kevorkian Erupts anew With Fourth Suicide." 1992. *Chicago Tribune,* 17 May, 14.

Cook, Timothy, and David Colby. 1992. "The Mass-Mediated Epidemic: the Politics of AIDS on the Nightly Network News." In *AIDS: The Making of a Chronic Disease.* Edited by Elizabeth Fee and Daniel Fox, 84–122. Berkeley: University of California Press.

Crewdson, John. 1987. "Scientific Rivalry May Be Hurting AIDS Fight." *Chicago Tribune,* 16 August, 1, 22.

Crewdson, John. 1989. "Special Report: The Great AIDS Quest." *Chicago Tribune,* 19 November, sect. 5, 1–16.

Crewdson, John. 1990. "French Seek Way to End AIDS Pact." *Chicago Tribune,* 25 March, 6.

Crewdson, John. 1991a. "French Unravel AIDS Origin." *Chicago Tribune,* 5 May, 1–14.

Crewdson, John. 1991b. "Gallo Admits French Discovered AIDS Virus." *Chicago Tribune,* 30 May, 2.

Crewdson, John. 1991c. "Leftover Cells May Resolve AIDS Case." *Chicago Tribune,* 27 January, 21, 27.

Crewdson, John. 1991d. "Lies, Errors Cited in AIDS Article." *Chicago Tribune,* 15 September, 1, 18–19.

Crimp, Douglas. 1987. "AIDS: Cultural Analysis/Cultural Activism." *October* 43:3–16.

D'Adler, Marie-Ange. 1987. "SIDA: Course d'obstacles pour un vaccin." *Sciences et Avenir* 2667, no.484:20–26.

DaMatta, Roberto. 1984. "On Carnaval, Informality and Magic: A Point of View from Brazil." In *Text, Play and Story: The Construction and Reconstruction of Self and Society.* Edited by Edward Bruner, 230–246. Washington, DC: American Ethnological Society.

DelVecchio-Good, Mary-Jo. 1985. "Discourses on Physician Competence." In *Physicians of Western Medicine: Anthropological Approaches to Theory and Practice.* Edited by Robert Hahn and Atwood Gaines, 247–268. Dordrecht: D. Reidel.

Desenclos, J. C., G. Papaevangelou, and R. Ancelle-Park. 1993. "Knowledge of HIV Serostatus and Preventive Behavior Among European Injecting Drug Users: The European Community Study Group on HIV Injecting Drug Users." *AIDS* 7, no.10:1371–1377.

Des Jarlais, Don, Samuel R. Friedman, and Jo L. Sotheran. 1992. "The First City: HIV Among Intravenous Drug Users in New York City." In *AIDS: The Making of a Chronic Disease.* Edited by Elizabeth Fee and Daniel Fox, 279–295. Berkeley: University of California Press.

De Thé, Guy. 1987. "Au principe: Le virus." In *Le SIDA: Rumeurs et faits.* Edited by Emmanuel Hirsch, 71–86. Paris: Cerf.

Direction Générale de la Santé. 1990. "Surveillance du SIDA en France: Situation au 31 Mars 1990." *Bulletin Epidémiologique Hebdomadaire* 11 June, no.23:97–101.

Dormont, J., C. Bazin, J. F. Delfraissy, P. Dellamonica, P. M. Girard, C. Mayaud, J. F. Mettetal, B. Regnier, W. Rozenbaum, M. Seligmann, D. Smadja, R. Demeulemeester, and J. B. Brunet. 1990. *Recommandations du groupe d'experts sur la prise en charge et le traitement précoce de l'infection à VIH.* Paris: Ministère de la Santé.

Douglas, Mary. 1966. *Purity and Danger:an Analysis of Concepts of Pollution and Taboo.* London: Routledge and Kegan Paul.

Duesberg, Peter. 1989. "Human Immunodeficiency Virus and Acquired Immunodeficiency Syndrome: Correlation But Not Causation." *Proceedings of the National Academy of Sciences* 86:755–764.

Duesberg, Peter. 1990. "AIDS: Non-infectious Deficiencies Acquired by Drug Consumption and Other Risk Factors." *Research in Immunology* 141:5–11.

Dunagan, William, and Michael Ridner, eds. 1987. *Washington University Manual of Medical Therapeutics* 26th ed. Boston: Little, Brown.

Eisenberg, Leon, and Arthur Kleinman, eds. 1981. *The Relevance of Social Science for Medicine.* Dordrecht, Holland: D. Reidel.

El-Sadr, W., J. M. Oleske, B. D. Agins, K. Bauman, C. Brosgart, G. Brown, J. Geaga, D. Greenspan, K. Hein, W. Holzemer, R. Jackson, M. Lindsay, H. Makadon, M. Moon, C. Rappoport, W. Shervington, L. Shulman, and C. Wofsy. 1994. *Evaluation and Management of Early HIV Infection. Clinical Practice Guideline No. 7.* AHCPR Publication No. 94-0572. Rockville, MD: Agency for Health Care Policy and Research, Public Health Service, US Department of Health and Human Services.

Elsford, Jonathon. 1987. "Moral and Social Aspects of AIDS: A Medical Student's Project." *Social Science and Medicine* 24:543–549.

Escande, J. P. 1975. *Les médecins.* Paris: Grasset.

Essex, Max, M. F. McLane, T. H. Lee, L. Falk, C. W. S. Howe, J. I. Mullins, C. Cabradilla, and D. P. Francis. 1983. "Antibodies to Cell Membrane Antigens Associated with Human T-Cell Leukemia Virus in Patients with AIDS." *Science* 220:859–862.

Evans-Pritchard, E. E. 1940. *The Nuer.* New York: Oxford University Press.

Farmer, Paul, and Arthur Kleinman. 1989. "AIDS as Human Suffering." *Daedalus* 118, no.2:135–160.

Fee, Elizabeth, and Daniel Fox, eds. 1988. *AIDS: The Burdens of History*. Berkeley: University of California Press.

Fee, Elizabeth, and Daniel Fox, eds. 1992. *AIDS: The Making of a Chronic Disease*. Berkeley: University of California Press.

Feldman, Douglas. 1990. *Culture and AIDS*. New York: Praeger.

Feldman, Jamie. 1992a. "An American Anthropologist in a Paris Clinic: Ethical Issues in the French Doctor-Patient Relationship." Paper presented at the ninety-first American Anthropological Association Conference, 5 December 1992, San Francisco, CA.

Feldman, Jamie. 1992b. "The French Are Different: French and American Medicine in the Context of AIDS." *Western Journal of Medicine*, special issue, 157, no.3:345–349.

Feldman, Jamie. 1992c. "Gallo, Montagnier, and the Debate Over HIV: A Narrative Analysis." *Camera Obscura*, special issue, 28:101–133.

Feldman, Jamie. 1993. "French and American Medical Perspectives on AIDS: Discourse and Practice." PhD diss., University of Illinois.

Fielding, Jonathon, and Pierre-Jean Lancry. 1993. "Lessons From France—'Vive la différence': The French Health Care System and US Health System Reform." *Journal of the American Medical Association* 270, no.6:748–756.

The Fifth International Conference on AIDS: Abstracts. 1989. Montreal: International Committee on AIDS.

Fish, Stanley. 1980. *Is There a Text in This Class?* Cambridge, MA: Harvard University Press.

Fisher, Evelyn. 1993. *Physician's Guide to Treatment of Adults With HIV/AIDS*. 2d ed. Ann Arbor, MI: BMC Media Services, University of Michigan.

Fisher, Walter. 1987. *Human Communication as Narration: Toward a Philosophy of Reason, Value and Action*. Columbia: University of South Carolina Press.

Fleck, Ludwik. 1979. *Genesis and Development of a Scientific Fact*. Chicago: University of Chicago Press.

Foucault, Michel. 1972. *The Archaeology of Knowledge*. New York: Pantheon Books.

Fox, Daniel. 1988a. "AIDS and the American Health Polity: The History and Prospects of a Crisis of Authority." In *AIDS: The Burdens of History*. Edited by Elizabeth Fee and Daniel Fox, 316–343. Berkeley: University of California Press.

Fox, Daniel. 1988b. "The Politics of Physicians' Responsibility in Epidemics: A Note on History." In *AIDS: The Burdens of History*. Edited by Elizabeth Fee and Daniel Fox, 86–96. Berkeley: University of California Press.

Fox, Daniel. 1992. "The Politics of HIV Infection: 1989-1990 as Years of Change." In *AIDS: The Making of a Chronic Disease*. Edited by Elizabeth Fee and Daniel Fox, 125–143. Berkeley: University of California Press.

Fox, Daniel, Patricia Day, and Rudolf Klein. 1989. "The Power of Professionalism: Policies for AIDS in Britain, Sweden and the United States." *Daedalus* 118, no.2:93–112.

Fox, Daniel, and Elizabeth Fee. 1989. "The Contemporary Historiography of AIDS." *Journal of Social History* 23, no.2:303–314.

Fox, Renée, Linda Aiken, and Carla Messikomer. 1991. "The Culture of Caring: AIDS and the Nursing Profession." In *A Disease of Society: Cultural and Institutional*

Responses to AIDS. Edited by D. Nelkin, D. Willis, and S. Parris, 119–149. Cambridge: Cambridge University Press.

Freidson, Eliot. 1986. "Professional Dominance and the Ordering of Health Services: Some Consequences." In *The Sociology of Health and Illness: Critical Perspectives.* 2d ed. Edited by Peter Conrad and Rochelle Kern, 146–155. New York: St. Martin's Press.

Friedland, Gerald. 1989. "Clinical Care in the AIDS Epidemic." *Daedalus* 118, no.2:59–83.

Fujimura, Joan, and Danny Chou. 1994. "Dissent in Science: Styles of Scientific Practice and the Controversy over the Cause of AIDS." *Social Science and Medicine* 38, no.8:1017–1036.

Gaines, Atwood. 1982. "Cultural Definitions, Behavior and the   Person in American Psychiatry." In *Cultural Conceptions of Mental Health and Therapy.* Edited by A. Marsella and G. White, 167–192. Dordrecht: D. Reidel.

Gaines, Atwood. 1986. "Visible Saints: Social Cynosures and   Dysphoria in the Mediterranean Tradition." *Culture, Medicine and Psychiatry* 10:295–330.

Gaines, Atwood. 1987. "Medical Knowledge in France and America: Culture in History and Biology." Case-Western Reserve University, manuscript.

Gaines, Atwood. 1991. "Cultural Constructivism: Sickness Histories and the Understanding of Ethnomedicines Beyond Critical Medical Anthropologies." In *Anthropologies of Medicine.* Edited by G. Bibeau and B. Pfleidere, 221–258. Wiesbaden, Germany: Vieweg.

Gaines, Atwood. 1992. "Medical/Psychiatric Knowledge in France and America: Culture and Sickness in History and Biology." In *Ethnopsychiatry: the Cultural Construction of Professional and Folk Psychiatries.* Edited by A. Gaines, 171–201. Albany, NY: State University of New York Press.

Galavotti, C., and D. J. Schnell. 1994. "Relationship Between Contraceptive Method Choice and Beliefs About HIV and Pregnancy Prevention." *Sexually Transmitted Diseases* 21, no.1:5–7.

Gallagher, John. 1994. "Zero and Counting." *AIDS Patient Care* 8, no.1:13–15.

Gallo, Robert. 1991a. "Letter to Nature." *Nature* 351:358.

Gallo, Robert. 1991b. *Virus Hunting: AIDS, Cancer and the Human Retrovirus.* New York: Basic Books.

Gallo, Robert, and Luc Montagnier. 1987. "The Chronology of AIDS Research." *Nature* 362:435–436.

Gallo, Robert, Prem Sarin, E. P. Gelmann, Marjorie Robert-Guroff, Ersell Richardson, V. S. Kalyanaraman, Dean Mann, Gurdip Sidhu, Rosalyn Stahl, Susan Zolla-Pazner, Jacque Liebowitch, and Mikulas Popovic. 1983. "Isolation of Human T-Cell Leukemia Virus in Acquired Immune Deficiency Syndrome (AIDS)." *Science* 220:865–868.

Gallo, Robert, M. G. Sarngadharan, Mikulas Popovic, George Shaw, Beatrice Hahn, Flossie Wong-Staal, M. Robert-Guroff, S. Zaki Salahuddin, and Phillip Markham. 1986. "HTLV-III and the Etiology of AIDS." *Progress in Allergy* 37:1–45.

Geertz, Clifford. 1973. *The Interpretation of Cultures.* New York: Basic Books.

Gennep, Arnold van. 1960. *The Rites of Passage.* London: Routledge and Kegan Paul.

Gilman, Sander. 1987. "AIDS and Syphilis: The Iconography of Disease." *October* 43:87–107.

Gilmore, David. 1982. *Anthropology of the Mediterranean Area. Annual Review of Anthropology*. Palo Alto, CA: Annual Reviews.

Girard, Marc, and Louis Vallette, eds. 1987. *Retroviruses of Human AIDS and Related Animal Diseases: Second Colloque de Cent Gardes*. Lyon: Fondation Marcel Merieux.

Goedert, J. J., R. J. Biggar, M. Melbe, D. L. Mann, S. Wilson, M. H. Gail, R. J. Grossman, R. A. DiGioia, W. C. Sanchez, S. H. Weiss, A. William, M. D. Blattner. 1987 "Effect of T4 Count and Cofactors on the Incidence of AIDS in Homosexual Men Infected With the Human Immunodeficiency Virus." *Journal of the American Medical Association* 257:331–334.

Golden, L. L., and W. T. Anderson. 1992. "AIDS Prevention: Myths, Misinformation and Health Policy Perceptions." *Journal of Health and Social Policy* 3, no.3:37–50.

Goldstein, Jared. 1990. "Desperately Seeking Science: The Creation of Knowledge in Family Practice." *Hastings Center Report,* November–December, 26–32.

Good, Byron, and Mary-Jo DelVecchio Good. 1993. "Learning Medicine: the Construction of Medical Knowledge at Harvard Medical School." In *Knowledge, Power and Practice: The Anthropology of Medicine and Everyday Life.* Edited by Shirley Lindenbaum and Margaret Lock, 81–107. Berkeley: University of California Press.

Gougeon, M. L. V. Colizzi, A. Dalgleish, and L. Montagnier. 1993. "New Concepts in AIDS Pathogenesis." *AIDS Research and Human Retroviruses* 9, no.3:287–289.

Grmek, Mirko. 1990. *History of AIDS: Emergence and Origin of a Modern Pandemic.* Princeton, NJ: Princeton University Press.

Gullick, Muriel. 1985. "Common Sense Models of Health and Disease." *New England Journal of Medicine* 313:700–703.

Guo, Hong-Guang, Jean-Claude Chermann, David Waters, Leota Hall, Audrey Louie, Robert Gallo, Howard Streicher, Marvin Reitz, Mikulas Popovic, and William Blattner. 1991. "Sequence Analysis of Original HIV-1." *Nature* 349:745–746.

Hacker, Neville, and J. George Moore. 1992. *Essentials of Obstetrics and Gynecology.* 2d ed. Philadelphia: W. B. Saunders.

Hahn, Robert. 1985. "A World of Internal Medicine: Portrait of an Internist." In *Physicians of Western Medicine: Anthropological Approaches to Theory and Practice.* Edited by Robert Hahn and Atwood Gaines, 51–111. Dordrecht: D. Reidel.

Hahn, Robert, and Atwood Gaines, eds. 1985. *Physicians of Western Medicine: Anthropological Approaches to Theory and Practice.* Dordrecht: D. Reidel.

Hamburg, Margaret, and Anthony Fauci. 1989. "AIDS: The Challenge to Biomedical Research." *Daedalus* 118, no.2:19–39.

Hamilton, J. D., P. M. Hartigan, M. S. Simberkoff, P. L. Day, G. R. Diamond, G. M. Dickinson, G. L. Drusano, M. J. Egorin, W. L. George, F. M. Gordin, C. A. Hawkes, P. C. Jensen, N. G. Klimas, A. M. Labriola, C. J. Lahart, W. A. O'Brien, C. N. Oster, K. J. Weinhold, N. P. Wray, S. B. Zolla-Pazner, and the Veterans Affairs Cooperative Study Group on AIDS Treatment. 1992. "A Controlled Trial of Early Versus Late Treatment with Zidovudine in Symptomatic Human Immunodeficiency Virus Infection. Results of the Veterans Affairs Cooperative Study." *New England Journal of Medicine* 326, no.7:437–43.

Harden, Victoria, and Dennis Rodrigues. 1993. "Context for a New Disease: Aspects of Biomedical Research Policy in the United States Before AIDS." In *AIDS and*

Contemporary History. Edited by Virginia Berridge and Philip Strong, 183–202. Cambridge: Cambridge University Press.

Helman, Cecil. 1985. "Disease and Pseudo-Disease: A Case History of Pseudo-Angina." In *Physicians of Western Medicine: Anthropological Approaches to Theory and Practice*. Edited by Robert Hahn and Atwood Gaines, 293–332. Dordrecht: D. Reidel.

Herzlich, Claudine. 1973. *Health and Illness: A Social Psychological Analysis*. London: Academic Press.

Herzlich, Claudine. 1984. "Médecine moderne en quête de sens: La maladie signifiante sociale." In *Le sens du mal: Anthropologie, histoire, sociologie de la maladie*. Edited by Marc Augé and Claudine Herzlich, 189–215. Paris: Editions des Archives Contemporaines.

Herzlich, Claudine. 1985. "Sociology of Health and Illness in France, Retrospectively and Prospectively." *Social Science and Medicine* 20:121–122.

Herzlich, Claudine, and Janine Pierret. 1988. *Une maladie médiatisée: Le SIDA dans six quotidiens français*. Paris: CERMES-CNRS/INSERM/EHESS.

Hewitt, Bill. 1987. "The Politics of AIDS." *Newsweek*, 10 August, 12–20.

Hirsch, Emmanuel. 1987. *Le SIDA: Rumeurs et faits*. Paris: Cerf.

Hodgkinson, Neville. 1987. "1 in 10 AIDS Toll Looming Over America." *Sunday London Times*, 7 May.

Hollander, Harry. 1988. "Work-up of the HIV-infected Patient." In *The Medical Management of AIDS*. Edited by Merle Sande and Paul Volberding, 103–110. Philadelphia: W. B. Saunders.

Hunter, Kathryn. 1991. *Doctor's Stories: The Narrative Structure of Medical Knowledge*. Princeton, NJ: Princeton University Press.

"It's Over, Debbie." 1988. *Journal of the American Medical Association* 259, no. 2:272.

Jacobson, L. P., A. J. Kirby, S. Polk, J. P. Phair, D. R. Besley, A. J. Saah, L. A. Kingsley, and L. K. Shcrager. 1993. "Changes in Survival After Acquired Immunodeficiency Syndrome (AIDS): 1984–1991." *American Journal of Epidemiology* 138, no.11:952–964.

Joffrin, Laurent. 1987. "L'extrême droite étonne le grand air du SIDA." *Liberation*, 13 February, 24–25.

Juengst, Eric, and Barbara Koenig, eds. 1989. *The Meaning of AIDS: Implications for Medical Science, Clinical Practice, and Public Health Policy*. New York: Praeger.

Karp, Ivan, and Martha Kendall. 1982. "Reflexivity in Fieldwork." In *Explaining Human Behavior; Consciousness, Human Action and Social Structure*. Edited by Paul F. Secord, 249–273. Beverley Hills, CA: Sage.

Katz, D. H. 1993. "AIDS: Primarily a Viral or an Autoimmune Disease?" *AIDS Research and Human Retroviruses* 9, no.5:489–493.

Kleinman, Arthur. 1980. *Patients and Healers in the Context of Culture*. Berkeley: University of California Press.

Kleinman, Arthur. 1988. *The Illness Narratives*. New York: Basic Books.

Knorr-Cetina, Karin. 1981. *The Manufacture of Knowledge: An Essay on the Constructivist and Contextual Nature of Science*. Oxford: Pergamon Press.

Koenig, Barbara. 1988. "The Technological Imperative in Medical Practice: The Social
    Creation of a 'Routine' Treatment." In *Biomedicine Examined*. Edited by M. Lock
    and D. R. Gordon, 465–496. Dordrecht: Kluwer.

Koenig, Barbara, and Molly Cooke. 1989. "Physician Response to a New, Lethal and
    Presumably Infectious Disease: Medical Residents and the AIDS Epidemic in San
    Francisco." In *The Meaning of AIDS*. Edited by E. Juengst and B. Koenig, 72–85.
    New York: Praeger.

Kolata, Gina. 1991. "Ten Years of AIDS Battle: Hopes For Success Dim." *New York Times*,
    3 June, A11.

Koop, C. Everett. 1986. *Surgeon General's Report on Acquired Immune Deficiency
    Syndrome*. Washington, DC: US Department of Health and Human Services.

Kuhn, Thomas. 1970. *The Structure of Scientific Revolutions*. Chicago: University of
    Chicago Press.

Kuhn, Thomas. 1979. "Metaphor in Science." In *Metaphor and Thought*. Edited by Andrew
    Ortony, 409–419. Cambridge: Cambridge University Press.

Labov, William, and Joshua Waletzky. 1967. "Narrative Analysis: Oral Versions of Personal
    Experience." Unpublished manuscript.

Lakoff, George, and Mark Johnson. 1980. *Metaphors We Live By*. Chicago: University of
    Chicago Press.

Lang, Norris. 1989. "AIDS, Gays and the Ballot Box: the Politics of Disease in Houston,
    Texas." *Medical Anthropology* 10, nos. 2–3:203–209.

Lapierre, Dominique. 1990. *Beyond Love*. New York: Warner Books.

Latour, Bruno, and Steve Woolgar. 1979. *Laboratory Life: The Social Construction of
    Scientific Facts*. Beverly Hills, CA: Sage Publications.

Lecomte, Jeanne-Marie. 1987. "Science Has No Homeland." In *Retroviruses of Human
    AIDS and Related Animal Diseases: Second Colloque de Cent Gardes*. Marc
    Girard and Louis Vallette, vi–vii. Lyon:Fondation Marcel Merieux.

Lefevre, Christine. 1987. "SIDA: Les Raisons d'Esperer?" *Science et Vie*, no.838
    (July):44–48.

Leibowitch, Jacques. 1985. *A Strange Virus of Unknown Origin*.   New York: Ballantine.

Lemaître, M., D. Guetard, Y. Henin, L. Montagnier, and A. Zerial. 1990. "Protective
    Activity of Tetracycline Analogs Against the Cytopathic Effects of the Human
    Immunodeficiency Virus in CEM Cells." *Research in Virology* 141, no.1:5–16.

Levy, Jay. 1988. "The Human Immunodeficiency Virus and Its Pathogenesis." In *The
    Medical Management of AIDS*. Edited by Merle Sande and Paul Volberding,
    3–17. Philadelphia: W. B. Saunders.

Levy, Jay 1993. "Pathogenesis of Human Immunodeficiency Virus Infection."
    Microbiological Reviews 57, no.1:183–28.

Levy, Jay, A. D. Hoffmann, S. M. Kramer, J. A. Landis, J. M. Shimabukuro, and L. S.
    Oshiro. 1984. "Isolation of Lymphocytopathic Retroviruses from San Francisco
    Patients with AIDS." *Science* 225:840–842.

Lindenbaum, S., and G. Herdt. 1992. *The Time of AIDS: Social Analysis, Theory and
    Method*. London: Sage.

Lindenbaum, Shirley, and Margaret Lock. 1993. *Knowledge, Power and Practice: The
    Anthropology of Medicine and Everyday Life*. Berkeley: University of California
    Press.

Lynch, Michael. 1993. *Scientific Practice and Ordinary Action: Ethnomethodology and Social Studies of Science*. Cambridge: Cambridge University Press.

Makonkawkeyoon, S., R. N. Limson-Pobre, A. L. Moreira, V. Schauf, and G. Kaplan. 1993. "Thalidomide Inhibits the Replication of Human Immunodeficiency Virus Type 1." *Proceedings of the National Academy of Science of the United States of America* 90, no.13:5974–5978.

Mann, Jonathon, James Chin, Peter Piot, and Thomas Quinn. 1988. "The International Epidemiology of AIDS." *Scientific American* 259, no.4:82–89.

Marcus, George, and Michael Fischer, eds. 1986. *Anthropology as Cultural Critique*. Chicago: University of Chicago Press.

Marx, Jean L. 1986. "AIDS Virus Has New Name—Perhaps." *Science* 232:699–700.

Matthews, Thomas, and Dani Bolognesi. 1988. "AIDS Vaccines." *Scientific American* 259, no.4:120–127.

Maurice, John. 1983. "AIDS Investigators Identify Second Retrovirus." *Journal of the American Medical Association* 250, no.8:1010–1021.

Mavligit, Giora, M. Talpaz, F. T. Hsia, W. Wong, B. Lichtiger, P. W. Mansell, and D. M. Mumford. 1984. "Chronic Immune Stimulation by Sperm Alloantigens: Support for the Hypothesis that Spermatozoa Induce Immune Dysregulation in Homosexual Men." *Journal of the American Medical Association* 251:237–241.

May, Robert, Roy Anderson, and Sally Blower. 1989. "The Epidemiology and Transmission Dynamics of HIV–AIDS." *Daedalus* 118, no.2:163–201.

Mayaud, C. 1993a. "Synthèse des recommandations pour la prise en charge de personnes atteintes d'infection à VIH." *Revue de Pneumologie Clinique* 49, no.2:61–64.

Mayaud, C. 1993b. "Traitement par les antiviraux des personnes atteintes d'infection par le VIH." *Revue de Pneumologie Clinique* 49, no.2:71–74.

McCombie, S. C. 1990. "AIDS in Cultural, Historic, and Epidemiological Context." In *Culture and AIDS*. Edited by Douglas Feldman, 9–27. New York: Praeger.

Merck Manual of Diagnosis and Therapy. 1987. 15th ed. Rahway, NJ: Merck, Sharp and Dohme.

Mink, Louis. 1978. "Narrative Form as a Cognitive Instrument." In *The Writing of History*. Edited by R. Canary and H. Kozicki, 129–149. Madison: University of Wisconsin Press.

Mishler, Elliot. 1986. *Research Interviewing: Context and Narrative*. Cambridge, MA: Harvard University Press.

Moatti, J. P., L. Manesse, C. Le Galés, J. P. Pagès, and F. Fagnani. 1988. "Social Perception of AIDS in the General Public: a French Study." *Health Policy* 9:1–8.

Montagnier, Luc. 1986. "Lymphadenopathy Associated Virus: Its Role in the Pathogenesis of AIDS and Related Diseases." *Progress in Allergy* 37:46–64.

Montagnier, Luc, Jean-Baptiste Brunet and David Klatzmann. 1985. "Le SIDA et son virus." *La Recherche*, No.167(June):750–761.

Muller, Jessica, and Barbara Koenig. 1988. "On the Boundary of Life and Death: the Definition of Dying by Medical Residents." In *Biomedicine Examined*. Edited by M. Lock and D. R. Gordon, 351–374. Dordrecht: Kluwer,

Muraskin, William. 1993. "Hepatitis B as a Model (and Anti-model) for AIDS." In *AIDS and Contemporary History*. Edited by Virginia Berridge and Philip Strong, 108–132. Cambridge: Cambridge University Press.

Murray, Stephen, and Kenneth Payne. 1989. "The Social Classification of AIDS in
    American Epidemiology." *Medical Anthropology* 10, nos.2–3:115–128.
Nelkin, Dorothy, David Willis, and Scott Parris, eds. 1991. *A Disease of Society: Cultural
    and Institutional Responses to AIDS.* Cambridge: Cambridge University Press.
Newmeyer, J. A., H. W. Feldman, P. Biernacki, and J. K. Watters. 1989. "Preventing AIDS
    Contagion Among Intravenous Drug Users." *Medical Anthropology* 10,
    nos.2–3:167–175.
New York State Department of Health. 1987. *Acquired Immune Deficiency Syndrome: 100
    Questions and Answers.* Albany, NY: New York State Department of Health.
Norman, Colin. 1985. "AIDS Virology: a Battle on Many Fronts." *Science* 230:518–521.
Norton, Robert, Judith Schwartzbaum, and John Wheat. 1990. "Language Discriminations
    of General Physicians: AIDS Metaphors Used in the AIDS Crisis."
    Communication Research 17, no.6:809–826
Nowak, R. 1991. "New AIDS Definition." *Nature* 352, no.6337:653.
Ohnuki-Tierney, Emiko. 1984. *Illness and Culture in Contemporary Japan:an
    Anthropological View.* Cambridge: Cambridge University Press.
Oppenheimer, Gerald. 1992. "Causes, Cases, And Cohorts: The Role of Epidemiology in the
    Historical Construction of AIDS." In *AIDS: The Making of a Chronic Disease.*
    Edited by Elizabeth Fee and Daniel Fox, 49–83. Berkeley: University of
    California Press.
Ortony, Andrew. 1979. "Metaphor: Multidimensional Problem." In *Metaphor and Thought.*
    Edited by Andrew Ortony, 1–16. Cambridge: Cambridge University Press.
Ozawa, Martha, Wendy Auslander, and Vered Slonim–Neva. 1993. "Problems in Financing
    the Care of AIDS Patients." *Social Work* 38, no.4:369–377.
Packard, Randall, and Paul Epstein. 1992. "Medical Research on AIDS in Africa: A
    Historical Perspective." In *AIDS: The Making of a Chronic Disease.* Edited by
    Elizabeth Fee and Daniel Fox, 346–376. Berkeley: University of California Press.
Pappas, Gregory. 1990. "Some Implications for the Study of the Doctor-Patient Interaction:
    Power, Structure, and Agency in the Work of Howard Waitzkin and Arthur
    Kleinman." *Social Science and Medicine* 30:199–204.
Patton, Cindy. 1985. *Sex and Germs: The Politics of AIDS.* Boston: South End.
Patton, Cindy. 1990. *Inventing AIDS.* New York: Routledge.
Payer, Lynn. 1988. *Medicine and Culture: Varieties of Treatment in the United States,
    England, West Germany, and France.* New York: Henry Holt.
Pekkanen, John. 1987. "AIDS: The Plague That Knows No Bounds." *Reader's Digest*
    June, 49–60.
Pierret, Janine. 1984. "Les significations sociales de la santé: Paris, L'Essone, L'Herault." In
    Le sens du mal: Anthropologie, histoire, sociologie de la maladie. Edited by
    Marc Augé and Claudine Herzlich, 217–256. Paris: Editions des Archives
    Contemporaines.
Poirier, Suzanne, and Daniel Brauner. 1988. "Ethics and the Daily Language of Medical
    Discourse: Lessons from a Conference in Geriatrics." *Hastings Report* 18,
    no.4:5–9.
Pollak, Michael. 1988. *Les Homosexuels et le SIDA.* Paris: A. M. Métailié.
Popovic, Mikulas, M. G. Sarngadharan, Elizabeth Read, and Robert Gallo. 1984. "Detection,
    Isolation, and Continuous Production of Cytopathic Retroviruses (HTLV-III) from
    Patients with AIDS and Pre-AIDS." *Science* 224:497–500.

Rabinow, Paul. 1977. *Reflections on Fieldwork in Morocco*. Berkeley: University of California Press.

Rabinow, Paul. 1986. "Representations are Social Facts." In *Writing Culture: The Poetics and Politics of Ethnography*. Edited by James Clifford and George Marcus, 234–261. Berkeley: University of California Press.

Rabinow, Paul, and William Sullivan. 1979. "The Interpretive Turn: Emergence of an Approach." In *Interpretive Social Science: A Reader*. Edited by Paul Rabinow and William Sullivan, 1–21. Berkeley: University of California Press.

Rabson, A. B., and M. A. Martin. 1985. "Molecular Organization of the AIDS Retrovirus." *Cell* 40:477–480.

Ratner, Lee, William Haseltine, Roberto Patarca, Kenneth Livak, Bruno Sarcich, Steven Josephs, Ellen Doran, J. Antoni Rafalski, Erik Whitehorn, Kirk Baumeister, Lucinda Ivanoff, Stephen Petteway Jr., Mark Pearson, James Lautenberger, Takis Papas, John Ghrayeb, Nancy Chang, Robert Gallo, and Flossie Wong-Staal. 1985. "Complete Nucleotide Sequence of the AIDS Virus, HTLV-III." *Nature* 313:277–283.

Redfield, Robert, and Donald Burke. 1988. "HIV Infection: The Clinical Picture." *Scientific American* 259, no.4:90–98.

Redfield, Robert, D. C. Wright, and E. C. Tramont. 1986. "The Walter Reed Staging Classification for HTLV-III/LAV Infection." *New England Journal of Medicine* 314, no.2:131–132.

Rhea, Buford, ed. 1981. *The Future of Sociological Classics*. London: George Allen and Unwin.

Ricouer, Paul. 1976. *Interpretation Theory: Discourse and the Surplus of Meaning*. Fort Worth, TX: Texas Christian University Press.

Ron, Aran, and David Rogers. 1989. "AIDS in the United States: Patient Care and Politics." *Daedalus* 118, no.2:41–57.

Root-Bernstein, Robert. 1989. *Rethinking AIDS: The Tragic Cost of Premature Consensus*. New York: Free Press.

Rosenberg, Charles. 1989. "What Is an Epidemic? AIDS in Historical Perspective." *Daedalus*. 118, no.2:1–18.

Rothman, David, and Harold Edgar. 1992. "Scientific Rigor and Medical Realities: Placebo Trials in Cancer and AIDS Research." In *AIDS: The Making of a Chronic Disease*. Edited by Elizabeth Fee and Daniel Fox, 194–206. Berkeley: University of California Press.

Roy, Debra. 1991. "What is Kaposi's Sarcoma: an Interview with Marcus A. Conant, MD, Mark Illeman, NP, and Rene Etienn, NP." *Positively Aware* March, 20–25.

Rozenbaum, W. 1990. "Traitements." *Impact Médecin: Les Dossiers du Practicien—SIDA: Guide Practique 1990*. no.62 (1 June):41–48.

Sanchez-Pescador, R., M. D. Power, P. Barr, K. S. Steimer, M. M. Stempien, S. L. Brown-Shimer, W. W. Gee, A. Renard, A. Randolph, J. A. Levy, D. Dina, and P. Luciw. 1985. "Nucleotide Sequence and Expression of an AIDS-Associated Retrovirus (ARV-2)" *Science* 227:484–492.

Sapolsky, Harvey, and Stephen Boswell. 1992. "The History of Transfusion AIDS: Practice and Policy Alternatives." In *AIDS: The Making of a Chronic Disease*. Edited by Elizabeth Fee and Daniel Fox, 170–193. Berkeley: University of California Press.

Schafer, Roy. 1980. "Narration in the Psychoanalytic Dialogue." *Critical Inquiry* 7:29–53.

Schwartzman, Helen. 1984. "Stories at Work: Play in an Organizational Context." In *Text, Play, and Story: The Construction and Reconstruction of Self and Society.* Edited by Edward Bruner, 80–93. Washington, DC: American Ethnological Society.

"Settling the AIDS Virus Dispute." 1987. *Nature* 326:425–426.

Sharf, Barbara. 1990. "Physician-Patient Communication as Interpersonal Rhetoric: A Narrative Approach." *Health Communications* 2, no.4:217–231.

Shilts, Randy. 1987. *And the Band Played On: Politics, People and the AIDS Epidemic.* New York: St. Martin's Press.

Shulman, Lawrence, and Joanne Mantell. 1988. "The AIDS Crisis: A United States Health Care Perspective." *Social Science and Medicine* 26, no.10:979–988.

"SIDA: Ce que vous devez savoir." 1987. *L'Express*, Special edition, 20 February–March 19.

"Le SIDA change le sexe." 1987. *Liberation*, 1 June, 1.

Skinner, Quentin, ed. 1985. *The Return of Grand Theory in the Human Sciences.* Cambridge: Cambridge University Press.

Snow, C. P. 1963. *The Two Cultures.* Cambridge: Cambridge University Press.

Sontag, Susan. 1978. *Illness as Metaphor.* New York: Farrar, Strauss and Giroux.

Sontag, Susan. 1988. *AIDS and Its Metaphors.* New York: Farrar, Strauss and Giroux.

Starr, Paul. 1982. *The Social Transformation of American Medicine.* New York: Basic Books.

Steffen, Monika. 1993. "AIDS Policies in France." In *AIDS and Contemporary History.* Edited by Virginia Berridge and Philip Strong, 240–264. Cambridge: Cambridge University Press.

Stein, D. S., J. A. Korvick, and S. M. Vermund. 1992. "CD4 Lymphocyte Cell Enumeration For Prediction of Clinical Course of Human Immunodeficiency Virus Disease: A Review." *Journal of Infectious Disease* 165, no.2:352–363.

Strauss, Anselm, Shizuko Fagerhaugh, Barbara Suczek, and Carolyn Wiener. 1985. *Social Organization of Medical Work.* Chicago: University of Chicago Press.

Subcommittee of the International Committee on the Taxonomy of Viruses. 1986. "Letter to the Editor." *Nature* 321:10.

Susser, Mervyn. 1973. *Causal Thinking in the Health Sciences.* New York: Oxford University Press.

Tracy, David. 1987. *Plurality and Ambiguity: Hermeneutics, Religion, Hope.* New York: Harper and Row.

Treichler, Paula. 1987. "AIDS, Homophobia and Biomedical Discourse: An Epidemic of Signification." *Cultural Studies* 1, no.3263–305.

Treichler, Paula. 1992a. "AIDS and HIV Infection in the Third World: A First World Chronicle." In *AIDS: The Making of a Chronic Disease.* Edited by Elizabeth Fee and Daniel Fox, 377–412. Berkeley: University of California Press.

Treichler, Paula. 1992b. "AIDS, HIV, and the Cultural Construction of Reality." In *The Time of AIDS: Social Analysis, Theory and Method.* Edited by G. Herdt and S. Lindenbaum, 65–98. London: Sage.

Turner, Victor. 1969. *The Ritual Process: Structure and Anti-Structure.* Chicago: Aldine Publishing.

Turner, Victor. 1980. "Social Dramas and Stories about Them." *Critical Inquiry* 7, no.1:141–168.

Varmus, Harold. 1989. "Naming the AIDS Virus." In *The Meaning of AIDS*. Edited by E. Juengst and B. Koenig, 3–11. New York: Praeger.

Veldink, Connie. 1989. "The Honey-Bee Language Controversy." *Interdisciplinary Science Reviews* 14:166–175.

Velimirovic, B. 1987. "AIDS as a Social Phenomenon." *Social Science and Medicine* 25, no.6:541–552.

Volberding, Paul. 1988. "Caring for the Patient With AIDS: An Integrated Approach." In *The Medical Management of AIDS*. Edited by M. Sande and P. Volberding, 353–361. Philadelphia: W. B. Saunders.

Von Reyn, C. Fordham, and Jonathon Mann. 1987. "Global Epidemiology." In *AIDS—A Global Perspective: Special Issue Western Journal of Medicine* 147:694–701.

Wain-Hobson, Simon, Pierre Sonigo, Olivier Danos, Stewart Cole, and Marc Alizon. 1985. "Nucleotide Sequence of the AIDS Virus, LAV." *Cell* 40:9–17.

Wain-Hobson, Simon, Jean-Pierre Vartanian, Michel Henry, Nicole Chenciner, Rémi Cheynier, Sylvie Delassus, Livia Pedroza Martins, Monica Sala, Marie-Thérèse Nugeyre, Denise Guétard, David Klatzmann, Jean-Claude Gluckman, Willy Rozenbaum, Françoise Barré-Sinousi, and Luc Montagnier. 1991. "LAV Revisited: Origins of the Early HIV-1 Isolates from Institut Pasteur." *Science* 252:961–965.

Watney, Simon. 1988. "The Spectacle of AIDS." *October* 43:71–86.

Weber, Jonathon, and Robin Weiss. 1988. "HIV Infection: The Cellular Picture." *Scientific American* 259, no.4:100–109.

Webster's New Universal Unabridged Dictionary. 1992. New York: Barnes and Noble Books.

Whippen, Deb. 1987. "Science Fictions: The Making of a Medical Model of AIDS." *Radical America* 20:6.

WHO Collaborating Centre on AIDS. 1987. *AIDS Surveillance in Europe: Report No. 13: Situation by 31st March 1987.* Paris: Institut de Médecine et d'Epidémiologie Africaines et Tropicales.

WHO Collaborating Centre on AIDS. 1990a. *AIDS Surveillance in Europe: Quarterly Report No. 25, 31st March 1990.* Paris: Institut de Médecine et d'Epidémiologie Africaines et Tropicales.

WHO Collaborating Centre on AIDS. 1990b. *AIDS Surveillance in Europe: Quarterly Report No. 26, 30th June 1990.* Paris: Institute de Médecine et d'Epidémiologie Africaines et Tropicales.

The WHO International Collaborating Group for the Study of the WHO Staging System. 1993. "Proposed 'World Health Organization Staging Sytem for HIV Infection and Disease': Preliminary Teting by an International Collaborative Cross-sectional Study." *AIDS* 7, no.5:711–717.

Whorf, Benjamin. 1956. *Language, Thought and Reality.* Cambridge, MA: MIT Press.

Wilsford, David. 1991. *Doctors and the State: The Politics of Health Care in France and the United States.* Durham, SC: Duke University Press.

Winkler, Karen. 1992. "Debate Among Historians Signals Waning Influence of 'Discourse Theory' Outside Literary Studies." *The Chronicle of Higher Education* 22 April, A6–A10.

Winsten, Jay. 1985. "Science and the Media: the Boundaries of Truth." *Health Affairs*
    4:5–23.
Wintrebert, F., and A. Certain. 1990. "Evolution de la définition du SIDA: Principles
    classifications de l'infection par le VIH." *La Presse Médicale* 19,
    no.41:1892–1898.
World Health Organization (WHO). 1991. *Global Programme on AIDS: Guidelines for the
    Clinical Management of HIV Infection in Adults.* Geneva, Switzerland: World
    Health Organization.
Wright, Peter, and Andrew Treacher, eds. 1982. *The Problem of Medical Knowledge:
    Examining the Social Construction of Medicine.* Edinburgh: Edinburgh
    University Press.
Zuger, Abigail. 1991. "AIDS and the Obligations of Health Care Professionals." In *AIDS
    and Ethics.* Edited by F. Reamer, 215–237. New York: Columbia University
    Press.

Index

About the Author

JAMIE L. FELDMAN has a doctorate in anthropology and is a resident physician in Family Practice at Lutheran General Hospital in Illinois. She has published on the Gallo-Montagnier dispute over HIV and is currently researching patient models of AIDS/HIV. Her other publications have examined biomedicine from a cross-cultural point of view.

ISBN 0-89789-385-9

HARDCOVER BAR CODE